Eye Surgery in Hot Climates

Fourth Edition

William H Dean BSc MBChB MRCOphth MRCSEd
Specialist Trainee Ophthalmologist
Bristol Eye Hospital, Bristol, UK
CBM Ophthalmologist
Nkhoma Eye Hospital, Malawi

John Sandford-Smith MBE FRCS FRCOphth
Emeritus Consultant Ophthalmologist
Leicester Royal Infirmary, Leicester, UK
Ophthalmologist
Christian Hospital, Quetta, Pakistan
Senior Lecturer in Ophthalmology
Ahmadu Bello University Hospital, Kaduna, Nigeria

D1627791

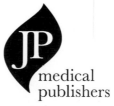

JP
medical
publishers

London • Philadelphia • Panama City • New Delhi

© 2015 William H Dean and John Sandford-Smith
Published by JP Medical Ltd
83 Victoria Street, London, SW1H 0HW, UK
Tel: +44 (0)20 3170 8910   Fax: +44 (0)20 3008 6180
Email: info@jpmedpub.com   Web: www.jpmedpub.com

First Edition published 1994
Second Edition published 2001
Third Edition published 2004

ISBN: 978-1-909836-23-5

British Library Cataloguing in Publication Data
A catalogue record for this book is available from the British Library

Library of Congress Cataloging in Publication Data
A catalog record for this book is available from the Library of Congress

Publisher:	Richard Furn
Editorial Assistant:	Sophie Woolven
Design:	Designers Collective Ltd

Indexed, typeset, printed and bound in India.

Preface

Unfortunately there are many people who still have no access to the basic eye surgery which could make such a difference to their lives. At present about 60% of patients requiring eye surgery in Asia receive it, whereas in some parts of Africa this figure is as low as 20%.

The purpose of *Eye Surgery in Hot Climates* is to describe simple, cost-effective procedures appropriate for countries with a low income. Eye surgery technology continues to advance in developed countries; however, much of this technology does not benefit patients in developing countries due to the expense. This book gives advice on those techniques which are within reach of health care professionals working in resource poor environments.

One of the main changes that has taken place since publication of the last edition is the reduction in cost of good quality intraocular lenses, the use of which has become standard practice worldwide. Moreover, global initiatives in support of blindness prevention have been scaled up enormously in recent years. Surgical training lies at the core of both of these developments. This book has been written with the goal of promoting these skills.

We hope that *Eye Surgery in Hot Climates, 4th Edition*, with its accompanying DVD demonstrating operative procedures, will prove invaluable to those in training and continue to provide practical advice for health care providers in developing countries.

William H Dean, John Sandford-Smith
October 2014

Dedication

We dedicate this book to Dr. Nick Metcalfe. He built up the Eye Hospital in Nkhoma, Malawi, to be the most productive department in Southern Africa, and a flagship for training and surgical excellence. If he had not sadly been stricken with a disabling disease four years ago, he would have been a co-author of this book.

WD

JS-S

Acknowledgements

There are many people we would like to thank for their help with the publication of *Eye Surgery in Hot Climates*: the co-author of the first edition, David Hughes, and the illustrator, Debbie Carmichael, for their hard work and encouragement. We would also like to thank the staff at the International Centre for Eye Health in London, especially Gordon Johnson, Allen Foster, Murray McGavin, Sue Stevens, Ann Naughton, Andy Richards, Keith Waddell and Isabelle Russell. Thanks must go to Parul Desai, the illustrator of additional figures in the second edition as well as Doonie Swales for her patient secretarial assistance.

This edition has had expert input from Dr Danielle Ledoux and Dr Nick Lees and, for the DVD, Dr Keith Waddell, Professor Andrew McNaught, Mr David Yorston, Dr Chris Williams, Dr Bansri Lakhani, Mr Tom Eke and Dr Albrecht Hennig.

The Ulverscroft Foundation in Leicester has been extremely generous from the very beginning and the continued publication of this book would not have been possible without their support.

WD

JS-S

Contents

DVD-ROM contents

All the operative video clips and quiz modules listed below are on the DVD-ROM attached to the inside front cover.

Suturing

Local anaesthesia

Cataract

Trabeculectomy

Trachoma lid surgery

Quiz module 1

Quiz module 2

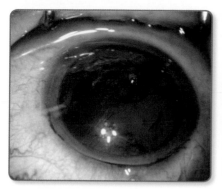

Plate 1

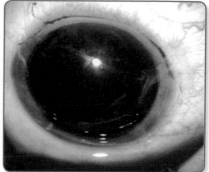

Plate 2

Plate 1 and 2. Extracapsular extraction. These pictures are taken through an operating microscope during the operation. In Plate 1 some pieces of cortical lens matter can be clearly seen against the red glow of light reflected from the back of the eye (the red reflex). In plate 2 the illumination has been changed so that it is no longer coaxial. Now the details of the lens cortex and capsule are no longer visible. Trying to perform extracapsular extraction without coxial illumination often results in complications.

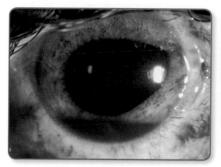

Plate 3

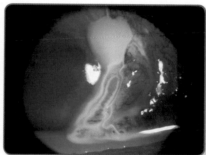

Plate 4

Plate 3 and 4 Siedel's test. This eye has a leaking wound at the limbus of the cornea at the 2 o'clock position. The iris is drawn up towards the leak and there is a small hyphaema. As soon as fluorescein dye is placed in the conjunctival sac (Plate 4) the fluorescein stains the leaking aqueous as it trickles down the surface of the eye. The effect is enhanced in blue light. The fluorescein dye usually appears yellow when dissolved in the tears. However, when aqueous is leaking into the tears it appears slightly green because the Ph of the aqueous is more alkaline.

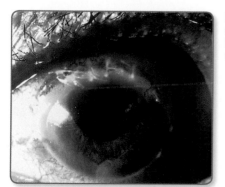

Plate 5 Iris prolapse. This patient had a cataract extraction with a broad iridectomy. However, the iris has prolapsed through the wound at 11 o'clock.

Plate 5

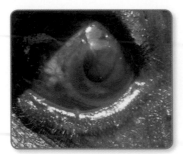

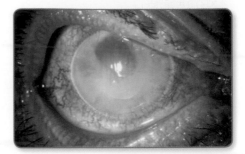

Plate 6

Plate 7

Plate 6 Striate keratopathy. Note the white opaque appearance of the cornea with a rather striped pattern deep in the corneal stroma. Only a part of the cornea is affected and so, hopefully, this cornea will clear in time.

Plate 7 Corneal oedema or bullous keratopathy. The end result of extensive damage to the corneal endothelial cells. The cornea is permanently oedematous. In this patient the pupil is also updrawn.

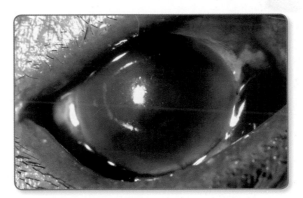

Plate 8

Plate 8 A total hyphaema. No details of the iris or pupils can be seen. If the intraocular pressure is raised as well, the hyphaema should be evacuated.

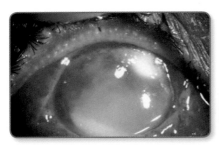

Plate 9

Plate 10

Plates 9 and 10 Post-operative endophthalmitis. Note the inflamed eye, the hazy cornea, the pus around the incision and the pus at the bottom of the anterior chamber (Hypopyon). In plate 9 the anterior chamber is still fairly clear, but in plate 10 it has become full of pus cells. Prompt and intensive treatment is essential to save these eyes.

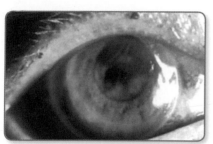

Plate 11 Retained cortical lens matter. This is seen as white fluffy material in the pupil. This eye also has striate keratopathy which are the faint white lines at the top of the cornea and a very small hyphaema, the faint red line across the pupil.

Plate 11

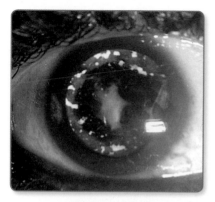

Plate 12

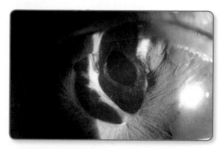

Plate 13

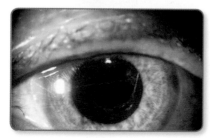

Plate 14

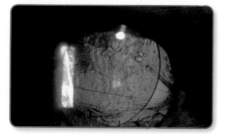

Plate 15

Plates 12, 13, 14 and 15 Thickening of the posterior lens capsule. Plate 12 shows a thickened lens capsule with a dense white plaque in the middle. Plate 13, a slightly thickened capsule with a hole in the centre following capsulotomy. Plates 14 and 15. These are two views of the same eye which has had an extracapsular cataract extraction with an intraocular lens implant. The pupil area appears normal in Plate 14, but on examining the red reflex (Plate 15) the thickened posterior capsule can be seen and so can the edge of the intraocular lens, which has become slightly decentered.

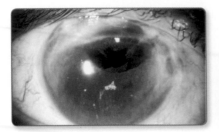

Plate 16

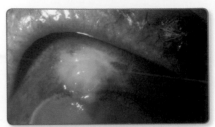

Plate 17

Plate 16 An updrawn pupil and corneal scarring. This is the end result of a rather poor cataract extraction, but the eye can still see.

Plate 17 An infected drainage bleb after glaucoma surgery. This requires urgent treatment.

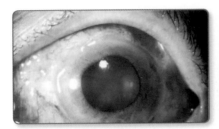

Plate 18

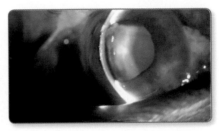

Plate 19

Plates 18 and 19 A flat anterior chamber following glaucoma surgery. The absent or flat anterior chamber can only be seen with the focal illumination of Plate 19. The iris is resting against the back of the cornea and the lens is almost touching the cornea. This eye should not be left for long without surgical treatment to reform the anterior chamber.

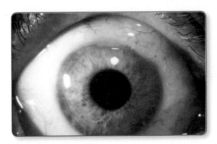

Plate 20

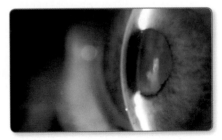

Plate 21

Plate 20 and 21 A shallow anterior chamber following glaucoma surgery. The glaucoma drainage bleb can be seen at the top of the eye in Plate 20. The shallow anterior chamber can only be seen with the focal illumination of Plate 21. There is a small gap between the iris and the lens and the back of the cornea (compare with Plate 19). This shows that the anterior chamber is present but shallow and so the eye can be left without surgical treatment.

Introduction

The world has entered the 21st century and our lives and health are being transformed more and more by modern technology. Many of us have access to things that our parents could only dream about, and our grandparents couldn't even imagine. This technology is changing the way eye surgery is performed and all the time this change is happening faster and faster.

Let us take a brief look backwards into history. The first clear description of eye surgery was in the code of Hammurabi, a king of ancient Babylon about 4,000 years ago. This was a set of laws which laid down the fees for eye operations and the penalties for unsuccessful ones. These could be rather severe. A surgeon could have his hand amputated for a failed operation. One wonders how any eye surgeon continued to practise.

Medical science and especially eye surgery did not advance very fast from Hammurabi's time for thousands of years. Eye surgery 200 years ago was probably not very different from 4,000 years ago. Even then changes only occurred very slowly. One hundred years ago there might be a significant advance in eye surgery about every 20 years. Now there are significant advances every year and almost anything is becoming possible in advanced modern eye surgery.

Unfortunately some aspects of medical care have not changed in the last 4,000 years. In Hammurabi's code it described how the fees for the treatment of a free man (ten silver pieces) differed from that for the treatment of a slave (two silver pieces). Today there is no slavery but it is still true for much of the world that the treatment, if available, depends mainly upon the patient's ability to pay.

Modern medical treatment is unfortunately very costly. It is therefore not available nor affordable for poor people living in low income countries whose governments cannot fund a comprehensive system of health care.

A study of world blindness shows some very disturbing facts. There are over 37 million blind people in the world although the exact number depends upon the definition of blindness. The accepted definition by the World Health Organisation is that a blind person is unable to count fingers at 3 metres distance with both eyes open (<3/60 in the better eye).

By far the most common cause of this blindness is cataract, for which surgery is the only treatment. Trachoma and glaucoma are also very important causes of blindness, and surgery has a big part to play in preventing blindness from both these diseases. Perhaps the most disturbing fact of all is that the numbers of avoidably blind people in the world who need surgery still seems to be increasing. This is happening despite all the advances in medical care and technology and the increasing numbers of doctors and medical schools throughout the world. Nearly all these blind people live in the rural areas of the poor countries of the world – the so-called "developing" countries. The reason for their blindness appears to be that the doctors and medical care are found mostly in the rich developed countries or crowded into the major cities in developing countries. In this way the rural poor remain untreated.

At present in most developing countries there is much debate and discussion about the relative importance of treating or preventing disease. Most medical workers are involved in treatment rather than prevention. However, the World Health Organisation and other expert international health agencies consider the prevention of disease should have priority over treatment. It is seen as a more effective and cheaper way of promoting health in the community, and has more chance of helping the poor.

As far as eye disease is concerned the debate is slightly different. All authorities agree that the basic aim in providing eye care is to prevent unnecessary blindness. This may require public health measures or medical or surgical treatment. The World Health Organisation (WHO) has identified five major causes of blindness and visual impairment world-wide which should be easily preventable. It has also identified two other important causes which are preventable but not so easily.

Easily preventable major causes of blindness and visual impairment	Cataract
	Trachoma
	Xerophthalmia
	Onchocerciasis
	Uncorrected Refractive errors
Other preventable major causes of blindness	Glaucoma
	Diabetic retinopathy

At present surgery is the only treatment for cataract and it is often the most appropriate treatment for glaucoma. It plays an important part in the prevention of blindness from trachoma. Therefore any plan to prevent unnecessary blindness must make basic low-cost surgical treatment available to all those who need it.

This book is written to describe appropriate surgical treatment to tackle this huge problem of avoidable blindness. It is about surgery in particular, and is written as a companion to "Eye Diseases in Hot Climates" which is about eye disease in general. In this opening chapter some of the basic problems in trying to provide surgical services will be discussed. The rest of the book is about surgical principles and techniques.

Why is there so much surgically treatable blindness in the poor hot countries of the world?

The first and obvious reason for this is the lack of medical facilities and personnel. The second reason is that many blinding diseases are much more common in these countries quite apart from any lack of treatment. Some examples of this are:

Cataract There is now plenty of evidence that cataract occurs at a younger age and is more common in hot climates and where hygiene is poor. The exact cause of this is not known for sure and there may be several causes. However episodes of severe dehydration in earlier life from previous gastro-enteritis, heat-stroke or fevers may increase the risk of cataract formation in later life. Life-time exposure to bright sunlight or high temperatures may also be factors. It therefore seems that poor people are more likely to go blind from cataract than rich people, and yet paradoxically the rich have a much better chance of getting treatment.

Trachoma occurs most severely in hot, unhygienic surroundings where flies, poor living standards and lack of water allow the passage of infection from person to person.

Glaucoma does not appear to be influenced by the environment, however certain ethnic groups have an increased risk of certain types of glaucoma. Open angle glaucoma is more prevalent and serious in blacks, and angle closure glaucoma is much more prevalent in mongoloid races.

Pterygium is probably caused by excessive exposure to ultra violet rays from the sun. It is a very common disease in hot climates but is of little significance elsewhere. It is more prevalent in rural areas where people live and work outdoors.

   Corneal scarring is a much more significant cause of blindness in poor countries and hot climates where the cornea is more exposed to trauma, infections and solar radiation. Malnutrition, especially vitamin A deficiency, also increases the risk of corneal scarring.

Consanguinity (marrying a close relative) may be common in certain communities, and may cause an increase of some surgically treatable conditions such as congenital cataract.

Infectious diseases can lead to blindness. Rubella in pregnancy can cause cataracts, and measles in childhood can lead to corneal ulceration and scarring. Both rubella and measles are easily prevented by immunisation, but some developing countries still have very poor immunisation rates.

How can appropriate surgical treatment be provided for those who need it?

This is a much more complex question and obviously no two countries are the same. In some countries there may be a desperate shortage of hospitals and specialist care, while in others the shortage of care may be only in rural areas. Often isolation or difficulty in travel may prevent people having access to medical treatment.

   By far the biggest challenge for eye surgery is to make cataract surgery available throughout the world. The initials of the word "cataracts" make nine convenient headings to describe nine principles for providing basic surgical treatment for all those who need it.

> C Commitment
> A Appropriate
> T Teamwork
> A Affordable
> R Rural outreach
> A Accountable by audit
> C Community-centred
> T Training
> S Specialisation

These principles mainly apply to cataract surgery but are relevant for every type of surgery.

*1. **Commitment*** In spite of all the advances in modern medical care, the number of blind people requiring surgical treatment has not yet decreased in many regions. What technically should be an easy problem to solve is in fact very difficult. Commitment and dedication is needed and major difficulties and problems must be identified.

Many of these difficulties are in the community. Most of the cataract blindness in the world is found in areas of poverty. There is not just a shortage of money but poverty of education, and community development as well.

However some of the difficulties come from the attitudes and limitations of those in authority. Governments, especially military governments, may not give a large share of the budget to health and education, and even then a health ministry may give cataract surgery a low priority when there are so many other health problems. Even those of us who are eye surgeons often find it hard to respond to the challenge of making basic surgical treatment available to all members of the community.

Most experts in world blindness prevention consider that it should be possible to solve the problem of treatable and preventable blindness even with the resources which are available. To this end the WHO and the International Agency for the Prevention of Blindness (IAPB) have launched the plan called "Vision 2020 the right to sight". 20/20 represents normal visual acuity recorded by the Snellen's method and measured in feet. (In fact it is usually measured in metres and recorded as 6/6). The hope is that by the year 2020 most of the avoidable blindness in the world should be eradicated, so that everyone in the world except those with untreatable and unavoidable disease should have a visual acuity of 20/20 by the year 2020. The surgical treatment of cataract blindness is one of the main aims of Vision 20/20.

A commitment to this plan and this ideal is obviously the first and most essential step in achieving it. Any commitment has two basic parts. Firstly, *awareness* of the problem and secondly, *action* to try to solve it. Most people involved in eye care are aware of the problem but unfortunately it is much harder to solve.

The need for commitment is shown by some statistics from India. In 1981 there were about half a million cataract operations performed in India. By 1999 this number had increased by about six times to 3 million, and by 2010 over 5 million cataract surgeries were being performed in India. This obviously demonstrates a very great commitment to eye care and the community. In spite of such a dramatic increase in surgery the numbers of blind people with cataract in India has apparently not yet fallen. The reasons for this are uncertain. One probable reason is that cataract is a disease of old age, and with people living longer the prevalence of cataract in the community is increasing. Another possible reason is that much of the increased cataract surgery is due to increased demand. Because the results of surgery are now so much better, many patients with early cataracts or with cataracts in only one eye are wanting treatment to improve their quality of life even though they have not gone blind.

It is hoped that some of the ideas in the rest of this chapter may encourage people to take appropriate action.

2. Appropriate The treatment given and the technology used must be appropriate for the needs and resources of the community.

The equipment used in medical care and especially in ophthalmology is becoming increasingly sophisticated. Phakoemulsification is now the standard treatment for cataract in the developed world and there are many different lasers and vitrectomy machines which can do much in the treatment of eye disease. Nearly all this technology has been developed by research in rich countries. It is expensive and the equipment needs servicing and maintenance.

Many different groups of people want to make this advanced technology available in developing countries as well :

1. All good doctors like to be up-to-date with the most modern techniques. It gives them professional satisfaction and benefits their patients as well.
2. The influential middle classes and the rich like to have every possible treatment available in their own country, so they don't have to travel abroad for it.
3. Governments feel a sense of pride if their country has the most modern facilities for medical treatment.
4. The organisations that manufacture and market high technology medical equipment are very anxious to sell it, and provide incentives and pressures to do so.
5. In private medical practice there is competition and commercial pressure to have the most modern equipment.

It is difficult for any conscientious and enthusiastic doctor working in a poor country to maintain a balanced view about expensive modern technology. It is difficult to balance enthusiasm for scientific excellence with a concern to provide effective treatment for as many patients as possible. The priority for high technology is to get an excellent result regardless of the cost, however small the number of patients treated or the longer time taken. The priority in treating the poor and needy is to be cost-effective and have a surgical department which can deal with large numbers of patients. Somebody has to pay for the treatment whether it is the government, a charity or the patients themselves or their relatives. The patients themselves usually cannot afford much, nor can governments, and charitable organisations are very concerned about cost-effectiveness with their donors in mind.

Nowadays, even rich countries are discovering that modern medical care is very costly, and there has to be a cash limit as to how much a country can afford to pay for its health care. If this is true for rich countries it is even more true for poorer ones. If a poor country invests in expensive sophisticated medical technology it means that resources have to be taken from possibly more important health needs in order to pay for it. Unfortunately, many hospitals in developing countries contain pieces of sophisticated, expensive equipment which are not being used. The usual reason is that they have broken down and cannot be repaired, or sometimes one small part is defective or missing.

There is an old saying, "*The best is the enemy of the good*". This is very true about providing medical care in poorer countries. If a poor country decides to make the best treatment available for a few it may at the same time prevent many others from receiving good treatment. Obviously everyone would like the best treatment for their own disease. However, people who have no access to medical care at all will accept any treatment as long as it is safe and effective, and it does not have to be the best.

The use of intraocular lenses in cataract surgery is a good example of the question "*What is appropriate technology?*". Intraocular lenses to restore the focus of the eye after cataract surgery instead of spectacles have now been used routinely in the western world for over 30 years. They provide better and much more natural restoration of the vision than spectacles, and if used correctly they don't cause any damage to the eye. The long-term results are good. They are obviously even more appropriate for cataract surgery in poor countries, because patients there have even more problems in looking after or replacing their spectacles. Until recently intraocular lenses (IOLs) were very expensive. The first edition of this book written twenty years ago did not promote the use of IOLs because of the problem of expense. At that time the cost of a good IOL was about 100 U.S.$ which meant it was not a technique which most poor people could afford. The price of IOLs has fallen dramatically since then. A good quality lens now costs 3 U.S.$ or less, and IOLs will become even cheaper in the future. This dramatic fall in price has come about because good quality IOLs are now manufactured in developing countries themselves. There is now no financial reason why IOLs cannot be recommended for all patients, although there are other reasons why their uses may not always be possible.

The development of low cost IOLs creates other subtle problems. The use of IOLs has meant that the indications for cataract surgery have changed. People are having surgical treatment at a much earlier stage in their disease. For instance a patient with a partial cataract in one eye and good vision in the other would not benefit much from the old-fashioned routine cataract extraction and giving spectacles. However he or she would benefit from an IOL. This may have the unfortunate effect of diverting medical resources away from more needy people towards the more privileged.

The problem of appropriate technology and health care should be considered quite carefully by doctors from developing countries who go to the western world for postgraduate medical training. Much of their training in advanced technology and expensive sophisticated medical care may not be what their fellow citizens most need or can afford.

The problem also concerns volunteers who go from the developed world to work or teach in poorer countries. Cheap and rapid air travel has now meant that these activities are becoming more frequent. What is needed in developing countries is a sustainable system of treatment which doesn't depend on visits from outside experts, but will continue to function and provide a service to the community on its own. If a specialist from overseas visits a developing country and carries out a few operations that is in itself is a very valuable service. However it is a very much more valuable service if a visitor from overseas can help to start a programme using available technology which can continue and grow of its own accord after he or she has left.

3. Teamwork Teamwork is an essential feature of a good surgical programme. With a team of people working together much more work can be done making the result more *effective* in terms of numbers of patients treated, and also more *efficient* because it means that everyone is working together and so the cost of the treatment is less.

Also teamwork brings about mutual *enthusiasm* and *encouragement*. Most people work much better and enjoy it much more when they are working in a team with others. One of the difficulties of medical care in poor countries is that so much activity is carried out by people working single-handed in small health centres or private eye clinics. It is an interesting thought that most people are happiest when they feel part of a group, and solitary confinement is one of society's worst punishments.

Teamwork is especially important in surgery. Surgical work is not carried out by just one individual, the surgeon, but by a team. This is especially true when there are large numbers of patients. *Everybody in the team is equally important although some may be more highly trained and skilled than others.* For example if an eye is not properly prepared for surgery or a local anaesthetic is not given correctly or the patient is not properly looked after post-operatively, the resulting complication may be just as serious as a major mistake by the surgeon during the operation.

Another important aspect of teamwork is the formation of local blindness prevention committees. These should involve a wide range of people in the community – eye surgeons, government health officials, local community leaders etc. as well as voluntary organisations like the red cross, the red crescent, rotary and lions clubs. In this way programmes to prevent blindness and provide surgical treatment can be started and maintained.

4. Affordable How is it possible to provide surgical treatment that poor people and poor countries can afford? The size of this challenge is shown by comparing the amount that is spent on health care in rich countries with that spent in poor countries. Rich industrialised western countries spend at least 1,000 U.S. $ per person per year on health care and in some countries much more than this. In poor countries the total expenditure both by government and by private individuals on health care is usually less than 10 U.S. $ per person per year. In such circumstances it is unrealistic to seek to give everybody the best and most modern medical treatment. However, there are ways in which the cost of medical care can be reduced without necessarily reducing its quality. The cost of intraocular lenses is a very good example of this. Increased efficiency and cost saving by manufacturing in developing countries has drastically reduced the price of IOLs, without any loss of quality. Great savings can be made by treating large numbers of patients where the overhead costs remain the same but are shared by the much larger numbers of patients treated.

In general there are three sources of funding for medical treatment: firstly the government, secondly what the patients themselves pay, and thirdly from charitable donations.

In poor countries the government finds it difficult to fund the entire cost of surgical treatment but it can provide incentives, support and encouragement, and may often pay the salaries of the staff.

Patients may have to be responsible themselves for paying for most or some of the treatment, a process which is called "*cost recovery*". Some ways of trying to reduce the cost of surgery have already been described. There is also the principle of "Robin Hood". (Robin Hood was a legendary bandit of long ago who stole from the rich in order to provide money for the poor). There are some treatment programmes in which the higher fees paid by richer patients subsidise those who are poorer.

One result of successful treatment for blindness is that the financial burden to the community of looking after a blind person is removed. If a person is blind or will become blind without treatment, then that treatment enables him or her to be self-supporting, to work and often to look after others. A blind person is not only unable to earn, but is also a great drain on the resources of the family and the community. Apart from all the other human and personal benefits of helping blind people to see, it makes good economic sense. It has been calculated that the total cost of looking after a blind person for one year is ten times the cost of a basic cataract operation.

Much medical treatment in poor countries is supported by local or international charities, or donations from rich people locally. Charitable donors are anxious that their donation should be really used to good effect. In this way well managed hospitals and programmes receive charitable support and so become even better and more effective, whereas badly managed programmes find it hard to get donors to support them.

5. *Rural outreach* In all poor countries most of the treatable and preventable blindness is found in rural areas. It is difficult and costly for people living in country villages to travel to big towns and cities for treatment. When they finally arrive, no cheap and effective system for treating them appropriately may be available. They may have to wait some time to be seen and for a hospital bed, even though they do not have the resources. So mobile teams or "eye camps" have developed as a response to this problem.

It may be much easier for a small surgical team and their equipment to travel to them, than for large numbers of elderly blind patients and their relatives to go to hospital. In countries where there is an effective cheap transport system the mobile team may only need to identify the patients who need surgical treatment, and can then refer them to a permanent base hospital. If transport is not cheap and easy then surgical treatment has to be provided locally. It is possible to carry out safe and effective eye surgery in any clean, well-ventilated building. All the necessary instruments and equipment for basic eye surgery can be transported easily, whereas equipment for high technology surgery cannot be moved and is not appropriate for this kind of work.

A programme of rural outreach is much more effective when there are also community based eye services (see below).

6. *Accountability by audit/quality control* Every doctor should know the effectiveness of the treatment that they give. In particular, a surgeon should know the results of his or her operations, how successful they were and what complications developed. The idea of "audit" is to give us a reasonably accurate assessment of the results of our surgery. This is often not easy to obtain, especially for people working in developing countries. Ideally all patients should be followed-up after eye operations, but many patients may not be able to come back for routine follow-up, or feel that such a visit is worthwhile. After successful surgery, patients may be content to stay at home. Patients who have had complications may not trust the surgeon and so may go to see a different person for follow-up. Therefore if a patient doesn't return for follow-up, there is no way of knowing whether the operation was successful or not. If we audit our work and keep up-to-date records of our successes and failures, this will help to identify the faults in our treatment and methods. In this way we can think creatively about how and what to change, in order to provide a better service and improve our techniques. Here are some examples of the importance of audit and accountability from both cataract surgery and other types of surgery:

- Monitoring visual outcomes of cataract surgery improves results: in other words, if you strictly record and review patients visual outcomes it will improve your results. It is very important to monitor every cataract patient's vision after surgery, and to record it.
- A community survey some years ago about cataract and cataract surgery mostly after "eye camps" showed that many people who had cataract surgery were still effectively blind.[2] This was either because of the complications of surgery, or because the cataract glasses they had been given were either lost or broken. This survey demonstrated firstly, the need for a reasonable quality of surgery to be carried out in "eye camps" and secondly, the need for low cost intraocular lenses as an alternative to spectacles.
- A community survey of patients after eye-lid surgery for entropion following trachoma showed that many patients had little benefit from the surgery, and also that certain operations were much more successful than others. Some surveys have also shown that the results of surgery by trained staff who are not fully medically qualified can be just as good as surgery by ophthalmic surgeons.[1]
- Glaucoma is a major cause of blindness and it is obvious that most people in poor countries cannot afford long-term medical treatment with drops for life. Glaucoma surgery unfortunately sometimes has complications and there is an urgent need of a good audit to assess the effectiveness of glaucoma surgery in preventing further loss of vision.

Accountability demands that the quality of our equipment, the quality of our surgical skill and the quality of our sterilisation and freedom from infection all achieve a certain basic standard.

7. Community centred Most medical staff, especially surgeons, see their work as being based in a hospital. However, programmes which are providing effective care in the rural areas also have primary health care workers who are based in the community. Community eye care is essential in preventing disorders like trachoma and xerophthalmia. It is also important in identifying patients with cataract or glaucoma who need surgery to prevent or cure blindness, and then continuing to look after them post-operatively. Many patients especially from villages need a lot of motivation and encouragement to come for treatment and community eye workers provide this. Surgical treatment, especially in remote areas, is both more efficient and more effective if there is a permanent infrastructure of primary health care in the community. Community based health workers can not only identify and encourage those who need treatment to come for it. They can also provide a vital follow-up service.

Some local communities do not always use the hospital services which are available for them. One of the problems seems to be that the community may feel alienated from the hospital service, they may feel it doesn't "belong" to them. "Ownership" is the word used to describe the way in which the community feels it has some responsibility in planning and delivering health care. Sometimes the people turn to traditional or unorthodox healers rather than trained and skilled doctors for the same reasons.

8. Training Training is one of the most important activities in trying to make basic surgical facilities available for all. It is also one of the main aims of the Vision 2020 programme.

In some countries there are considerable problems in obtaining a good and comprehensive surgical training. Any surgical training programme must have three essential components:

1. *Knowledge and information.* This can usually be obtained from text books and libraries, or nowadays electronically, although lectures and seminars are often more helpful for the student.
2. *Clinical skills.* This requires more person-to-person contact between the trainer (teacher)and the trainee (student).
3. *Surgical skills.* These can only be acquired by an apprenticeship training.

(There are of course other important skills to learn in a postgraduate training programme,such as communication skills, teaching skills and management skills, as well as having a professional and caring attitude.)

Apprenticeship training is the most difficult and time consuming part of a surgical training programme. Trainees can usually acquire knowledge and information relatively easily and clinical skills without too much difficulty. However it is often very hard to find the trainers who have the time available and the expertise to teach surgical skills. There are four stages in a surgical apprenticeship:

1. The student must acquire the necessary background knowledge to perform surgery. This means a detailed knowledge of relevant basic medical science: anatomy, physiology, pathology, medicine etc. as well as a knowledge of surgical technique.
2. The student should then assist the teacher while he explains each step of the operation and how to do it.
3. The student then performs the operation with the teacher assisting. This is usually done in stages, the student performing the easier parts of the operation first and then progressing to the more complex parts.
4. Finally the student performs the operation alone but the teacher is available in case problems or difficulties arise.

Once the student has acquired both theoretical knowledge and practical ability, he or she can work without supervision. Sometimes post-graduate training in surgery can consist of a great deal of theory and a considerable amount of observation but very little practical experience. Theory can be learned from a book but the practical experience cannot. This does not mean that surgical textbooks have no value. They do have a value in explaining principles and techniques and discussing likely problems that may arise and how to deal with them. However a textbook cannot replace practical instruction and an apprenticeship training. There is general agreement about the way that surgeons should be trained. There is however great controversy about who should be selected for training.

Much time and money is invested in training doctors and especially postgraduate specialists. Apart from general education there are usually six years at medical school and about six years of postgraduate training after medical school. After such a costly and lengthy training a specialist needs to support and repay a wide circle of family and dependants. There are therefore strong economic reasons why he or she may have to work in major cities and concentrate on private medical practice. It is very hard to see how a health care system which is mostly dependent on this type of specialist will be able to provide effective surgical treatment for the poor, especially in the rural areas of less developed countries.

It is now well recognised that appropriate people who are not graduate doctors can be taught to carry out basic eye care, and to diagnose and treat eye disease. Those with the right motivation and skill can be given further training and taught to operate. The whole question: "What is the place of non-doctors in delivering health care?" is unfortunately very controversial. In some developing countries there are very comprehensive training programmes for such staff who are called Ophthalmic Clinical Officers or Ophthalmic Assistants, but in other countries there are strong objections to anyone other than doctors being taught to give treatment. Provided such trainees are given appropriate support and encouragement, they are much more likely to remain in the rural areas. It is obvious that in any training programme of this nature the people being trained must be properly selected, trained, accredited and supervised.

Proper *training* will ensure that he (or she) is able to be of real help to the community.

Proper *accreditation* will ensure that the government and medical authorities recognise and approve of the work, and that there is a career structure.

Proper *supervision* will keep up the morale and support of someone who may be working in isolated and difficult situations.

Most international organisations concerned with preventing blindness recognise the need for training Ophthalmic Clinical Officers, Ophthalmic Surgical Assistants, or Non-Doctor Cataract Surgeons. Sometimes the established medical profession or government is opposed to this type of training, especially if it is specific training in surgery. However for countries with a serious problem of avoidable blindness and a shortage of specialist skills there is really no other way forward. There is an ever increasing problem of cataract blindness especially in the rural areas, and few specialists who are able or willing to leave the big cities. Usually graduate doctors who are not specialists have received very little training in ophthalmic diagnosis and treatment, so eye care is often better when given by a "specialist" who is not a doctor than by a doctor who is not a "specialist". Unfortunately in many developing countries there is great enthusiasm and competition for training as a doctor but often little interest in giving training at a more practical level.

9. Specialization Certain surgically treatable diseases may require special expertise in particular paediatric, retinal detachments and difficult cases of glaucoma. Wherever possible these should be referred to someone with particular training and expertise. Many eye surgeons and cataract surgeons are very capable of treating the main blinding eye diseases. In some eye units, where training and subsequent expertise is available, specialization is taking place. Sometimes a surgeon will have special training in paediatric, retinal, or other surgery; and if this is available it may be best to refer a challenging patient to the specialist.

This textbook is not meant to be comprehensive. It is meant to focus on basic surgical techniques for common and important causes of blindness or disabling eye conditions. Therefore most of the book concerns cataract, glaucoma and trachoma surgery. In particular there are some aspects of eye surgery which are deliberately omitted. Squint surgery is not described at all, nor is retinal detachment surgery. Retinal detachments can cause blindness and can be treated surgically, but because of the more complex nature of the operations which need both extra equipment and skills they are definitely techniques for the fully qualified specialist. Corneal diseases and corneal scarring are both very important, and in many cases corneal grafting could improve or restore the sight. Some aspects of corneal surgery are included, but corneal grafting is also a treatment which requires special training and of course some donor corneal tissue.

Modern ophthalmic surgery, even when carried out in fairly basic conditions should be effective with very few serious complications. If serious complications do occur they are usually from a failure to observe basic surgical principles and not from any lack of sophisticated or advanced technology. The five most common causes of serious complications from intraocular surgery are:

1. A bad local anaesthetic block.
2. Intraocular infections.
3. Damage to the corneal endothelium or other intraocular structures during surgery.
4. Failure to suture the wound securely and accurately.
5. Poor post-operative care.

All these complications should be avoidable simply by keeping to basic surgical principles.

Throughout the book there is an emphasis on trying to provide practical help for someone working in difficult circumstances and without the aid of expensive modern technology.

References

1. Kapoor H, Chatterjee A, Daniel R et al. Evaluation of visual outcome of cataract surgey in an Indian eye camp. Br J Ophthalmol. 1999; 83:323-326.
2. Rajak SN, Collin JR, Burton MJ. Trachomatous trichiasis and its management in endemic countries. Surv Ophthalmol 2012;57(2):105-35.

Surgical training and learning

Objectives
- Learning
- Assessment
- Before starting surgery
- An approach to learning
- Educational resources

This chapter focuses on general principles in the learning of surgical skills. A number of educational resources are also highlighted for further reading.

Learning

Everyone learns differently, and surgical training opportunities and courses will differ around the world. There are however some central principles to keep at heart when learning surgical techniques and throughout your career as an eye surgeon. We learn in a progression of stages. From the stages of novice and beginner, then competent and proficient, and finally we aim for expertise. From the stage of novice or beginner to competency, we rely on our surgical trainer. Simulated surgical training and sustained deliberate practice of techniques can play a huge part in the early stages of training. Gaining proficiency in a surgical procedure requires a lot of guidance, and deliberate and motivated practice;[1] perhaps within a fellowship or apprentice training. The final stage of expertise requires constant self-monitoring and self-evaluation, which results in constant self-improvement.

This five-stage model of acquiring a skill through formal instruction and practice, developed by Dreyfus in 1980 for the US Air force, is illustrated below.

Novice
A novice has incomplete knowledge and understanding, and approaches tasks mechanistically (in other words, with a rigid adherence to rules or plans that have been taught). They always need supervision to complete the tasks and have very limited ability for discretionary judgement.

Advanced Beginner
An advanced beginner possesses some situational perception and a working understanding. They tend to see actions as a series of separated steps, and can complete some simpler tasks without supervision.

Competent

Someone who is competent has a good working and background understanding, and sees actions in relation to goals, at least partly in context. They are able to complete work independently to a standard that is acceptable, though it may lack refinement. They are capable of deliberate planning and can formulate routines.

Proficient

Someone who is proficient now has a deep understanding, sees actions and situations holistically. They can prioritize the importance of different aspects and can achieve a high standard routinely.

Expert

An expert has an authoritative or deep holistic understanding, deals with routine matters intuitively and is able to go beyond existing interpretations. They achieve excellence with ease, and can transcend reliance on rules and guidelines. They have developed an analytical approach to new situations and complications or problems.

Motivation[2]

Being well motivated and developing a strong will to learn is critical. If you do not want to learn, then no-one will be able to teach you. Furthermore, if you are not self-motivated to learn and strive to be a good surgeon, you will miss out on a lot, it will take a lot longer, and ultimately it is unlikely that you will progress from being a novice/advanced beginner towards competence and proficiency. Learning continues throughout life, not just in a training period. From starting surgery, until the point of expertise, motivation is central. You have to be motivated to learn, motivated to monitor your surgery and surgical outcomes, and motivated in yourself to continually learn and improve your surgery.

Some motivation is external and this may include, for example, "learning this surgery will allow me to get a better job with a higher salary". It is, however, internal motivation that often leads to deeper learning and understanding. Motivations such as "to prove to myself", "to be the best surgeon I can be", to "develop skills and develop as a person and professional", are sometimes more powerful and can lead to deeper learning.

Learning and performing eye surgery is exciting and challenging. Developing the skills, professionalism and knowledge to help people see is an incredible privilege and motivation in itself. However, there are some ways that you, together with your trainer, can develop your motivation:[3]

1. Self-efficacy is the strength of your belief in your own ability to complete tasks and reach goals. Make sure you have clear and achievable goals, and celebrate when you achieve them.
2. Understand that learning is a process and does not happen instantly. Your own effort and taking control of your own learning is very valuable for motivation.
3. Embrace the value and importance of what you are learning. There is an incredibly great value in learning eye surgery: you are learning to help prevent sight loss and restore vision for the patients you serve in the future.

Audit and assessing your outcomes is something every surgeon should do, from the beginning to the end of their career. A simple system monitoring outcomes can lead to less complications and better results. We all need to carry out quality control.[4, 5, 6]

Assessment

Assessment drives learning. This means that if there is some sort of test as part of the learning then people will learn better. There are two sorts of assessment:

- **Assessment by others.** This may be a formal test like an exam, or it may be informal, when a surgical teacher gives feedback to the surgical trainee. (The International Council of Ophthalmology have developed a series of Ophthalmology Surgical Competency Assessment Rubrics (OSCAR) which show in detail how to assess an ECCE operation while in training.[3] http://www.icoph.org/resources/230/Surgical-Assessment-Tool-ICO-OSCAR-in-English-and-Spanish.html).
- **Assessment by oneself.** Every surgeon, whether he or she is at the beginning of their career or the end, should assess their results. This is often called **audit.**

Table 2.1 shows an example of a simple but very effective table for monitoring outcomes of your cataract surgeries. Consecutive operations are recorded in successive rows. **The key points to record are:**

- Operation number
- IOL power inserted
- VA (pre-operative)

Table 2.1 Self-audit form

Operation number	IOL	VA pre-op	Surgical complications	Good VA: 6/6–6/18	Borderline VA: 6/24–6/60	Poor VA: <6/60	Cause of poor outcome		
							Selection	Surgery	Spectacles
1923W	21.5	HM		(6/18)	6/24				
1924W	22.0	6/60	Microhyphaema	6/18					
1925W	24.5	1/60	PXE-PCT at nucleus exraction. VL. Vity. Sulcus IOL	(6/18)	6/36				
1926W	20.5	5/60		6/18 (6/12)					
1927W	22.5	PL				3/60	Macular hole		
1928W									
1929W									
1930W									
1931W									
1932W									
N	I		C	G	B	P	P1	P2	P3

- Surgical complications (these would be of course in the patients notes/ surgical records)

The outcome is coded good, borderline or poor, according to the VA. Also recorded, if VA is <6/60, is the reason for the poor outcome:

- Selection (In other words another eye disease not noted before surgery; e.g. maculopathy)
- Surgery (in other words a surgical complication that caused the poor outcome)
- Spectacles (a high refractive error post-operatively resulting in the poor outcome)

   Post-operative complications are also recorded.

There is a software CD version of the monitoring of cataract outcomes available from the International Centre for Eye Health: (www.cehjournal.org/ files/mcso/MCSOv2.4%20Manual.pdf).

If you encounter a surgical complication during any surgical procedure, you **must** stop at the end of the operation and think:

1. Why did it happen?
2. When did it happen?
3. What could I have done to avoid it?
4. Did I manage it correctly?
5. What can I change in my technique to learn from it?

> All surgeons make mistakes. A good surgeon learns from their mistakes, a bad surgeon just repeats them.

Before starting surgery

Knowledge of surgical anatomy

It is essential as an eye surgeon that you understand the anatomy of the eye.

   For example, for lid surgery you need to know: blood supply and nerves of the lids; the tear drainage anatomy; and the layers of tissues of the lids.

   Another example, for cataract surgery you have to understand the anatomy and thickness of the sclera and cornea; the anatomy of the limbus, the lens dimension, the iris anatomy etc.

   For enucleation, you have to understand the anatomy of the extraocular muscles etc.

Surgical videos and training manuals

This book aims to provide practical help and guidance for someone working in difficult and challenging circumstances without the aid of modern technology. Of course it can also be used by the training ophthalmologist or ophthalmic clinical officer/medical assistant. It is not however aimed as a substitution to hands on surgical training.

Observe senior surgeons first

Starting surgery is exciting, but can be stressful. Spend as many hours as you can observing. Make notes on the procedures you see: what are they doing at each step? How are they doing it? If you can, when surgery is finished ask the surgeon to go through your notes with you to discuss, elaborate and make further notes and corrections.

Observe the surgical team

Eye surgery relies upon a great team effort. The nursing staff preparing the patient for theatre, the anaesthetist, the surgical scrub nurse, the theatre assistants, and the administrative staff, all work together for the patient. Observe how the theatre team works, for example how does the surgeon communicate well with the scrub nurse?

Simulated surgical training: wet/dry lab, and practicing techniques

It is hard to over-emphasise how useful time spent in a wet/dry laboratory can be, or creating your own laboratory with some simple pieces of equipment. Simulated surgical training and practise is invaluable, and is proven not only to increase the learning curve, but reduce complications when subsequently starting to operate on real patients. A wet/dry laboratory is a place where surgical skills can be learnt and practised, not on a living patient. A wet laboratory may use animal eyes or artificial tissue. Time spent in a wet laboratory is extremely important as it gives the trainee surgeon both skill and confidence. When practising a specific surgical technique (for example hand movements during a scleral tunnel, suturing, capsulorrhexis, etc.) the opportunity of perfecting this in your own time, many times over, in a wet laboratory or in the theatre when operations are finished for the day, can be very rewarding.

Remember

* A good amateur will practise in order to be able to do something right.
* A professional will practise something to such an extent that they cannot get it wrong. Even a surgeon at the beginning of their training has to be a professional because every mistake is serious to the patient.

In the same way, if you can practise a good scleral tunnel technique on an apple many times with the operating microscope in theatre, with no pressure, you will be much better at performing the procedure than if you had performed it on ten eyes under supervision and stress. Of course it is only useful to practise the correct technique so ask your surgical trainer to supervise you and most importantly give you feedback.

You do not necessarily need expensive laboratory equipment and models for a wet laboratory. The skin of an apple is perfect to practise scleral incision and scleral tunnelling. The skin of an orange and banana are very much like eyelids, and perfect for practising suturing techniques. The skin of a grape is very good at simulating a lens capsule.

Practice with equipment and instruments

Get used to handling instruments and looking through operating glasses/microscope, before you ever touch a patient.

Be familiar with the operating microscope and know how the hand or foot controls work magnification or zoom, the focus, and 'x&y' axis. Be familiar before you start operating on patients. Spend 30 minutes at the end of the first few days practising how to focus, refocus, move the microscope into place and change the 'x&y' axis. Doing these again and again, when theatre is free, will be invaluable when you are then operating, as you won't have to think too much about the microscope and you will be very used to how to handle it. Also make sure that you have a comfortable operating chair or stool.

More general principles

While learning surgery, remember:
- Practice makes perfect, but total perfection can be the enemy of the very good. This means that when performing surgery, it is important to aim for a good outcome, but absolute perfection might be counter-productive. For example, chasing all the small soft lens matter in a cataract operation might lead to a posterior capsule rupture, whereas leaving a little of it might have been fine
- Perform surgery in a relaxed atmosphere, with no time pressure on you. It is very important to create and have a relaxed atmosphere around you when operating
- Aim for precision and consistency, not speed, when you are training and operating. The aim when training and operating is to learn and perform the best surgical procedure with the minimum risk of complications. Speed should never be a motivation and in fact only comes after mastery of a good procedure, efficiency of movement, and with avoiding complications
- If in doubt, ask for advice from your trainer or a senior surgeon. Embrace the advice from your trainer; they are there to instruct and guide you, to help you, and to provide valuable feedback
- Listen well to your surgical instructor
- Be patient. Learning a craft skill such as eye surgery takes time. Be focussed, motivated, but patient when you are operating
- Draw pictures and write about everything you see in operations (especially complications) in an exercise book that you keep with you

An approach to learning surgery

An approach to learning a surgical skill is illustrated below. This is only a suggestion and you should, with your trainer, adapt your own style of learning to the teaching opportunities available and to your own previous experience and personal expectations, as well as the expectations of your surgical trainers.

1. Basic principles, concepts and knowledge provide the basis for further learning.
    a. Re-read about basic surgical principles; practise suturing techniques; revise the concepts of the surgical procedure you are going to learn and make sure that you thoroughly understand and know the relevant surgical anatomy.

b. This prior understanding and knowledge needs to be activated when you are learning.

2. Plan your learning.
    a. With your surgical trainer, discuss and specify your learning outcomes, ensuring that these are achievable. "Learning eye surgery" is not a specific objective and cannot be achieved in one teaching session or course. A better learning outcome would be, "learn releasable sutures for trabeculectomy to a level of competence", or "understand the importance of audit and monitoring of outcomes of cataract surgery", or "practise and know the dilution protocol for intra-cameral Cefuroxime" are much more specific and achievable objectives.

3. Engage in your learning.
    a. Focus and pay great attention when observing, practising and learning under supervision and instruction. 'Passive' learning will not work. You have to engage.
    b. Understand and question the 'why' of surgery and surgical procedures and practice. Why is this step important? Why is this done this way? Etc.
    c. It is only through active engagement with what you are learning that you will internalise it and it will transform you to be a better surgeon.
    d. Write about and draw pictures of what you are leaning in theatre and beyond. Go through these with your surgical trainer from time to time.

4. Feedback and discussion are very important. Make sure you have adequate time for this with your surgical trainer. Whether it is feedback on the parts of a procedure that you did well or others aspects that you can improve upon; discussion on the specific or general principles of surgery; feedback for simulated surgical training or with a patient in the theatre, feedback is critical to your learning experience.
    a. Feedback acts to check that you have correctly grasped the lessons and new understanding.
    b. You will be able to reflect better on your learning.

5. Reflection.
    a. Take time at the end of the day to reflect on your learning and what you have been taught. Reflective practice is a great way to internalise, understand and remember the valuable lessons of that day. Simply going to theatre, doing something a few times, then leaving and forgetting about it will be of little benefit.

6. Assessment.
    a. There is a saying, "Assessment drives learning". It means that if you know that there will be an assessment at the end of a learning period, you will be more driven to learn. This is often true and can be true for a surgical learning experience.
    b. Plan with your trainer to have a formal assessment at the end of a training period.

c. One such assessment could be the 'OSCAR' (ophthalmology surgical competency assessment rubric) from the International Council of Ophthalmology. This is an excellent assessment tool for a number of ophthalmic surgical procedures. They are available from the ICO website, www.icophth.org.[9]

Educational resources

There are a number of free resources available via the internet which may prove helpful. Many of these can be accessed even when the download speed is not very fast.

TALC UK

Teaching Aids at Low Costs aim to provide health materials – including low cost health text books, videos, and CDs etc to health care workers.
Address: TALC, PO Box 49, St Albans, Herts, AL1 5TX, UK.
Telephone: +44 (0) 1727 853869. Fax: +44 (0) 1727 846852.
Email: info@talcuk.org
Web: www.talcuk.org
http://www.talcuk.org/books/eye-disease-and-opthamology.htm

International Centre for Eye Health

Address: London School of Hygiene & Tropical Medicine, Keppel Street, London, WC1E 7HT, UK.
Telephone: +44(0)20 7958 8359.
Email: iceh@iceh.org.uk
https://www.iceh.org.uk/display/WEB/ICEH+Publications+List

American Academy of Ophthalmology

Eye Care America is a public service foundation of the American Academy of Ophthalmology
Address: International Assistance Program, 655 Beach Street, San Francisco, CA 94109-1336, USA
Telephone: +1 415 561 8500 Fax: +1 415 561-8533
Web: www.aao.org
     www.eyecareamerica.org
http://www.aao.org/international/upload/Publications-on-Ophthalmology.pdf

International Council of Ophthalmology

The International Council of Ophthalmology provides educational resources via their website
www.icoph.org

Simulated Ocular Surgery

A new and innovative website which provides excellent simulated surgical training resources. There are instruction videos for simulated surgical training in cataract, glaucoma, strabismus, and retinal surgery.
www.simulatedocularsurgery.com

Global Sight Alliance

Wonderful online network of eye care professionals, agencies, corporations, eye clinic/hospitals and like-minded individuals who collaborate for the purposes of:

1. Prioritizing curing preventable blindness world-wide, cataract blindness in particular
2. Advocating for effective international partnership and health care delivery models
3. Connecting and collaborating on global eye care needs, efforts, progress and outcomes. (OPEN communication)
4. Educating and equipping eye care providers with the best techniques, tools, and teaching resources available.
   www.globalsight.org

References

1. Ericsson KA. Deliberate practice and the acquisition and maintenance of expert performance in medicine and related domains. Acad Med 2004;79(10 Suppl):S70-81.
2. Prozesky DR. Teaching and learning. Community Eye Health 2000; 13:60-1.
3. Fry H, Ketteridge S, Marshall S. A Handbook for Teaching and Learning in Higher Education: Enhancing Academic Practice. 3rd Edition ed. New York: Routledge, 2009.
4. Cook C. Monitoring cataract surgical outcomes: 'hand written' registration method. Community Eye Health 2002; 15:54-6.
5. Limburg H. Monitoring cataract surgical outcomes: methods and tools. Community Eye Health 2002; 15:51-3.
6. Limburg H, Foster A, Gilbert C, et al. Routine monitoring of visual outcome of cataract surgery. Part 2: Results from eight study centres. Br J Ophthalmol 2005; 89:50-2.
7. Golnik KC, Beaver H, Gauba V, et al. Cataract surgical skill assessment. Ophthalmology 2011;118:427 e1-5.
8. Golnik KC, Haripriya A, Beaver H, et al. Cataract surgery skill assessment. Ophthalmology 2011; 118:2094- e2.
9. The Information Commissioner's Office. http://www.icoph.org/resources/230/Surgical-Assessment-Tool-ICO-OSCAR-in-English-Spanish-Chinese-Portuguese-Vietnamese-and-French.html

| 3 | **Surgery and the eye** |

Objectives

The main aim of this chapter is to look at surgical principles, which are:

- Knowledge of basic sciences
- Knowledge of surgical techniques
- Practical surgical skills & principles of intra-ocular surgery:
  – Magnification and illumination
  – Prevention of tremor
  – Prevention of infection
  – Surgical access
  – Haemostasis
  – Protection of the corneal endothelium
  – Avoiding damage to the lens
  – Handling the iris
  – Management of the vitreous
  – Wound closure
  – Reducing post-operative inflammation

This chapter is about basic surgical principles and techniques, and how a delicate and specialised organ like the eye reacts to surgery. It is obvious that a surgeon must know all this in detail. However nurses and theatre assistants looking after eye patients should also understand these basic principles.

Basic surgical principles

There are three areas of knowledge and experience required to practise any kind of surgery. These are listed below:

1. *Knowledge of basic sciences*
   - *Anatomy.* This describes the structure of the body.
   - *Physiology.* This describes the function of the body.
   - *Pathology.* This describes diseases that affect the body, and how they alter the structure and function.
   - *Microbiology.* This describes micro-organisms, and how they affect the body.
2. *Knowledge of surgical techniques*
   - Sterility and prevention of infection.
   - Handling instruments.
   - Basic surgical method.
   - Haemostasis.
   - Wound closure and sutures.
3. *Practical surgical skills*
   Surgery on a small and delicate organ such as the eye is obviously different from other types of surgery. There are therefore several other vitally important principles specific to eye surgery. These will be discussed later in the chapter.

Knowledge of basic sciences

It is not possible in this book to provide all the necessary details of the anatomy, physiology and pathology of the eye. However, important points will be mentioned in the text.

Anatomy

It is essential for a surgeon (and anyone involved in surgical care) to be familiar with the detailed anatomy of the region where he is operating, in particular its blood and nerve supply.[1]

Physiology

The surgeon must know how each tissue and structure works when it is healthy. He should also know how the tissues react to surgical injury and what effect the operation will have upon the function of the tissues.

Pathology

The surgeon must know the causes of disease and the effects each disease will have in altering both the anatomy and the physiology of the diseased structures.

Microbiology

The surgeon must understand about prevention of infection; and the detection and treatment of infection.

Knowledge of surgical technique

Eye surgeons should understand the basic science and technical skills of surgery. These include:

1. *Sterile technique.* This is essential in order to limit the risks of bacterial contamination and to prevent subsequent infection.
2. *Correct handling of surgical instruments.* It is important that the surgeon knows the exact purpose for which each instrument was designed and how to use it correctly. This ensures that tissues are grasped, cut, divided and retracted properly. Also the working life of instruments is extended by using them properly.
3. *Basic surgical method.* The surgeon should have a methodical approach, completing each step of the operation before progressing to the next. He must ensure good exposure and haemostasis at each stage. In this way the surgeon can see what he is doing and knows the exact structure he is touching. Complications frequently occur because inadequate attention has been paid to these details.
4. *Haemostasis (see also p.38).* Bleeding obscures the surgical field and makes an operation difficult. Blood may collect post-operatively and result in haematoma formation which delays wound healing and encourages infection. The surgeon should know how and where to place incisions so as to minimise bleeding and also how to manage bleeding. This can be controlled by compression, artery forceps and ligature, cautery or diathermy.

Compression or pressure effectively stops bleeding. Venous bleeding requires only gentle pressure, arterial bleeding requires firm pressure. If the pressure is maintained for a few minutes the cut blood vessels will constrict and the bleeding will lessen. Blood may also clot in the vessel. It is not sensible to rely on pressure alone to control bleeding from large vessels, because the blood vessel may well stop constricting, or the clot may give way and so cause post-operative haemorrhage.

Artery forceps and ligature should be used to secure medium or large blood vessels. However compression for three to four minutes is a helpful way of lessening blood loss from a large vessel so that it can then be more easily identified and clamped.

Surgical diathermy if available is the best way of stopping bleeding from small blood vessels, or bleeding from the surface of the eye. However, if diathermy is not available pressure or applying artery forceps for a few minutes without ligature is usually effective for small blood vessels.

Cautery is used mainly on the surface of the sclera. However it is not very effective in soft tissues. Both diathermy and cautery should not be used excessively on the surface of the eye, or they will cause burning and tissue destruction followed by excessive scarring. Minimal diathermy or cautery is all that is needed to seal off the small blood vessels.

5. *Wound closure and sutures.* It is essential to close wounds securely by bringing together each layer of tissue in the correct plane and without undue tension. It is most important to suture each layer to itself, epithelium to epithelium, fascia to fascia, skin to skin and so on. Good bites of the tissues are taken by rotating the needle holder along the curve of the needle. Care must be taken not to overlap edges nor to tie the sutures too tight which may cause death of the intervening tissues (necrosis) and poor healing.

    The surgeon should be able to tie surgical knots using instruments and not fingers. Although the suture itself should not be too tight, the knot must be tight and tied correctly to prevent it slipping or coming undone. A working knowledge of the different suture materials and an understanding of how they behave in the body will allow him to make an appropriate choice. Sutures for extraocular surgery are usually 4-0 to 6-0 gauge, sutures for intraocular surgery are usually finer (see page 42). There are two types of suture: absorbable and non-absorbable.

    Absorbable sutures have traditionally been made of "catgut" or collagen and dissolve after about 4 weeks. They are used for suturing deeper structures. Synthetic absorbable sutures such as polyglactin (vicryl) is stronger than catgut and therefore finer gauges (5-0, 6-0 or even as small as 10-0) can be used. They also cause less tissue reaction than catgut. Absorbable sutures can be used for skin closure if the patient cannot easily return to have the sutures removed or in small children who cannot easily cooperate. However absorbable sutures on the skin may cause some inflammation while they slowly dissolve. Very fine absorbable sutures are the best way of closing the conjunctiva.

Non-absorbable sutures can be made of many different materials: cotton, silk, nylon etc. They are normally used for closing the skin and are removed after 5–10 days. They can however be used to close deeper layers when they will remain buried in the tissues. 4-0 to 6-0 is an appropriate gauge for most extraocular surgery. Monofilament suture material (nylon or polypropylene) has only one strand and is only used for skin closure. It causes less tissue reaction but is harder to handle than braided sutures. Most modern ophthalmic sutures are fused to a needle by the manufacturers. However threaded reusable needles can be used which save money. Needles may be cutting, for skin or tough tissues like the tarsal plate, or round bodied, for muscle and connective tissue. Very fine corneal or scleral needles have a flat lancet point which is a variation of the cutting needle. All ophthalmic needles are curved. The correct way of tying knots in sutures is described on pages 47 to 49.

Practical surgical skills

This is the final stage of learning as an apprentice with a trainer. Much useful advice can be learned from books and also from videos, but surgery is essentially a practical skill and needs to be taught as an apprenticeship training.

Eye surgery may be divided into two distinct categories:-extraocular and intraocular surgery.

Extraocular surgery is performed on the structures surrounding the eye itself such as the eyelids and the conjunctiva. These tissues have an excellent blood supply. They therefore heal very well and rarely become seriously infected. They are on the surface of the body so surgical exposure is usually not a problem. They can be anaesthetised easily by infiltrating the tissues with local anaesthetic. Adrenaline (called epinephrine in the U.S.A.) (1 in 100,000) is always used in the local anaesthetic to lessen bleeding because these tissues are so vascular. For all these reasons the principles of extraocular surgery are the same as those for general surgery. However the extraocular tissues are rather small and some magnification is usually helpful for the surgeon.

Intraocular surgery is performed on the eye itself. The eye structures as well as being very small are very specialised and delicate. There are therefore several other basic rules or principles for any sort of intraocular surgery. Because it is specialised the eye has only limited powers of recovery from injury including the injury from the surgeon's operation. Other parts of the body will often recover completely from rough handling at operation or from complications like infection. Alternatively it may be possible to do another operation to correct any post-operative complications. Unfortunately this is not true of the eye. Bad surgery or post-operative complications will often lead to permanent loss of sight. It is a sad but true fact that there are some parts of the world where operative and post-operative complications of eye surgery are a significant cause of blindness in the community. Even the best surgeon has complications but with care and correct technique serious complications should be rare.

> **Principles of intraocular surgery**
>   1. Magnification and illumination.
>   2. Prevention of tremor.
>   3. Prevention of infection.
>   4. Surgical access.
>   5. Haemostasis.
>   6. Protecting the corneal endothelium.
>   7. Avoiding damage to the lens.
>   8. Handling the iris.
>   9. Management of the vitreous.
>   10. Wound closure.
>   11. Reducing post-operative inflammation.

Magnification and illumination

The eye is small and delicate. It is important that the surgeon has a good clear view of the various fine structures and can see exactly what he is doing and touching. Therefore some magnification and good illumination are essential.

Magnification

This can be achieved in one of three ways:

1. *Simple convex spectacles.* These shorten the focal length of the surgeon's eye and so reduce the working distance. There are obvious disadvantages to this method; the surgeon's head is very close to the patient's eye and the degree of magnification is limited. However these lenses are cheap, robust and simple.
2. *Telescopic operating glasses.* (**Figure 3.1**) These can be designed to any working distance which the surgeon finds comfortable. The degree of magnification can be varied from X2 to X5. To magnify more than X5 is difficult since small movements of the surgeon's head will make the object appear to move. In addition the field of view reduces with

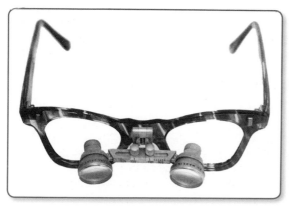

Figure 3.1 Telescopic operating glasses

increased magnification. Telescopic operating glasses are generally better than spectacle lenses but are more expensive and require a period of training in order to get used to them. Each model varies slightly and a surgeon will develop a preference for one particular type. In the end choice depends on preference, price and availability.

3. *Operating microscope.* Binocular operating microscopes are now used for nearly all intraocular surgery in developed countries, and this is rapidly becoming standard practise in developing countries also. The magnification and clarity are much greater than with telescopic glasses, and this means that intraocular surgery can be done to a higher standard with a microscope. Indeed for some intraocular operations a microscope is essential.

However, microscopes have some disadvantages. They are relatively expensive even if purchased second-hand. Most are large and difficult to transport although portable microscopes are available (see appendix page 348). If the patient does not lie completely still, the focusing and positioning has to be constantly changed. The training period is longer and many surgeons find that operating with a microscope takes longer.

Top tip Before scrubbing up and starting surgery, make sure that the seat position, the interpupillary distance (IPD), magnification and focus of the microscope is all correct for you

Illumination

Good illumination is obviously required as well as magnification. Since only a small area needs to be lit the overall power of the light does not have to be great. There are satisfactory lamps available that work on mains electricity or 12 volts DC (see appendix page 349). Correct positioning is important to avoid shadows.

Nearly all modern operating microscopes have a *co-axial illuminating system*. This means that the light travels along the same path as that used to view the eye. It is difficult to achieve this using telescopic operating glasses. However some operating glasses are available with a head mounted light source which can provide rather poor quality coaxial illumination. The advantage of co-axial illumination is that the bright red reflex is seen emerging from the pupil against which details of the lens structure are clearly seen (see colour plates 1 and 2). Whilst this is extremely important when performing modern extracapsular cataract surgery it has little advantage for most other procedures.

Prevention of tremor

All surgeons must have steady hands and this is particularly important for eye surgeons. During early training anxiety and nervousness may cause a slight tremor. This should settle as experience and confidence are acquired. If it does not the trainee should be counselled to change to another career.

Some very simple suggestions to avoid tremor:

- Make sure the whole atmosphere in the operating room is calm and relaxed for both staff and patients. Some people find that having quiet background music is helpful.
- Make sure the patient is not restless, that the drapes are not obstructing the airway, and that the local anaesthetic block is satisfactory. The patient needs to be comfortable and not too hot or cold. A restless patient or a poor nerve block creates tension and anxiety in the surgeon. If possible someone should hold the patient's hand which is very reassuring and relaxing.
- The surgeon should obviously avoid alcohol and sometimes even coffee and other stimulants before operating. Try to avoid physical and emotional stress before operating, such as heavy manual work or driving long distances.
- A comfortable position with the operating table and the surgeon's chair at the right height makes a big difference for the surgeon. A bad posture for the surgeon can not only cause tremor but backache and cramps. In particular there must be support for the surgeon's elbows, forearms and wrists. The best way of ensuring this is to have an operating pillow with a deep hole for the patient's head (**Figure 3.2**). If it is not available pillows or sandbags beside the patient's head will help support the surgeon's arms and the patient's head.

Prevention of infection

A good sterile technique is absolutely essential for intraocular surgery. Post-operative infections elsewhere in the body are a serious complication but in the eye are a total disaster. Pathogenic bacteria multiply with ease inside the eye where they are out of reach of the body's defenses. The delicate intraocular structures are rapidly damaged and even vigorous treatment frequently fails. The result is a partial or total loss of sight. Intraocular infections following surgery are usually the result of poor surgical technique or operating theatre practice. The incidence of this tragic complication should be very low, hopefully less than 1 in 1,000. An incidence higher than this should suggest a breakdown of correct procedures which needs to be identified and corrected. Good sterile technique is important for any operation but is absolutely vital for intraocular operations. In particular there are three specific precautions to take:

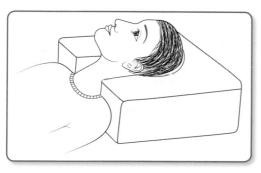

Figure 3.2 A head pillow for eye surgery

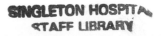

1. Patients with infection of the conjunctiva, lacrimal sac or eyelids, or with trichiasis must have this treated before intraocular surgery.
2. During surgery a "*no touch*" technique should be used. Each instrument should be held correctly by its handle. The "working" end that goes into the eye should not touch the surgeon's or the assistant's hand or the patient's skin or eye lashes. After use it should be placed on the instrument table avoiding other instruments. Wet instruments can destroy a "no touch" technique with moisture running down to the working end or contaminating other instruments. A good "no touch" technique is extremely important and must be practised by the assistant and anyone else handling the instruments as well as the surgeon. The routine use of surgical gloves may reduce the risk of infection. Some surgeons think that gloves reduce the delicate sense of touch from instruments. Therefore they do not use them unless performing more major surgery where significant blood loss is expected or the case is infected. In theory gloves should reduce the risk of a patient transmitting diseases such as Hepatitis B or AIDS to the surgeon. Although it remains important to observe a "no touch" technique, wearing gloves is a sensible precaution both to reduce the risk to the patient of infection and to protect the surgeon.
3. *Irrigating fluids.* When irrigating the eye there is a risk of introducing infection with contaminated fluids. This is more likely if irrigating fluids are taken from a multi-dose container. If possible, use a fresh single dose container or a new infusion bag for each case. Any fluid used to keep the cornea moist must also be sterile. As a general rule never irrigate any fluid inside the eye unless it is essential.

This vital subject of preventing infection is discussed more fully in chapter 4.

Surgical access

The eye is a surface structure but the eye-lids must be held open. Although this can be achieved with sutures, a speculum is more nearly always used. A solid speculum (**Figure 3.3**) is quite heavy and presses a little on the eye. It provides excellent exposure and is used for procedures where there is no risk that the ocular contents will prolapse e.g. pterygium or trabeculectomy.

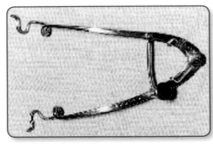

Figure 3.3 A solid adjustable speculum – this is known as "Lang's"

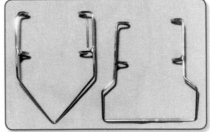

Figure 3.4 Two types of wire speculum – the right hand one is adjustable and the left hand one is not

However a trained assistant can adjust the speculum so as to overcome any pressure on the eye (see pages 109 and 127).The wire speculum (**Figure 3.4**) is lighter but the exposure is not quite so good. It is used where there is a risk of the intraocular contents being pressed out of the eye at the time of surgery e.g. at cataract operations or repairing penetrating injuries. If the patient is nervous or squeezing the eyelids a facial block may be necessary to stop the eyelids contracting and pressing on the eye.

Canthotomy procedure to enlarge the palpebral fissure (Figure 3.5) In the normal patient, once the eyelids are held open with a speculum, there is enough space to gain access to the eye. Occasionally a patient may have rather contracted eyelids or a very deep set eye, causing some difficulty in getting good exposure of the eye. In such cases the palpebral fissure can be easily and quickly enlarged with a lateral canthotomy procedure.

1. Inject a small amount of local anaesthetic with adrenaline into the lateral canthus.
2. Apply an artery forceps to clamp the lateral canthus for a few seconds to produce haemostasis (**Figure 3.5a**).
3. Remove the artery forceps and cut with scissors along the line of the tissue clamped by the artery forceps (**Figure 3.5b**).

It is never necessary to re-suture or repair a lateral canthotomy at the end of the operation.

Superior rectus stay suture

Most intraocular operations are performed on or near the upper limbus. In order to gain access to this the eye must be rotated downward. This is usually done by using a superior rectus stay suture. Insert this as follows:

1. Place a lens expressor or similar blunt instrument (such as the flat end of a squint hook) into the lower fornix and press gently to rotate the eye down (**Figure 3.6**).
2. Grasp the eye through the conjunctiva with toothed forceps 6 mm above the upper limbus. This is where the superior rectus muscle is inserted into the globe. Check that the forceps have grasped the muscle insertion by moving them downwards and the eye should rotate downwards at the same time. Now pass a 4-0 suture beneath the forceps and through the muscle insertion (**Figure 3.7**), but obviously it must not be placed too deeply so that it penetrates the sclera. Gentle upward traction on this suture should rotate the eye downward and expose the limbus.

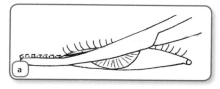 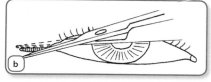

Figure 3.5 Lateral canthotomy. a. Applying the artery forceps to the lateral canthus; b. Cutting the lateral canthus with scissors

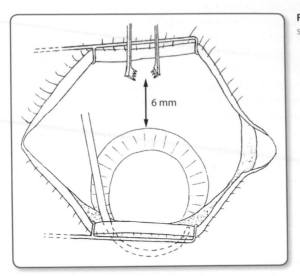

Figure 3.6 Grasping the superior rectus insertion

6 mm

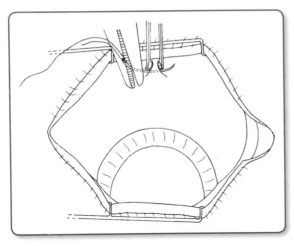

Figure 3.7 Inserting the superior rectus suture

3. If the suture has not been placed through the muscle the eye will not rotate downwards but the conjunctiva will be tented up instead.
4. Once correctly positioned the suture is clamped lightly to the drapes to hold the eye rotated downwards. It should not be used to force an eye down when the superior rectus muscle is still contracting.

Where exposure is a problem, an inferior rectus suture as well as a superior rectus suture provides even better exposure. The two sutures together will also displace the eye forwards without causing any pressure on it. The inferior rectus suture is inserted in just the same way as the superior rectus suture.

Incisions into the eye

These can be made through the cornea, the sclera or the limbus. The limbus is the zone where the cornea and sclera meet.

The advantage of *corneal incisions* is they do not bleed, and they can be made quickly. However the disadvantages are that they do not heal quickly, and they may cause astigmatism from distortion to the cornea. A badly sutured corneal incision can cause serious astigmatism.

The sutures will cause irritation because they are on the surface of the eye, unless monofilament sutures are used with buried knots. Nearly always corneal sutures will need to be removed later on.

The advantage of *scleral incisions* is that they heal well and the sutures can be buried under the conjunctiva. The disadvantage is that they bleed from the wound surface and edges, and they cannot be made so quickly.

A good site for incisions is at the *limbus* which avoids the worst complications of both corneal and scleral incisions. The incision may bleed a little from the surface but this can be prevented with cautery. However the blood vessels are very small and will usually stop bleeding spontaneously. Limbal incisions heal fairly well and the sutures can be buried under the conjunctiva.

The anatomy of the limbus

Most incisions into the eye are made in or near the limbus. This is where the transparent cornea joins the opaque sclera. The surgeon must know this part of the anatomy of the eye particularly well, and also to understand exactly what he (or she) sees when looking at the eye.

Figure 3.8 is a diagram representation of the limbus and **Figure 3.9** shows what the surgeon sees. At the limbus there are three different changes taking place.

1. On the surface of the cornea, the *epithelial layer*. This becomes the conjunctiva
2. In the substance of the cornea, the stromal layer. This becomes the sclera
3. On the inside of the cornea, the *endothelial layer*. This finishes at the angle of the anterior chamber

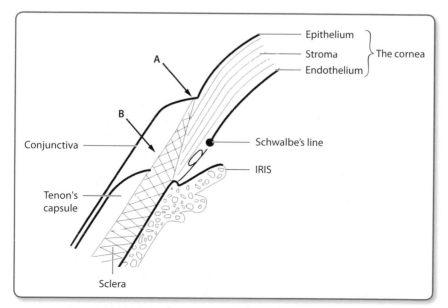

Figure 3.8 The anatomy of the limbus

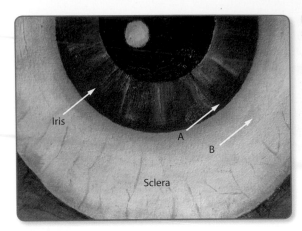

Figure 3.9 How the surgeon sees the limbus

- At the surface the corneal epithelium changes to become the conjunctival epithelium. The basement membrane for the corneal epithelium is called Bowman's membrane. It is firmly attached to the cornea so the corneal epithelium cannot be picked up with forceps. Bowman's membrane changes to become the basement membrane of the conjunctiva. This is very loosely attached to the sclera and so the conjunctiva can be picked up with forceps. This takes place at point **A** in **Figure 3.8**.
- The stroma of the cornea is transparent and it gradually changes into the opaque white sclera. The cornea is said to be held in the sclera rather like a watch glass inside a watch. This means that the anterior layers of the corneal stroma change to become the sclera at point **A** but the posterior layers of the cornea do not change into sclera until point **B**.
- On the inside of the cornea there is the corneal endothelium, which rests on Descemet's membrane. This finishes in a distinct line called Schwalbe's line. There is then a space of about 1 mm where the trabecular meshwork drains the aqueous out of the eye, and then the base of the iris is attached to the sclera. This is called the scleral spur, and is found in line with point **B** in **Figure 3.8**.

So the limbus stretches all the way from point **A** to point **B** and this is a distance of about 2 mm. Finally just posterior to point **B** the Tenon's capsule is inserted into the sclera. Tenon's capsule is a thin layer of fascia which joins the conjunctiva to the sclera.

We will now look at the limbus from the viewpoint of the surgeon – **Figure 3.9**. At one end is the transparent cornea and at the other the opaque sclera. The surgeon can easily identify point **A** where the conjunctiva is attached to the corneal epithelium, and the limbus stretches for 2 mm back from this point. At first there is a blue-grey area about 1 mm thick which gradually becomes completely white like the rest of the sclera. This marks the position of Schwalbe's line, "Where the white meets the blue – Schwalbe's line waits for you!" There is nothing special to identify point **B** where the iris joins the sclera at the scleral spur but it is 2 mm posterior from point **A** which can be identified.

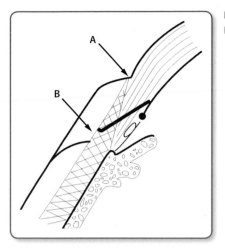

Figure 3.10 The limbus to show the ideal position for the incision into the eye

If an incision is planned at the limbus, it should enter the sclera at point **B** where the sutures will be well covered by the conjunctiva , and it should enter the anterior chamber at point **A** where it will be well clear of all the important structures in the angle,and it will not damage the iris.The ideal position for the incision is shown in **Figure 3.10**.

Dissecting the conjunctiva

The conjunctiva must be cut and reflected back before surgery either at the limbus or on the sclera. It can be used to cover and protect the wound at the end of the operation. The conjunctival flap can be raised with its base at the fornix (**Figure 3.11**) or the limbus (**Figure 3.12**). The fornix based flap is cut along the limbus and undermined upwards. The limbus based flap is raised by cutting the conjunctiva approximately 5 mm above the limbus and reflecting it downwards. Both techniques are satisfactory. Tenon's capsule is a layer of connective tissue which lies between the conjunctiva

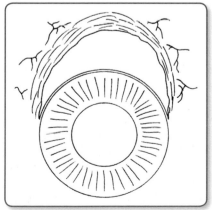

Figure 3.11 A fornix based conjunctival flap

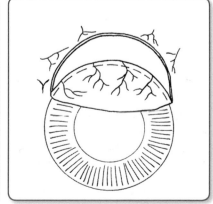

Figure 3.12 A limbus based conjunctival flap

and the sclera. It is particularly thick and obvious in younger patients, but tends to atrophy in old age. It must be dissected from the eye together with the conjunctiva.Failure to dissect it properly from the sclera results in poor haemostasis and difficulty in placing the incision accurately, as well as potential difficulty in visualising and judging the depth of a scleral tunnel. Excessive post-operative fibrous reaction in Tenon's capsule has been suggested as a cause of failure after trabeculectomy procedures.[2]

The fornix based flap seems to be becoming increasingly popular nowadays because:

- It does not cut through any of the conjunctival blood vessels, and so the conjunctiva heals quicker and better.
- Less dissection is needed to bare the limbus where the incision into the eye will be made.
- Tenon's capsule is more easily cleared.
- With a fornix based flap, any cautery to the limbus is less likely to cause burns of the conjunctiva as well.
- The conjunctiva can be secured at the end of the operation with one or at the most two sutures. Often this Is not necessary as it will seal Itself spontaeneously

Haemostasis

Even small quantities of blood obscure the details of the eye and make surgery difficult. Most troublesome bleeding usually occurs from the episcleral blood vessels on the surface of the eye. It is difficult to deal with haemorrhage once it has occurred and so it is best to try to prevent it. This is usually done with very light cautery or diathermy. Take great care not to apply too much cautery or diathermy which will cause death (necrosis) of the tissues and delay wound healing and then later cause scarring. Bleeding from small vessels on the surface of the eye usually stops by itself after a short time as the blood clots and the cut end of the vessels contract.

The cautery is applied on the surface of the eye along the line where the incision is going to be made. This will be at the limbus for most cataract operations but further back on the sclera for a trabeculectomy operation. For surgery to the sclera try to avoid the penetrating branches of the anterior ciliary arteries or the major veins and plan the incision accordingly.

Types of cautery or diathermy

- A hot point cautery (see **Figure 6.12**) can be heated over a small spirit lamp or a butane/cigarette lighter, and is very simple and effective. Alternatively an old squint hook or a glass rod may be used.
- A battery cautery is an alternative. (See **Figure 4.6K**)
- Diathermy works by passing a high frequency low voltage electrical current through the tissues to cause a localisedburn.The diathermy terminals remain cool but the tissues through which the current passes become hot. Most diathermy machines are bipolar, the current passes across the two jaws of a pair of forceps. For diathermy on the surface of the eye the two jaws of the forceps must be slightly apart and the surface

of the eye must be moist to allow the current to flow through the tissues and heat them.

The most important fact about using the cautery or diathermy is to apply the **minimum heat possible** that just shrinks the superficial blood vessels and blanches them without causing any charring. Excessive use of the cautery will cause necrosis in the sclera. This will prevent the wound from healing and also cause post-operative inflammation. If the cautery is applied to the edge of the incision, the edges will shrink and contract. It may then be difficult to achieve a water-tight wound closure. For this reason, cautery should only be applied very lightly to the surface of the eye *before* any incision has been made to the limbus or sclera. In cataract surgery particular attention should be given to the ends of the incision at 3 o'clock and 9 o'clock. These are often more vascular than the rest of the incision especially if a pterygium is present.

Haemorrhage from the iris is not usually a problem although there may be a small amount of bleeding when an iridectomy is performed. This is really very surprising because the iris is an extremely vascular structure. If the iris does bleed the best treatment is patience. The bleeding will nearly always stop quickly and cautery should never the used on the iris or inside the eye. Blood can be washed out with gentle irrigation to the anterior chamber before it clots. If it has clotted a cellulose sponge will usually adhere to the clot and it can be gently lifted out of the anterior chamber, but this should be done with great care as the clot often adheres to the iris as well. If there is persistent bleeding, holding an irrigating simcoe cannula in the eye for a few minutes will apply hydrostatic pressure to stop the bleeding.

Damage to the corneal endothelium

The corneal endothelium is a single layer of cells lining the inner or posterior surface of the cornea. These cells remove water from the substance (stroma) of the cornea and are very active metabolically, keeping the cornea dehydrated. If they are damaged, the cornea swells as its water content increases, a condition known as corneal oedema. The cornea loses its transparency and becomes hazy and cloudy. The endothelial cells are unable to multiply and are not replaced once injured or destroyed. However neighbouring endothelial cells can hypertrophy and migrate to fill a small gap if only a few endothelial cells are damaged.

During any intraocular surgery but particularly cataract surgery some of the endothelial cells may be damaged. Patches of corneal oedema occur post-operatively, and appear as irregular white opaque lines in the deeper parts of the corneal stroma. The condition is called *striate keratitis* or *striate keratopathy* (see colour plates 6 and 11). It usually occurs on the upper part of the cornea because this is the part where surgical trauma is likely to occur. In most cases the other endothelial cells will take over the function of the damaged ones, and after a week or so the cornea becomes clear once again.

However in serious cases many endothelial cells may be damaged or the endothelial cells may not have been healthy in the first place. If this happens the remaining cells are unable to take over the function of the ones damaged at surgery, and so the entire cornea will become swollen (oedematous) and hazy. Fluid-filled blisters develop in the epithelium on the surface of the cornea, these are called bullae. As each blister bursts there is a shallow corneal ulcer so the patient experiences recurrent episodes of sharp pain. The vision is greatly reduced because of the corneal haze. The condition is called *bullous keratopathy* (see colour plate 7). It usually comes on quite soon after the operation but it may be delayed for a few months or even years.

It is extremely important to preserve the corneal endothelium and to limit any damage to endothelial cells at surgery. The surgeon should be aware of the different ways in which this damage may occur. The corneal endothelium is susceptible to both mechanical and chemical injury.

1. *Mechanical injury.* The endothelial cells are very fragile and can easily be rubbed off if an instrument touches the inner corneal surface. They can be damaged by a clumsy incision. Great care must be taken during any intraocular procedure to avoid touching the inside of the cornea. It is best to maintain a deep anterior chamber when instruments are being introduced into the eye. Excessive folding of the cornea by the assistant can cause damage as can vigorous irrigation in the eye. Massaging the cornea so that it rubs against the lens or the iris will also damage the endothelial cells. The golden rule of all intraocular surgery is "avoid any unnecessary or excessive manipulation inside the eye".

2. *Chemical injury.* Take great care when choosing an irrigating fluid to be used in the anterior chamber. Ideally its composition should match that of the aqueous. Hartmann's or Ringer's solutions are best but physiological saline is acceptable. Solutions of the wrong osmotic strength or composition and particularly solutions containing preservatives can destroy the endothelial cells and cause permanent corneal oedema. Locally sold preparations are sometimes manufactured without proper quality control or are incorrectly packaged. Bacterial or chemical contamination may be present. It is very important to ensure that irrigating fluids come from a reliable source or are freshly prepared in one's own hospital pharmacy. There may be chemical residues on surgical instruments if chemical solutions are used to sterilise the instruments. These must be very thoroughly rinsed. Take particular care to rinse very carefully the insides of any tubes, irrigation lines or cannulas. These may contain chemicals, boiled water or other residues which can seriously damage the corneal endothelium.

   In the middle of an intraocular operation think twice before asking for drops to be put into the eye. The drops will almost certainly contain preservatives and these will damage the corneal endothelium.

Avoiding damage to the lens

The lens capsule is another sensitive structure and, if the capsule is damaged or punctured, fluid will enter the lens and a cataract will form later. It is very easy to puncture the lens, and so great care must be taken not to touch it during operations such as iridectomy or trabeculectomy in which the lens is not to be removed from the eye.

Handling the iris

The iris is involved in many intraocular operations, and is often damaged in penetrating injuries.

The iris is probably less affected by surgical trauma than any other intra-ocular structure. Pieces of it can be excised without damaging the rest of the eye or the rest of the iris. If a complete segment of the iris is removed then of course the pupil sphincter will no longer function normally.

The iris is very vascular but surprisingly enough there is usually very little bleeding following surgery on it. However like all intraocular tissues it should be treated with great gentleness and care. There are certain situations in which the iris may create surgical problems during intraocular operations:

- If it is grasped or pulled too firmly, it may become torn off from where it is attached to the ciliary body. This is called the root or base of the iris, and it is where the main artery supplying the iris runs right round the iris at its base. An iris tear here will cause a brisk intraocular haemorrhage. When performing an iridectomy, try not to pull it away from its attachment to the ciliary body or it will bleed profusely. A peripheral iridectomy should leave a small hole in the middle of the iris and a full iridectomy will also divide the pupil margin (see pages 151–53).
- During surgery the iris easily becomes adherent to adjoining structures especially to the edges of the limbal incision. These adhesions should be freed before finishing the operation.
- Post-operatively the iris may adhere to the back of the cornea (anterior synechiae), or to the lens surface or to the face of the vitreous (posterior synechiae). Some degree of inflammation in the iris (iritis) is very common postoperatively and will contribute towards these adhesions.

The vitreous

The vitreous is a gel-like substance that fills the bulk of the eye behind the lens. It has complex and delicate attachments to the retina. In youth these are strong and the gel has a firm consistency. As the vitreous ages it degenerates and becomes more fluid. This occurs more readily in myopic eyes and following ocular inflammation.

Because of its attachment to the retina any disturbance or damage to the vitreous has a significant risk of causing damage to the retina, particularly a retinal detachment. Until comparatively recently the vitreous was a "no go" area for eye surgeons. Nowadays operations can be carried out inside the vitreous, and the vitreous can be removed and replaced. However the equipment is very delicate, sophisticated and expensive and not routinely available in developing countries.

For the surgical procedures described here every attempt should be made to avoid any contact with the vitreous.

However the vitreous may occasionally prolapse from the eye either as a complication of cataract extraction or following a penetrating injury. If this happens it is very important to manage the vitreous loss correctly and so reduce the risk of further complications (see page 129–31).

Wound closure

Obviously the eye must be closed properly at the end of an intraocular operation. The use of fine sutures and accurate, secure wound closure has greatly lowered the incidence of post-operative complications. However all suture materials are foreign bodies and they can in themselves cause complications if they are used incorrectly. Sutures on the surface of the eye can cause severe irritation to the cornea, which can progress to corneal scarring and vascularisation. Just occasionally corneal sutures can cause infected corneal ulcers, and even endophthalmitis.

Suture materials

For intraocular surgery sutures must be very fine, 8-0 or finer. Several different materials are used as sutures, and the surgeon must know how these sutures behave both at the time of operation and also into the future postoperatively.

The most commonly used sutures for intraocular surgery	
Non absorbable sutures	*Size*
Virgin silk (braided)	8-0 or 9-0
Nylon (monofilament)	9-0 or 10-0
Polyester or mersilene (monofilament)	10-0 or 11-0
Absorbable sutures	
Collagen	8-0
Polyglactin or vicryl	8-0 or 9-0

Braided sutures are made of many different strands of material and have the advantage of being easier to handle and knot. Monofilament sutures have just one strand. They are stronger for their size and cause less tissue reaction, but are harder to handle and knot.

1. "Virgin silk" is the usual name for very fine 8-0 or 9-0 silk. This is very popular, it is easy to handle and knots well because it is braided.
    On the surface of the eye it is fairly soft and doesn't cause too much irritation. Some delayed tissue reaction occurs because the suture dissolves very slowly over the course of some months or even years. Virgin silk is always used as interrupted sutures. About five sutures are recommended to close a standard cataract incision. It can also be used to suture the conjunctiva and the scleral flap of a trabeculectomy.
    If virgin silk sutures are buried under the conjunctiva they can usually be left for ever, but they can occasionally cause a foreign body reaction. If they are used to suture the conjunctiva they will usually fall out by themselves after a few weeks. If they are used on the cornea they **must**

be removed after a few weeks, because they act like a foreign body and will cause inflammation and possibly infection.

2. Fine monofilament nylon of 9-0 to 10-0 gauge is by far the most commonly used suture for intraocular surgery. Polyester and polypropylene are much less common and many people never use them. Nylon is strong and extremely fine. It is so fine that the 10-0 gauge is hard to work with unless using an operating microscope. Nylon is inert and causes hardly any tissue reaction or inflammation in itself. Because it is so fine and inert a nylon suture on the cornea will become covered by the corneal epithelium. In this way it doesn't cause any inflammation. However if the knots and the suture ends are left on the surface of the eye, they will not become covered by the epithelium. Nylon is much harder than virgin silk ,and so these knots and suture ends lying on the cornea will act like sharp and hard foreign bodies. Even when a nylon suture is used under a conjunctival flap, the stitch ends can protrude through the conjunctiva and cause irritation. Therefore using nylon sutures on the cornea, the knots **must** be buried in the tissues and not left on the surface. Even under the conjunctiva the knots should be buried if possible. If not the ends should be cut very short so there is no risk of the ends coming through the conjunctiva. There are two ways of burying the knots with nylon sutures:

    - Insert the needle from the inside of the wound outwards so the two ends and the knot are inside the wound (see **Figure 3.13**).
    - Alternatively tie the knot on the surface of the cornea as normal and using suture-tying forceps twist the stitch so that the knot then becomes buried (see **Figure 3.14**). (This technique will not work for 9-0 nylon, as the knot is too thick to pass into the cornea).

    Nylon sutures are not as easy to work with as virgin silk, and the knots tend to slip or come undone. The knots must be tied correctly (see previous page). Interrupted monofilament sutures can be used to close a cataract incision or to suture the scleral flap after a trabeculectomy. Monofilament nylon is very popular as a continuous or running suture

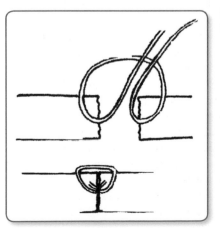

Figure 3.13 Placing the suture with the knot buried

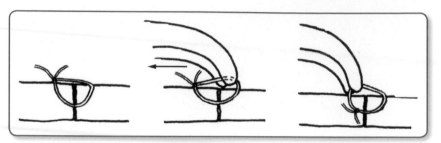

Figure 3.14 Rotating the suture to bury the knot

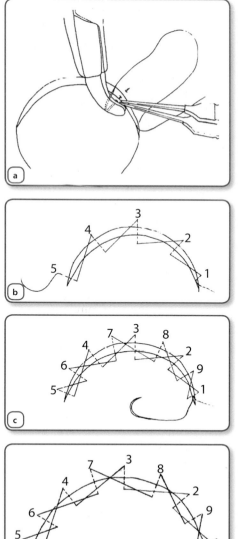

Figure 3.15 The technique of closing a wound with a running monofilament suture

to close cataract incisions (**Figure 3.15**). It provides a very quick and secure wound closure with minimal inflammatory reaction but the knot should be buried in the tissues. The way to do this is to start the suturing from inside the tissues and also finish the suturing inside the tissues so the knot is automatically buried.

There is another problem with monofilament nylon sutures on the surface of the cornea. After about a year the suture material "bio-degrades", so that it weakens because of the action of the tissue fluids and will eventually break. This means that the ends come to the surface, so they are no longer covered with corneal epithelium. They then act as foreign bodies causing irritation and a risk of corneal abscesses. After some time the sutures may also become loose and in this way act as foreign bodies. Therefore if nylon sutures are used on the surface of the cornea *they must be removed*. The ideal time for this is about six months after the operation. If they are removed before this there is the possibility of causing astigmatism because it takes up to six months for a corneal wound to heal completely.

3. Polyester or mersilene sutures are also monofilament and are fairly similar to nylon. Polyester is even harder and stronger than nylon, and so even finer gauges can be used, 10-0 to 11-0. However it is slightly more difficult to handle. Polyester sutures do not "biodegrade" at all. As long as they do not become loose they can be left indefinitely in the cornea, which is an advantage if the patient is not coming back after the operation.

4. Collagen or polyglactin sutures are absorbable. Absorbable sutures usually cause some inflammation in the surrounding tissues during the process of absorption. Collagen is rarely used now for intraocular surgery because polyglactin is much stronger, and causes less inflammation. 8-0 polyglactin (vicryl) is braided and handles very much like virgin silk, except the knots are not quite so secure so have to be tied more carefully. It should only be used as interrupted sutures, and should be used in the same way as virgin silk. That means:-to close a scleral or limbal incision under a conjunctival flap, or to suture the conjunctiva itself. Absorbable sutures should not be used on the cornea, because they will cause a foreign body reaction. Polyglactin is more expensive than virgin silk. It has the advantage of not causing delayed foreign body reactions in the tissues because it is always absorbed after a few weeks.

5. Other suture materials are used occasionally. Polypropylene is very similar to polyester but more elastic. Very fine stainless steel can be used. It is inert, but the ends must be buried. In an emergency human hair can be used, if there is a fine needle to thread it on.

Summary of recommended sutures for intraocular use
1. Incisions at the limbus or in the sclera
Either	a:	interrupted virgin silk or polyglactin
Or	b:	continuous nylon or polyester
Or	c:	interrupted nylon or polyester
2. Corneal incisions or repairing corneal wounds
Either	a:	interrupted or continuous polyester (buried knots)
Or	b:	interrupted or continuous nylon (buried knots and remove after 6 months)
3. Conjunctiva   interrupted polyglactin or virgin silk. Fine nylon can be used but the knots should be buried

Loose sutures are not performing any useful function and should always be removed. Once any suture becomes loose it will work its way to the surface of the eye and cause irritation. Loose suture material on the conjunctiva causes some irritation, but will fairly soon falls out. However loose sutures on the surface of the cornea cause severe irritation and may become infected forming a corneal abscess. They must therefore be removed immediately.

Needles

The needles used for suturing the eye are obviously fine and small and can be easily damaged. They have a flat lancet point. Nowadays nearly all needles come with the thread attached. Since the cornea and sclera are tough tissue, blunt needles are very difficult to use. If handled incorrectly the needles can bend or even snap. The needle should be held between the tips of a needle holder half-way along its length (**Figure 3.16**). Don't handle the tip of the needle with any instrument, as it will become blunt very quickly.

Suture technique

For intraocular surgery it is very important to adjust the tension of the sutures correctly. If tied too tightly they can cause astigmatism; too loosely and the wound may leak. The needle point should enter the tissue with the needle tip pointing straight downwards approximately 1 mm from the wound edge. Countertraction is applied by holding the wound edge with forceps and this helps to hold the tissues in place. These forceps should be either

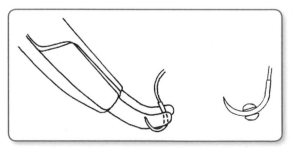

Figure 3.16 The correct position to hold the needle

fine toothed forceps (**Figure 3.17**) or fine cupped forceps (**Figure 3.18**). The cupped forceps are more practical because they are less likely to get damaged. As the needle passes through the tissues the needleholder is rotated and this applies force along the curve of the needle to avoid bending it. The tip of the needle will come out into the wound and should pass through at least half the total thickness of the cornea or the sclera (**Figure 3.19a**). The needle is allowed to carry on into the opposite side so that the depth of the suture is equal to avoid a step in the wound. The needle is advanced until the tip is well clear before it is grasped with the needle holder to pull the suture through. In this way the tip is avoided and so the risk of blunting it is reduced. Some people find it easier to take separate bites with the needle on each side of the wound. The sutures are placed perpendicular to the incision passing the needle from mobile tissue to fixed tissue, i.e. from cornea to sclera. Try to take bites of equal size on each side of the wound.

If the stitch is not deep enough it will fail to hold the wound edges together securely and the wound may leak (**Figure 3.19b**). If the stitch is too deep the suture material may pass right into the anterior chamber. The stitch will then become a wick" which may allow aqueous to leak out of the eye, or it may become a track which allows infection to enter the eye (**Figure 3.19c**). This "wick" effect is more of a problem with virgin silk sutures than monofilament sutures.

Tying knots

Suture materials vary in their ease of handling and knotting. Tying knots is made easier if the suture end is kept short. This also reduces wastage of the suture material. Suture-tying forceps are available but in general any blocked

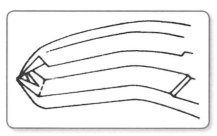

Figure 3.17 Toothed forceps

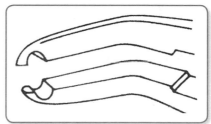

Figure 3.18 Cupped forceps

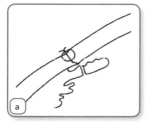

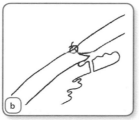

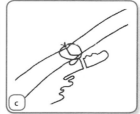

Figure 3.19 Suturing the wound. a. Correct depth of suture; b. Too shallow, poor healing and risk of wound leak; c. Too deep, risk of a "wick" effect especially with braided sutures

tissue holding forceps and the needle holder are adequate. Using the forceps the suture is wound twice around the jaws of the needle holder (**Figure 3.20**). The suture end is then grasped with the needle holder. The knot is then pulled off the holder and tensioned so that the wound edges are brought together but not too tightly. A second single hitch is applied this time winding a loop into the needle holder in the opposite direction. The original direction is used for the third hitch thus ensuring a surgical knot (**Figure 3.21**). It is important

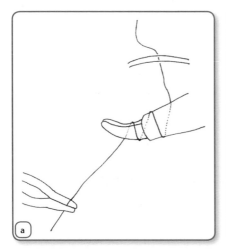

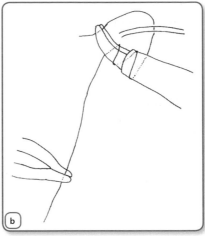

Figure 3.20 Winding the suture around the needle holder. a. The suture is wound twice around the needle holder or suture tying forceps; b. The needle holder or forceps grasps the end of the suture; c. The two instruments are crossed over to complete the first half of the knot (a double half hitch)

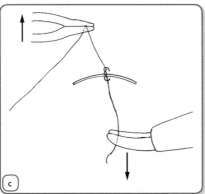

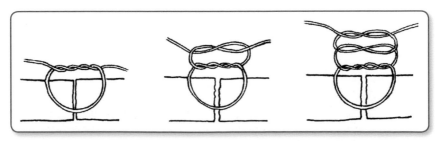

Figure 3.21 The complete knot

to lay the hitches properly so as not to twist the knot. The knot should always be left on the scleral side of the incision where it can be more easily buried under the conjunctiva. The ends are cut short. (With monofilament sutures the knots may slip or come loose. Some surgeons therefore wind the thread three times round the needle holder on the first hitch).

The conjunctiva heals very rapidly and does not require extensive suturing. However it is helpful to use one or two fine sutures to hold it in place. One great advantage of the fornix based conjunctival flap is that it can be secured with one or at most two sutures to tighten it (see **Figure 6.52**, page 137).

Poor wound closure can cause many problems post-operatively. The most common are:

- Excessive leakage of aqueous causing a delay in the reformation of the anterior chamber.
- Prolapse of the iris or vitreous through the wound.[3]
- Bleeding into the anterior chamber a few days after the operation from the rupture of small blood vessels trying to bridge the gap in the wound.
- Astigmatism from the irregularity of the curvature of the cornea.

These complications are all discussed in greater detail on page 172.

Reducing post operative intraocular inflammation

There is always some inflammation following any intraocular operation. This will be increased if the surgery was difficult or complicated. Post-operatively topical steroids, are applied to the eye routinely to diminish post-operative intraocular inflammation. Usually topical antibiotics are given together with the steroids, and sometimes mydriatic drops to dilate the pupil are also given. (Post-operative inflammation and its treatment is discussed in more detail on pages 169).

References

1. Snell, R.S. and M.A. Lemp, Clinical Anatomy of the Eye. 2nd ed. 1998: Wiley, John & Son.
2. Sandford-Smith, J.H., The surgical treatment of open-angle glaucoma in Nigerians. Br J Ophthalmol, 1978. 62(5): p. 283-6.
3. Naylor, G., Iris prolapse; who? When? Why? Eye (Lond), 1993. 7 (Pt 3): p. 465-7.

4 Operating theatre procedures and equipment

Objectives

The main aims of this chapter are to look at:

- Teamwork, and the equal importance of everybody in the surgery team.
- Theatre routine, and the important jobs that must be done to keep a theatre running smoothly, well stocked and maintained, and clean.
- Sterility, as the most essential thing in theatre.
- Instruments, and how to care for and maintain them.

Two things are essential for an operating theatre to run effectively and efficiently.

The first and most important is **sterility**. The purpose of all the precautions and care taken in operating theatres is to prevent infection occurring at the time of operation. This is particularly important for eye surgery where infection is not just a complication but a disaster. An additional risk in eye surgery is that intraocular damage may be caused by chemicals or inappropriate irrigating solutions entering the eye.

The second is **teamwork**. Surgery is not the work of one important person, the surgeon, with a few other people who are not so important doing what they are told. It is the work of a whole team. Everybody in the team is equally important although obviously the surgeon has had a longer training than the others.

The old proverb "the strength of a chain is its weakest link" is particularly true for operating theatre staff and procedures (see **Figure 4.1**).

- It only needs one dirty instrument to introduce infection to the eye and destroy it.
- It only needs one person in theatre to make a mistake with fluids which are irrigated in the eye, to cause destruction of the corneal endothelium and blindness.
- Everyone must share the responsibility for safety and sterility.

The reason for all good surgical practice is to make the operating theatre a **safe place**.

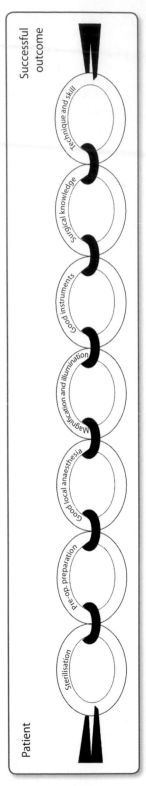

Figure 4.1 The chain of successful surgery – if any one link is broken, the surgery will not be successful

1. Safe for the *patient* who must be protected from infection and other harm. (The patient is the most important person who needs protection.)
2. Safe for the *staff* from the risk of needle-stick and other injuries. These can spread Hepatitis, HIV and other infections. In those parts of the world where hepatitis and HIV infections are common, *every used needle and sharp instrument can be as dangerous as a loaded gun.*
3. Safe for the *community* by careful and safe disposal of soiled materials, especially sharp instruments and needles.

In developed countries most eye surgery takes place in very sophisticated operating theatres dedicated to eye surgery alone, with staff who are fully trained.

In developing countries eye surgery often takes place in general theatres, and some takes place in buildings which may have other uses and are only temporary operating theatres. Often the staff are not fully trained and accredited as nurses or theatre technicians. In spite of these short-comings many surgical teams have to cope with a large volume of work and often with very limited resources. While safety and sterility are obviously the most important aspects of all theatre work, efficiency is also important because of the large volume of work.

Another aspect of safety in operating theatres concerns looking after unconscious patients receiving general anaesthesia, or resuscitating a patient who may have collapsed. Everyone working in a theatre team should know about basic life support. This is how to care for an unconscious patient or one who has collapsed. Basic life support means how to maintain a clear airway and how to give artificial respiration to a patient who has stopped breathing, and how to check the pulse and give cardiac massage to a patient who has no heart beat. All theatre staff should regularly practise these skills, so as to be ready if and when an emergency occurs. At least one member of the theatre team should be trained in advanced life support, which involves taking and interpreting ECGs, the use of a defibrillator and giving appropriate intravenous fluids and drugs.

Theatre procedures depend on many different factors: the work-load; the equipment available; the choice of the surgeon; etc. Eye surgery is practised in many different ways especially in developing countries. There are some highly effective units with a massive through-put of cases. On the other hand, there are some surgeons who are only part-time ophthalmologists, and there are many mobile teams working in temporary accommodation. Therefore this chapter only discusses basic principles and guidelines.

The theatre team

It is important to have an adequate number of motivated and enthusiastic staff. If they are dedicated to eye surgery they will have a better understanding of the requirements of both the surgeon and the patient. A happy relaxed atmosphere and good working relationships in the theatre team makes the work much more pleasant and mistakes less likely.

The theatre team should have a leader who takes responsibility for organising the work and making sure all the routine jobs are done regularly. This ensures both the safety and efficiency of theatre work.

For a regular operating list the basic personnel required are:

1. A scrubbed assistant to look after the sterile instruments and assist the surgeon.
2. An anaesthetic assistant to give the local anaesthetics, prepare the patients and if required help with any general anaesthetics.
3. A circulating nurse to clean and sterilise the instruments and apply the dressings.
4. A general assistant, to help in theatre and assist the patient into and out of theatre.

It is often appropriate that the team leader assumes a fairly basic position, such as being the general assistant, in this way he or she can supervise all the other team members.

Operating theatre routine

There are a variety of important jobs that must be done to keep a theatre well stocked and maintained. Many of these are rather obvious, but without maintenance equipment will break down, and without planning spare parts and consumable materials will run out and take a long time to be replaced. The general routine will include:

1. Building maintenance.
2. Cleaning.
3. Maintenance of equipment and instruments.
4. Manufacture of dressings and drapes.
5. Sterilisation and disinfection procedures.
6. Stock-keeping, storage and security.

Building maintenance

A good sound building is an obvious requirement for safe surgery. Eye surgery can be performed in a great variety of buildings, which are not purpose built operating theatres. However the room should be as insect-proof as possible and well ventilated. It does not have to be blacked-out, although the windows should be shaded. Paint work should be in good condition and a secure water supply present. The room should have doors that can be closed during surgery. Regular inspections of the insect-proofing is important.

Cleaning

General cleaning should be carried out regularly in addition to preparations on the day of surgery. Floors and sometimes walls and ceilings must be washed in all rooms used as part of the operating theatre suite. Any furniture including instrument tables, operating tables and cabinets must be wiped clean to avoid the build up of dust. Spilt blood or other debris should be wiped up as soon as possible, because once dried it may be difficult to remove. A weak solution of bleach is adequate for cleaning purposes and will kill most micro-organisms including the HIV virus.

Anyone who washes drapes and surgical instruments MUST wear gloves to protect themselves from the risk of infection.

Maintenance of equipment and instruments

Equipment can only function if it is regularly maintained.[1] A schedule needs to be drawn up for items such as sterilisers, operating lights and air conditioners. The importance of having spares to enable quick repairs to be carried out locally cannot be stressed too much. Surgical instruments need to be looked after carefully and checked that they are working properly.[2]

Manufacture of dressings and drapes

Eye pads

With modern surgery and small self-sealing incisions, patients are no longer routinely given an eye pad postoperatively. However many patients still require an eye pad postoperatively and outpatients may also be padded as part of their treatment. The purpose of the eye pad is to protect the eye in the immediate post-operative period. It also prevents the patient or his attendants from interfering with the eye and keeps flies out. It prevents eye-lid movements against the eye and applies gentle pressure, which will encourage haemostasis and wound closure. An eye-pad is not a substitute for poor surgery, and it is rarely necessary to keep an eye padded for more than 1-2 days postoperatively.

The cost of buying ready-made pads is high and there are inevitable delays as a result of ordering supplies. Eye pads can be manufactured locally using cotton wool and gauze. A layer of gauze is placed on a table and onto this is put a layer of cotton wool about 2 cm thick. A further layer of gauze goes on top of the cotton wool making a cotton wool sandwich enclosed in gauze. Then, using a simple card shape as a guide, eye pads can be cut out. These are placed into an autoclave box or bin for sterilization.

The technique for applying pads is simple but important. The pad needs to be placed so that the eyelids will not be able to open. If the eyelids open under the pad, the pad will rub against the cornea and this will harm the eye and not protect it. The pad is placed diagonally over the closed lids.

If the eye is very deeply set it is best to fold the pad in half and place it so that the folded edge fits below the eyebrow. The pad is taped firmly in place using three strips of adhesive tape, ideally 1 cm wide and positioned as shown in **Figure 4.2**. Added protection can be provided by a plastic eye-shield. These can be bought or made locally from old X-ray plates or cardboard (see **Figure 4.3**).

In most surgical cases it is safer to bandage the eye with elasticated or crepe bandage after applying the pad. The bandage is applied across the forehead and around the head above the ear (**Figure 4.4**). On the second turn the bandage is taken across the eye pad and below the ear. This is repeated alternating so that the bandages passes above and below the ear on the affected side. The bandage should pass just below the occiput otherwise it will tend to slide off the head. It must not be too tight as this may damage the eye. Elasticated bandages can be reused after washing. Alternatively the pad may be secured with adhesive strapping or tape.

Swabs

Swabs used externally on the eye can be made easily from cotton wool and gauze and then autoclaved. *For intraocular surgery it is essential to use*

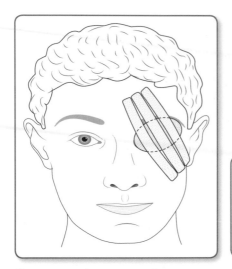

Figure 4.2 Applying an eye pad

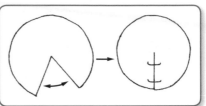

Figure 4.3 How to make a simple eye shield from X-ray plates

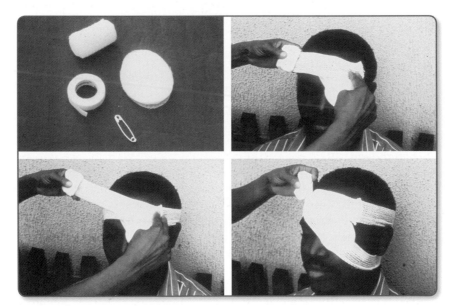

Figure 4.4 To show how to apply a bandage after applying the pad

swabs which will not leave any particles inside the eye, also any sponge or small swab which goes in the eye must be sterile and free of contamination. Cellulose is better than cotton because it will not leave residues. Small packets of pre-sterilised sponges can easily be purchased. Often an automated vitrector is not available, and a 'sponge and scissors vitrectomy' is necessary.

Surgical drapes

These can also be made locally out of close woven cotton preferably in a dark colour which reduces glare. The drape should be large enough to extend from the chest of the patient over the head and to the top of the operating table. The drape should have a hole in its centre for the eye about 3x4 cm in size. Special sterile adhesive plastic drapes can be used to cover up the eyelids and eyelashes leaving just a gap for the speculum, but these single-use drapes are more expensive. A much cheaper alternative is to autoclave a piece of plastic cellophane "clingfilm" spread out on paper. This can be placed across the eyelids and lashes and a small hole cut in the middle for the speculum. After use the drapes should be washed in soapy water and sun dried before packing and sterilizing.

Ideally all the theatre staff and the patient should have special clothes to wear in theatre but this may not be possible. As a minimum the surgeon should wear a theatre mask and hat and have a sterile gown and gloves for operating.

Sterilisation and disinfection procedures

The sterilising of instruments, swabs, linen and eye-pads is by far the most important step in safe surgery. *Sterilisation* means that all living micro-organisms, bacteria, viruses, fungi etc. including spores have been killed. Disinfection means that bacteria which are likely to cause infection have been killed, but spores and some very resistant micro-organisms may survive disinfection. Obviously sterilisation is better than disinfection. There are four common ways of sterilising or disinfecting.[3, 4]

Methods of sterilisation and disinfection

1. Autoclave
2. Dry heat oven
3. Boiling
4. Immersion in chemical solutions

Autoclaving and the dry heat oven will sterilise, and boiling and chemical solutions will only disinfect. However the methods of sterilisation may only disinfect if the treatment is not applied for long enough, and a chemical which disinfects may sterilise after a long period of immersion. Instruments must first be carefully cleaned before sterilising. **The best time for cleaning instruments is immediately after they have been used,** otherwise blood and secretions may become dried and encrusted. Dried blood and secretions are much more difficult to remove, and they prevent spores and bacteria from being killed by the sterilisation process. They can also shorten the life of some instruments. Instruments should be washed with soap and water using a soft brush (a soft tooth-brush is often sufficient) or cloth, paying particular attention to the joints of scissors, artery forceps and needle holders. They should then be rinsed in clean water. If instruments are going to be stored or sterilised using dry heat or chemicals they should also be carefully dried.

Autoclave

Autoclaving is by far the safest, best and most reliable way of sterilisation.
It is the only effective way of sterilising surgical drapes and dressings, and is

the best way to sterilise surgical instruments. If used properly it is guaranteed to kill both bacteria and spores. The autoclave produces water vapour at pressures in excess of 1 atmosphere, and this enables temperatures up to 134 degrees Centigrade to be achieved. The higher the pressure, the higher is the temperature at which the water boils to form water vapour or steam. Steam is more efficient than either dry heat or boiling water at killing microorganisms, and it will not damage dressings and drapes. The time to achieve sterility will vary with the temperature as shown in the following table:

Autoclave Times
134-138 degrees at   3 minutes
126-129 degrees at 10 minutes
121-123 degrees at 15 mintues
115-116 degrees at 30 minutes

(The total time for the autoclave cycle will be longer than these times, because the autoclave has to first heat up and drive out all the air, and then vent off the steam and cool down.)

The higher temperatures can safely be used for instruments, but linen, rubber gloves and cryoprobes should not be sterilised at temperatures greater than 115 degrees. Autoclaves are made in different shapes and sizes. Large ones may be very expensive and need spare parts, but simple pressure cookers are quite cheap, and the running costs for all autoclaves are very low.

Large autoclaves are used for bulk sterilisation of gowns and dressings in between lists. They can be powered by electricity, gas or kerosene.

Small electric bench top autoclaves are ideal for sterilising instruments between cases. (One very popular model is called the "little sister").

Small pressure-cooker type autoclaves heated by a kerosene or butane gas stove or are easily portable and can be used where facilities are very basic. Sterility can only be achieved if steam is able to circulate around all the compartments and if all the air has been evacuated and none is trapped. There are specially designed autoclave bins for sterilising linen and dressings and specially designed autoclave trays for sterilising instruments. These have holes or vents in the side which can be opened to allow steam to enter and drive out all the air. At the end of the sterilisation they can be closed again so as to keep their contents sterile. It is convenient to have an intraocular tray and an extraocular tray, which contain all the basic instruments for intraocular or extraocular surgery. The number of these trays will depend upon the work-load of the unit, and the exact instruments will obviously depend upon the surgeon's preference. A basic intraocular and a basic extraocular set are illustrated in **Figures 4.5** and **4.6**. Setting out the instruments on trays before sterilization will limit damage to the instruments so that they will last longer. It also lessens the handling of instruments once they have been sterilised, and this will lessen the risk of infection. If it is necessary to handle instruments after sterilisation this should be done using the *no touch technique,* so that the instruments are neither lifted nor touched by the end that enters the patient's eye.

Autoclave tape may be applied to each article or alternatively to one package in a load. This special tape has stripes that change colour when the right conditions for sterilisation have been reached. It acts as a simple test for the efficient working of the autoclave.There are also autoclave indicators which change colour when the autoclaving has been completed satisfactorily. Special care should be taken when using an autoclave with attention to correct procedures and safety. The reservoir should be checked and kept at the right level. Only distilled or rain water should be used. Correct venting is essential although many autoclaves vent themselves at the end of the cycle. All staff using the autoclave require training and must strictly adhere to the instruction manual.

Different autoclaves may be calibrated in various units. Below is an approximate conversion table for the units of pressure which may be helpful.

Bar	Pounds/square inch	g/cm²	Temperature
bar	psi	kPa	°C
2	30	200	120
3	40	270	130

Dry heat oven

A hot air oven is quite expensive but requires very little maintenance and is a very effective way of sterilising instruments. It will preserve the edge of delicate cutting instruments better than an autoclave. However instruments must be scrupulously clean and dry first, and the process is very slow. It takes 1 hour at 180 degrees Centigrade to sterilise instruments, and then the instruments must be left to cool.

Boiling

The great advantage of boiling is that it is very quick, simple, easy and cheap. However boiling does not sterilise, it only disinfects. Boiling for 10 minutes will kill all bacteria but it will not kill spores. Although this is a problem in theory it is not a real problem in practice. However boiling has two particular disadvantages:

1. Repeated boiling will cause tarnishing and corrosion of instruments and will certainly damage the cutting edge of fine instruments. Corrosion is lessened by adding 2% sodium carbonate to the solution. If possible, distilled water should be used and not tap water. This is available commercially from garages as water for car batteries. Distilled water will not cause corrosion.
2. After boiling the instruments are wet. They can be dried with a sterile gauze but this might compromise sterility and will break the "no touch technique" rule of not touching the instrument end that enters the eye. If they are used when wet, water from the handle of the instrument will drip down on to the working end and again compromise the no touch

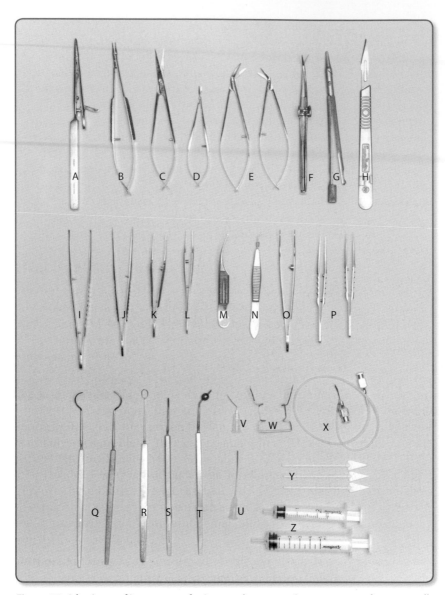

Figure 4.5 A basic set of instruments for intraocular surgery (most surgeons do not use all of these). Some surgeons may also prefer a few other instruments

A. Heavy needle holder for large needles; B. Fine needle holder for fine needles
C. Conjunctival scissors; D. Intraocular scissors (Vannas); E. Right and left corneal scissors; F. Iridectomy scissors (De Wecker's); G. Razor blade fragment holder; H. Scalpel blade (Bard-Parker); I. Heavy toothed forceps; J. Conjunctival forceps; K. Fine corneo-scleral forceps with teeth at the tip (see page 34); L. Fine corneo-scleral forceps with cups at the tip (see page 34); M. Curved fine corneo-scleral forceps; N. Intraocular forceps for handling the lens capsule (Kelman McPherson); O. Capsule forceps for intracapsular extraction (Arruga); P. Fine suture tying forceps; Q. Right and left lens expressor; R. Lens loop; S. Iris repositor; T. Hot point cautery for use with spirit lamp (a battery cautery is shown in Fig. 3.6); U. Cannula; V. Cystotome; W. Adjustable speculum; X. 2-way irrigating/aspirating cannula for extracapsular extraction ('simcoe' cannula); Y. Intraocular swabs ; Z. 2 cc and 5 cc syringes

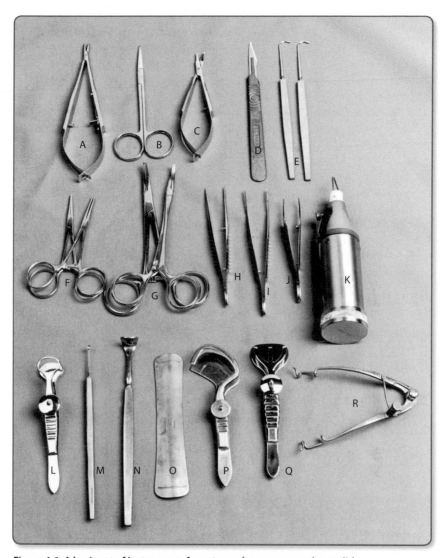

Figure 4.6 A basic set of instruments for extraocular surgery on the eyelids
A. Needle holder; B. Straight scissors; C. Curved spring scissors; D. Scalpel blade; E. Squint hooks;
F. Fine straight artery forceps; G. Curved artery forceps; H. Conjunctival forceps without teeth; I.
Heavy toothed forceps; J. Fine toothed forceps; K. Battery cautery; L. Meibomian cyst lid clamp;
M. Small curette; N. Eyelid retractor (Desmarres); O. Eyelid guard; P. Large eyelid clamp; Q. Eyelid
clamp (Cruikshank or Erhardt); R. Adjustable speculum (Laing)

"technique". If the instruments are placed in the boiler in a perforated rack or tray, then they will dry automatically and not require handling. In emergencies, drapes can be sterilised by boiling and then squeezed dry, although this is certainly not a technique to be recommended.

Chemical solutions

Most chemical solutions are effective against bacteria but not against spores, and so they only disinfect but do not sterilise. However if the instruments are left in the chemical for long enough they may indeed sterilise. Chemical sterilisation and disinfection is good at preserving sharp instruments but there are two main disadvantages.

1. These chemical disinfectants are very toxic especially to the inside of the eye, and the instruments must be thoroughly rinsed in sterile water and dried very carefully after immersion in the chemical. This again will break the "no touch technique" rule.
2. With time or use, the solution may lose some of its potency, or may become chemically inactivated, or the alcohol in alcohol based chemicals may evaporate.

The most commonly used solutions are *Chlorhexidine* (trade name Hibitane) or *Chlorhexidine* and *Cetrimide* combined (trade name Savlon).

Hibitane is available as a 5% concentrate and needs to be diluted 10 times with 70% alcohol to make a solution which is 0.5% Chlorhexidine (Hibitane) in 70% alcohol and 30% water (i.e. one part of concentrate for 9 parts of 70% alcohol).

Savlon is available as a concentrate containing 1.5% Chlorhexidine and 15% Cetrimide and needs to be diluted thirty times in 70% alcohol (1 part of concentrate for 29 parts of 70% alcohol).

(The stock bottles should have clear instructions about how they should be diluted).

Both of these solutions should disinfect instruments after 10 minutes. After prolonged usage some of the alcohol may evaporate and the solution may lose its strength. If alcohol is not available concentrated Savlon diluted 1:30 in boiled water will disinfect instruments after 30 minutes.

Povidone Iodine is another widely used disinfecting agent, which is effective against most micro-organisms. A 10% solution can be made as follows:

• Take 500ml of distilled water (cooled, boiled rain water is an alternative)
• Add sodium phosphate 16.6 g and citric acid 3.4g (these act as a chemical buffer)
• Then add 50 g of Povidone Iodine, thus making a 10% solution. This will also disinfect instruments after 10 minutes.

A 10% solution of Povidone Iodine can be used for cleaning the eyelids and the conjunctival sac preoperatively, but if it is left in the conjunctival sac for some time, some people think that 5% is safer.

Formalin vapour is an effective sterilising agent against all micro-organisms and spores. It is supplied as formalin tablets, which are placed in an airtight container at a warm room temperature. 12 hours are required for sterilisation.

99% sugar cane alcohol is often found as an affordable and readily available product in many parts of the world. It is a very effective chemical sterilizer, but as with all chemicals instruments should be thoroughly rinsed with sterile water before intraocular use.

Cryoprobes are not very often used nowadays because intracapsular cataract extraction has become obsolete and most people now recommend extracapsular cataract extraction. However, the sterilisation of cryoprobes often presents a problem. They can only be autoclaved at lower temperatures and so will take half an hour for the cycle. Cryoprobes are quite often sterilised by immersion in chemical solutions between patients on the same list. As the probe actually enters the eye great care must be taken both to wash off all these chemicals, and also to make sure that the probe is not in any way contaminated. A small portable cryoprobe used with freon gas can however be safely boiled. (Do not boil the cylinder of gas itself, as it will explode!)

Sterilised instruments, drapes and dressings can be safely stored and transported in sealed autoclave bins and trays. If such bins or trays are not available all items must be double wrapped in linen before sterilisation and can then be safely stored or transported.

Stock keeping, storage and security

Good stock keeping to maintain essential supplies is often overlooked. However its importance cannot be over emphasised especially when there may be long delays between ordering supplies and their arrival. A system of monitoring stores and the rate at which consumables such as medicines, dressings, sutures etc. are used will allow for ordering and budgeting.[5] Money is always limited so there is no place for holding excessive quantities. The only way to be aware of annual usage and any seasonal variations in consumption is to have a strict system of stock keeping. This important part of theatre management should be the responsibility of the person in charge of the theatre.

It is obvious that equipment and supplies should be stored in a place where they will not deteriorate, and where they are safe.

Managing with limited resources

In many circumstances the volume of surgical work or financial limitations mean that correct theatre procedures cannot be followed strictly. In correct theatre procedures everybody who enters the operating theatre and all the staff and patients should wear a complete change of clothes. All those operating scrub up completely between cases with fresh gloves and a fresh gown. Often it may not be possible to maintain these standards. The patients may have to come to the operating theatre wearing their own clothes. The surgical staff should always scrub up completely at the beginning of a list, but may be obliged just to change their gloves in between cases or even to wipe their gloves in alcohol between cases. In order to maintain surgical through put it may be necessary to have more than one operating table in the same operating room.

Sometimes instruments which are designed for single use and then to be thrown away, may be resterilised and reused. Make sure that they are resterilised correctly and in an appropriate way.

To ensure safe surgery there are four areas in which "cutting corners" and compromises are strictly forbidden. These are:

1. Correct preparation of the patient for surgery, with a thorough cleaning of the face and skin preparation around the eye (see pages 70–71). This includes "marking" the eye for surgery to avoid mistakes.
2. Sterilisation of all instruments, drapes and dressings. If an item like an intraocular lens or a pre-sterilised disposable instrument comes from the manufacturer in a sterile wrapping, then make sure that the packaging has not in any way been damaged.
3. Sterilisation and purity of all solutions used in intraocular irrigation.
4. The correct handling of instruments and dressings and the use of a "no touch technique". Nothing that enters the eye should touch the eyelids or lashes.

People working in small units, or on tour in rural areas may have to rely on boiling and chemicals as the only means of disinfecting between cases. Although this is not the best way it appears to be safe as long as everyone sticks to the rules. Some people will boil the blunt instruments and use chemicals for the sharps.

*   Don't try to shorten the time needed for immersion in chemicals or boiling.
*   Make sure that the chemical solution is fresh.
*   Make sure that the instruments are dried with a sterile swab and there is no chemical residue on the instruments. This should be done by someone who understands how important this is.
*   *Never rely on just wiping the instruments between cases with spirit, ether or acetone. It isn't safe enough.*

Infection control strategy

Post-operative infections do sometimes occur, even with the most careful and well-trained surgical team. Good units have an infection rate of about one case in a thousand or less. It is reasonable to assume that any infection developing within the first post-operative week has been contracted at the time of the operation. Even an isolated case of post-operative infection should make the surgeon and the surgical team review all their techniques, equipment and procedures. If several infections occur close to each other an even more radical overhaul of theatre procedures is required. Any irrigating fluids should be discarded and a new batch obtained. All made up disinfectant solutions should be discarded and new ones made, and the steriliser changed or a new method of sterilisation tried. If available an infection control officer or a microbiology department will help to trace the source of an infection. The following is a list of the more common possible sources of infection during surgery:

Sources of infection

From the patient:

- Skin and eye not properly cleaned or draped.
- Conjunctivitis.
- Blepharitis.
- Dacrocystitis.
- Septic lesion near the eye.

Infection from the patient is usually due to either poor preparation or poor case selection.

From the staff:

- Septic lesions.
- Poor scrubbing up.
- Contaminated gloves.
- Failure to observe the "no touch technique" by the surgeon or assistant, or touching the lids or lashes with instruments entering the eye.
- Prolonged manipulation during the operation.

Infection from the staff is usually due to poor surgical technique by the surgeon or assistant

From the theatre equipment:

- Contaminated irrigating fluid.
- Faulty steriliser.
- Faulty sterilising technique.
- Contamination of sterile trolleys e.g. from flies.
- Contamination or inactivation of disinfectant solutions.
- Broken or defective packaging for an IOL or instrument which is factory sterilised.

References

1. Walia D, Huria J, Cordero I. Equipment maintenance and repair. Community Eye Health 2010; 23:26-9.
2. Cox I, Stevens S. Care of ophthalmic surgical instruments. Community Eye Health 2000;13:40-1.
3. Heaton R. Sterilization of surgical instruments. Community Eye Health 1998;11:14-5.
4. Singh KM, Stevens SM. Sterilization of surgical instruments. Community Eye Health 1998; 11:15.
5. Thulasiraj R. Managing your eye unit's supplies. Community Eye Health 2011; 24:32-5.

5 Anaesthesia of the eye and preparing the patient for surgery

Objectives

Principle objective:

For intraocular surgery a careful preoperative preparation and a good local anaesthetic block are just as important as the operation itself.

In this chapter, the following are covered:

- Preparation, including pre-operative assessment of the patient and the eye; and pre-operative cleaning and preparation of the face and eye.
- The pupil, and its treatment before surgery.
- Sedation.
- Local anaesthesia.
- Complications of local anaesthesia and how to deal with them if they occur.
- General anaesthesia, a brief summary.

It is essential that a patient is given a satisfactory anaesthetic and is correctly prepared for intraocular surgery.

These preparations are almost as important as the operation itself. A badly anaesthetized or badly prepared patient is likely to cause serious problems during the operation and have an increased risk of post-operative infection. Anaesthesia and preparations for extraocular surgery are very much simpler.

Anaesthesia aims to produce a pain-free surgical field. When operating on the eye it is best to paralyse the extraocular muscles, so the eye doesn't move; and the orbicularis oculi muscle, so the eyelids don't squeeze.

Anaesthesia can be produced in 2 ways, general anaesthesia (GA) in which the patient is unconscious, or local anaesthesia (LA) in which only certain nerves are blocked and the patient remains conscious. Even in ideal circumstances where first-class general anaesthesia is readily available, many surgeons will operate under LA by choice. Most eye surgery can be done under LA, especially if GA facilities are not ideal.

The advantages of local anaesthesia

Safety

Nowadays both GA and LA should be safe. However complications do occur even in the best of hands, but these complications are less common and less serious with LA than GA. Many eye patients are elderly and may have chronic respiratory or cardio-vascular disease. These may deteriorate with GA. After GA there is always a risk of post-operative confusion especially in the elderly, and coughing and vomiting may cause complications after an intraocular operation. After GA there is also a slight risk of post-operative chest infection or deep vein thrombosis developing.

Speed

LA is quicker than GA because less time is required to give the anaesthetic. In particular a patient after LA can go straight out of the operating room, but after GA the patient must be carefully nursed by skilled staff until full consciousness has returned.

Cost

The cost of the equipment and anaesthetic agents is obviously much less with LA. There is also saving because the services of an anaesthetist and an-aesthetic nurse or technician are not required.

However in certain situations GA is either necessary or desirable.
These are:

- *Children.* Young children must be given a GA, and in older children GA is preferable for all except very minor procedures.
- *Penetrating eye injuries.* LA is difficult to give effectively. There is often orbital haemorrhage, and there is a risk of raising the pressure in the eye and expelling some of the ocular contents after LA. When a patient with a penetrating injury or an open eye is given a GA, it is usually recommended that Suxamethonium Chloride (Scoline) is not used as a paralysing agent. There is some evidence that it causes contractions of the extraocular muscles and may lead to extrusion of ocular contents.
- *Major surgery or long operations* such as exenteration or retinal detachment surgery.
- *Confused or demented patients.* These patients are better operated upon under GA.
- *Inflammation or infection of the orbit.* It is often difficult to achieve a good anaesthetic block in these situations, and the injection may spread the infection.

Local anaesthesia can be achieved in 3 ways:

1. Topical drops.
2. Local infiltration.
3. Nerve block.

Topical drops

If local anaesthetic drops are applied to the conjunctival sac they will anaesthetise the conjunctiva and corneal surface. This is all that is required for minor surgical and diagnostic procedures like removing corneal foreign bodies or checking intraocular pressures. Various agents are available:

Amethocaine 1%
Oxybuprocaine 0.4%
Proxymetacaine 0.5%

Lignocaine 4%
Tetracaine 4%

The anaesthesia will last for about 15 minutes. The effect of topical drops can be increased if a small swab is soaked in the local anaesthetic agent and left for a minute on the conjunctiva. In this way sub-conjunctival or sub-Tenon's injections can be given painlessly.

Local infiltration

If local anaesthetic is injected into the tissues it will produce anaesthesia in the region where it is injected. This is the usual method of anaesthesia for surgery to the eyelids or conjunctiva. Lignocaine 1% to 2% is the most popular agent.

It is recommended that dilute adrenaline (1 in 100,000) should be used in the local anaesthetic solution. (Adrenaline is called epinephrine by medical staff trained in the U.S.A.) If the lignocaine solution is being made up in a local pharmacy or operating room this means adding the equivalent of 1mg of adrenaline (or a 1ml. Ampoule of 1/1000 adrenaline) to 100 cc of lignocaine solution. The eyelids and conjunctiva are vascular tissues. The adrenaline constricts the blood vessels and lessens bleeding at surgery. It also prolongs the action of the local anaesthetic and slows its absorption time, so that the risk of systemic side effects is lessened.

Nerve blocks

With this technique the anaesthetic agent is injected close to the main trunk of a nerve or its branches so that its sensory or motor function is blocked. This is the usual way of giving LA for intraocular surgery. With a nerve block a relatively small injection can achieve a large effect. However a stronger solution of anaesthetic may be necessary and lignocaine 2% is the usual agent. Also the surgeon must know the anatomy of the nerves to place the injection correctly.

Preparing a patient for an extraocular operation is very straightforward. The tissues are infiltrated with local anaesthetic and adrenaline. The area is cleaned and the surgical drapes applied. For intraocular surgery much more preparation is necessary.

This will be discussed under the following headings:

Preoperative assessment of the patient's general health.
Preoperative assessment of the eye.
Cleaning and preparing the face and eye.
Treatment to the pupil.
Sedation.
Local anaesthesia.

Preoperative assessment of the patient's general health

it may not be possible to carry out a full medical examination, but the patient's heart and lungs should be examined to make sure there are no signs of heart failure, breathing difficulties, or uncontrolled coughing. The blood pressure should be measured to check for *hypertension*, and the urine tested for sugar to exclude *diabetes*.

Patients in rural areas may not be able to receive long-term treatment for heart failure, chronic cough, hypertension or diabetes, but if possible these disorders should receive some treatment before surgery. The patient must be able to lie still and fairly flat for the duration of the surgery. Coughing and breathlessness can cause serious complications in the middle of an eye operation. Severe hypertension has an increased risk of expulsive haemorrhage during intraocular surgery, and diabetes has an increased risk of post-operative infection.

Preoperative assessment of the eye

The eyelid, lacrimal apparatus and conjunctiva protect the eye and should be free from infection. If they are themselves diseased there is a serious risk of post-operative infection or irritation to the eye. In particular look for the following conditions:-

Entropion or trichiasis The in-turned eyelashes will constantly irritate the eye postoperatively, and entropion should be corrected before doing any intraocular surgery. In cases of mild trichiasis where just a few eyelashes are turning in, it is reasonable to epilate the offending eyelashes, carry out the intraocular operation, and treat the eyelashes later.

Mucopurulent conjunctivitis If there is a mucopurulent or sticky discharge from the conjunctiva it means there is a bacterial infection of the conjunctiva. There is a great risk of this infection spreading into the eye during intraocular surgery. The conjunctivitis must be treated with intensive local antibiotics, until the eye appears free from inflammation and infection. Chloramphenicol drops every two hours and ointment at night is an effective local antibiotic, but there are many others that can be used. Bacterial conjunctivitis may occur in an otherwise healthy eye, but usually there is a reason for it. Examine the eye carefully for entropion, ectropion, facial palsy, blepharitis or dacryocystitis. If any of these conditions are present the conjunctivitis will not resolve until they are corrected.

Septic spots Make sure the patient has no septic spots on the face or scalp. Many patients having intraocular surgery may have other abnormalities such as a pterygium, conjunctival or corneal scarring. These conditions are not a contraindication to surgery, although they might make it a little harder to perform.

Cleaning and preparing the face and eye

The importance of keeping pathogenic bacteria from the eye and conjunctiva is obvious. It is not possible to clean the eye with strong disinfectants because they would irritate the conjunctiva and corneal epithelium. Fortunately the healthy eye has various mechanisms which prevent pathogenic bacteria surviving in the conjunctival sac. The production and drainage of tears and the act of blinking will wash away any bacteria that may land on the eye, and the tears contain lysozyme, an enzyme which inactivates many bacteria.

A standard regime for cleaning and preparing the patient's face and eye should be as follows:

- Wash the face and hair the evening before the operation, and then wash the face thoroughly with a medicated soap or 1% aqueous Cetrimide on the morning of the operation.
- Many surgeons recommend trimming the eyelashes carefully some time before the operation. This will lessen the risk of instruments or an intraocular lens touching the eyelashes and becoming contaminated during the operation. Even better is to use sterile cellophane drapes which stick to the skin and cover the eyelids and lashes. These can be bought as sterile units or made as described on page 57. Their use obviously makes cutting the eyelashes unnecessary.
- Topical antibiotics. The healthy eye usually remains free of bacteria, but there is some evidence that the very slight risk of post-operative infection is lessened by the routine use of pre-operative topical antibiotics. It is usual to apply antibiotic drops to the eye shortly before intraocular surgery, and many surgeons like to apply antibiotic ointment the night before the operation as well.
- Preoperative skin preparation. This is usually done after the local anaesthetic nerve block has been given and before applying the sterile drapes at the beginning of the operation. The eyelids, eyebrows, cheek and side of the nose should be prepared.[1] Various solutions can be used. They should be effective in killing bacteria and yet be non-irritant to the eye, therefore they must be water-based and contain no alcohol. Beware! Many general surgical skin preparations contain alcohol. The following can be recommended:
  i. Aqueous solutions of organic iodine compounds such as 10% povidone iodine. (This is certainly the most popular skin preparation at present)
  ii. Aqueous solutions of Cetrimide and/or Chlorhexidine such as 1% "Savlon".

Usually the skin preparation is applied on a swab held in a sponge-holding forceps. Start at the nose and loop outwards around the eyelids, ending with the surface of the eyelids and lashes. Some surgeons deliberately allow some of the povidone-iodine solution to go into the conjunctival sac. It should not be left there too long before being washed out, because the strength recommended for applying direct to the conjunctiva is 5%. Clean the area twice and then use a third sterile dry swab to dry the skin. As soon as the skin has been prepared, the drapes are applied and a speculum inserted to hold open the eyelids. At this stage some surgeons like to leave a few drops of 5% povidone-iodine in the conjunctival sac for about half a minute. Finally the conjunctival sac should be irrigated with sterile saline to wash away any debris, mucus or residual skin preparation present.

Treatment to the pupil

For cataract surgery the pupil must be dilated with mydriatic drops. There are two types of mydriatics.

Parasympathetic blocking agents will paralyse the iris sphincter muscle. Cyclopentolate 1% or tropicamide 1% are the drugs of choice. Cyclopentolate acts for about one day and tropicamide for a few hours and they both start working within a few minutes. Homatropine may also be used as an alternative. Atropine 1% causes mydriasis for up to a week and acts rather slowly so is not usually recommended.

Sympathetic stimulating agents cause the iris dilator muscle to contract. They also constrict the conjunctival blood vessels which helps to limit bleeding during the operation. Phenylephrine 10% is the drug most commonly used. (A weaker strength of 2.5% is recommended for young children and adults with hypertension.) Adrenaline 1% and cocaine 4% are also effective, but are not such powerful mydriatics.

The usual dose is to give one drop each of a parasympathetic blocking drug and a sympathetic stimulating drug one hour or half an hour an hour before the operation, and repeat this just before surgery if the pupil is not fully dilated. **Don't start putting dilating drops in the eye more than one hour before surgery because their effect will start to wear off. Further drops will then not be so effective.**

During extracapsular extraction the manipulations inside the eye may make the pupil start to constrict. *It is very important to maintain pupil dilatation throughout the whole operation, and there are several ways of achieving this.*

- By the use of topical prostaglandin inhibitors preoperatively. (Diclofenac, ketorolac and flurbiprofen are all available as eye drops although they may not be marketed in some areas).These drugs will not dilate the pupil, but help to counteract the pupil constriction or miosis which often occurs during the operation.
- A very small amount of adrenaline added to the intra-ocular infusion bottle (0.5mg added to 500ml of infusion) is even more effective and should be used routinely for all extracapsular cataract extractions.
- The infusion bottle should not be too cold as this can provoke pupil constriction.

For operations on the iris or for glaucoma, mydriatics should not be given and many surgeons prefer the pupil to be constricted with Pilocarpine drops. Many glaucoma cases will already be receiving Pilocarpine. The only exception is an iridectomy for pupil block glaucoma in which case mydriatics should be used.

Sedation

Any patient having intraocular surgery under local anaesthetic will be frightened and anxious. By far the best way to relieve fear and anxiety is to spend a little time reassuring the patient and explaining the purpose of the operation and the effect of the local anaesthetic injection. Reassurance and explanation is much more valuable than any amount of tablets or injections. Usually the patient will not need any further sedation and will relax and lie still for the operation. However some sedation given after this reassurance and explanation may be helpful for anxious patients. It is most important not to over-sedate patients. Too much sedation is much worse than none at all. The patient, especially if they are frail may fall asleep or become confused and restless and will then not co-operate during the operation. The most popular sedative drugs are the benzodiazepines. Diazepam (Valium) is most commonly used, the oral dose being 5 mg for a frail person and 10 mg for a robust person one or two hours before the operation. There are many other alternative sedatives. Some surgeons like to give multivitamin tablets at the same time, as it helps to prevent poor wound healing in patients who may be malnourished or deficient in vitamins.

The patient must lie still during the operation and in particular must not move their head. The best way to keep the head still is to use a special pillow of foam rubber with a large hole in the middle of it to fit the head. (see Figure 2.2, page 19) Alternatively two small foam pillows or sand bags can be placed on either side of the head. Patients must keep their arms and hands by their sides throughout the operation. The best and most pleasant way to ensure this is to have someone hold the patient's hands, this also provides comfort and reassurance. If no one is available then the patient's hands should be gently tucked under their buttocks as they are lying flat. Some people restrain the patient's hands with a strap tied gently around their wrists but this may alarm and frighten them more. If such a restraint is used, the patients must be told why they are being "strapped down".

Local anaesthesia

The LA injections have the four following aims:
1. Anaesthesia of the eye.
2. Paralysis of the extraocular muscles.
3. Paralysis of the orbicularis oculi muscle.
4. To block the patient's vision.

Anaesthesia of the eye so that no pain is felt

The sensory fibres from the eye pass in the ophthalmic branch of the trigeminal nerve (the 5th. cranial nerve).The cornea, iris and sclera are extremely sensitive to pain, while the conjunctiva is less sensitive.

Paralysis of the extraocular muscles so that the eye does not move during surgery (akinesia)

The extraocular muscles are supplied by the oculomotor (3rd), trochlear (4th) and abducens (6th) cranial nerves. A moving eye makes surgery very difficult. In addition the pull of the muscles on the sclera once the eye has been opened will increase the intraocular pressure and make prolapse of the contents much more likely.

With the use of modern phakoemulsification equipment, cataracts can be removed through a very small watertight incision. So some expert surgeons are happy to perform phakoemulsification without even paralysing the extraocular muscles. They recommend just applying local anaesthetic drops to anaesthetise the corneal and the conjunctiva. The anaesthesia can be supplemented by instilling lignocaine directly into the anterior chamber during the operation. (This must be free of all preservatives and isotonic.)

However, these techniques are only used by very expert surgeons, and good nerve blocks make the operation very much easier. For an inexperienced or trainee surgeon or in a difficult case a good block is essential.

To block the vision by anaesthetising the optic nerve (2nd cranial nerve)

In this way the patient is not upset by the bright operating theatre light.

Paralysis of the orbicularis oculi muscle which closes the eyelids

This muscle is supplied by the facial nerve (the 7th cranial nerve). If the patient is squeezing his eye shut during the operation surgical exposure will be difficult. There is also a serious risk that once the eye has been opened the pressure of the eyelids trying to close will force out the ocular contents. This is obviously a very serious complication.

The first three aims may be achieved by a single nerve nerve block, the **retrobulbar** block. Alternatively two separate injections into the orbit called the **peribulbar** block may be given. Recently a **sub-Tenon's** block using a blunt cannula has been described which is becoming increasingly popular.

The fourth aim, to paralyse the orbicularis oculi muscle is achieved by a **facial block.**

Lignocaine 2% is the most popular agent for nerve blocks. It has a rapid onset of action and will usually last for an hour. An alternative is **Bupivacaine** (Marcain) 0.5% or 0.75%. It is more expensive, its onset of action is not so rapid but it lasts for up to 3 hours or longer. Some surgeons use a 50/50 mixture of Lignocaine and Bupivacaine to try to get the advantages of each.

Adrenaline (Epinephrine) 1:100,000 should always be added to the facial block and most people add it to the peribulbar block. Its addition slows the absorption time so that the anaesthetic lasts longer and the risks of the systemic toxic side-effects from rapid absorption of local anaesthetic are less. Many people also add adrenaline to the retrobulbar injection, but there is in theory a possible risk of causing vasoconstriction in the retinal or choroidal arteries. However these arteries are probably not very sensitive to adrenaline.

(In some countries 5% lignocaine is available. This produces an excellent nerve block but because of its strength can have complications. It should always be used with dilute adrenaline to delay its absorption and the maximum overall dose is 5 ml–2.5 ml for the facial block and 2.5 ml for the retrobulbar block).

Hyaluronidase (Hyalase) in a strength of approximately 25 to 50 units/ml may be added to the retrobulbar or peribulbar injections only. (One ampoule of hyalase containing 1500 units is usually added to a 20 ml or 50 ml bottle of 2% lignocaine. Once it has been diluted the hyalase becomes ineffective after a few days). The hyaluronidase helps the local anaesthetic to spread through the tissues, and so increases the effectiveness of the nerve block, especially with a retrobulbar injection where so many nerves need to be blocked by a single injection. Adding hyaluronidase means that a smaller amount of injection has a better effect. It is expensive and is unavailable in many countries.

The retrobulbar block

Principle

The retrobulbar space lies inside the extraocular muscle cone behind the eye (**Figure 5.1** and **5.2**). The 2nd, 3rd, 6th and branches of the 5th cranial nerves are all found in this space and the 4th nerve passes very near. Therefore all the nerves supplying the eye and extraocular muscles are blocked by one injection of local anaesthetic into the retrobulbar space. After a successful block there is no sensation, no movement and no vision in the eye.

Indications:

- Intraocular surgery
- Evisceration or enucleation
- As a supplement to ketamine general anaesthesia (see page 84).

Method

1. Prepare the injection–3 to 5 ml of 2% lignocaine is used. If hyaluronidase is available 2 to 3 ml is usually sufficient.(Whether or not to add adrenaline has already been discussed). In the past a long (50 mm), fine (26G) retrobulbar needle has been used to deliver the injection to the apex of the orbit, where the nerves are all close together. However the further back into the orbit the injection is given, the greater is the risk of the needle entering a nerve or blood vessel, and causing potentially serious complications. Also with very fine needles there may be some uncertainty as to which direction the tip is pointing.

   For this reason it is better to give the injection in the anterior part of the retrobulbar space, placing the tip of the needle 30 mm deep to the skin. A standard 23G needle is satisfactory. The hyaluronidase in the injection will help it to spread through the tissues. If hyaluronidase

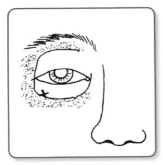
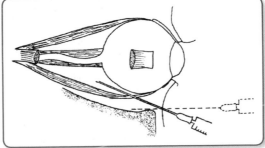

Figure 5.1 The retrobulbar block, to show the entry point for the needle

Figure 5.2 The retrobulbar block, to show the direction of the needle for the first 15 mm (dotted line) and second 15 mm (full line)

is not available, it is safer to give a larger volume of injection (5 ml) anteriorly in the retrobulbar space than to give the injection at the apex of the orbit. Many people use a needle for retrobulbar injection that does not have an acute bevel (see **Figure 5.3**). This lessens the risk of perforating the eyeball. However it is most important that the tip of the needle is sharp and not blunt and the best way to avoid penetrating the eye is to know the anatomy and advance the needle in the correct direction.

2.   The patient lies flat and is asked to look straight ahead. This may be difficult if the patient cannot see but is best achieved by holding the patient's hand in front of his eye and asking him to look at it. Both the eyelids are swabbed clean.

3.   The lower orbital rim is felt and the needle passed through the skin just above the orbital rim and about one-third of the way from the lateral end of the eyelid (**Figure 5.1**). It is passed straight back below the eye for 15 mm It is best to have the bevel pointing upwards towards the globe as shown in **Figure 5.2**. Often some resistance is felt as it passes through the orbital septum. The tip of the needle may hit the hard bone on the floor of the orbit.

4.   The direction of the needle is now changed so that the tip is pointing slightly upwards and inwards towards the opposite occiput (**Figure 5.2**). This ensures that the tip enters the retrobulbar space and lies within the muscle cone. Some resistance is felt as the needle passes through the muscles and this may rotate the eye downwards slightly. The needle should be advanced no more than 30 mm in all from the skin.

5.   The plunger is first withdrawn slightly to ensure that a blood vessel has not been entered, and then the injection given. There should not be any significant resistance. The needle is withdrawn, the eyelids closed with a pad and *immediate firm but gentle* pressure is applied. This may be applied with a special pneumatic balloon (the Honan balloon) inflated to 30 mm Hg or more simply with a spongy ball or a round weight designed to fit neatly into the orbit. The most simple way of applying pressure is with the hypothenar eminence of the patient's or assistant's hand which will fit nicely into the orbit. This gentle but firm pressure should be maintained for 5–10 minutes.

6.   After this time the retrobulbar blocks (and the facial block if it has been given) are assessed to ensure that they are adequate. There is often

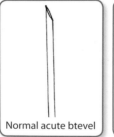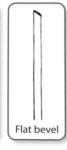

Figure 5.3 The bevel of needles

Normal acute btevel   Flat bevel

some residual movement of the eye and lids but as long as most of the muscle action is blocked the operation can proceed. If movement is excessive the blocks can be repeated once only.

Complications of retrobulbar anaesthesia

1. Inadequate anaesthesia and akinesia.
2. Retrobulbar haemorrhage.
3. Injection into a blood vessel or into the cerebrospinal fluid.
4. Injection into the eyeball.
5. Permanent neurological damage.
6. Toxic reaction from excessive anaesthetic.

The first two complications are quite common but are rarely of any serious significance. The last four complications are all serious but should be extremely rare.

Inadequate anaesthesia and akinesia

The best test of success of a retrobulbar block is to examine the ocular movements. If these have been blocked, there will almost always be adequate anaesthesia. If there is almost a full range of eye movements then the block may be repeated once. Sometimes the block fails because of poor technique. Either the needle is passed along the orbital floor and not into the muscle cone or alternatively the needle is not advanced far enough out of fear of penetrating the eyeball.

Despite an otherwise adequate block the eye may rotate upwards due to the continued action of the superior rectus. In these cases the superior rectus may require further anaesthesia. 1 ml of 2% lignocaine is injected above the eye either through the conjunctiva or through the upper eye lid. The eye may rotate slightly upwards if the needle tip enters the superior rectus muscle itself.

Retrobulbar haemorrhage

slight retrobulbar haemorrhage is quite common and is caused by a small blood vessel being pierced by the retrobulbar needle. Often it is only noted post-operatively, when there may be bruising of the eyelids or a subconjunctival haemorrhage as the blood tracks forward. Severe or marked retrobulbar haemorrhage causing proptosis should occur in less than 1% of cases. If there is proptosis the operation must be postponed as the raised orbital pressure will increase the risk of serious complications during surgery. A firm pad and bandage should be applied and the operation can be repeated when the haemorrhage has completely subsided. It is very unusual for any permanent damage to occur from a retrobulbar haemorrhage, but there is always the possible risk of optic nerve compression and subsequent optic atrophy. The risk of haemorrhage can be reduced by:

*   Checking that the retrobulbar needle has a smooth sharp tip. Damaged or hooked tips can tear delicate blood vessels.
*   Holding the needle steady after advancing and whilst injecting the anaesthetic. Excessive movement of the needle increases the risk of haemorrhage.

- Applying *gentle pressure* on the eye *immediately* after withdrawing the needle will limit any blood leaking from small vessels.
- Some surgeons suggest that the anaesthetic should be injected as the needle advances to move the tissues away from the tip of the needle.

Injection into a blood vessel or into the cerebrospinal fluid

In either case this can be very serious and there is a risk that the patient may die. Injection into a blood vessel is best avoided by slightly withdrawing the plunger of the syringe before injecting. Injection into a vein can cause cardiac irregularities, collapse or convulsions. Injections into a retinal or ciliary artery can cause temporary or permanent visual defects.

The optic nerve is surrounded by dura mater containing cerebro-spinal fluid and it is possible to put the needle through the dural sheath and thus inject lignocaine into the cerebrospinal fluid. This can cause loss of consciousness, respiratory arrest and convulsions. The risk of injecting into the cerebrospinal fluid is reduced by taking 2 precautions. Firstly, by not advancing the retrobulbar needle more than 30–35 mm from the skin. Secondly when giving the retrobulbar injection, making sure the patient is looking straight forward and not looking up. If the patient looks up this brings down the back of the eyeball and the optic nerve and thus nearer to the path of the retrobulbar needle.

If the patient's airway is protected and artificial ventilation and cardiac resuscitation given, the patient should usually recover completely from unconsciousness or collapse caused by intravenous or cerebrospinal injection of local anaesthetic.

Anyone giving local anaesthesia to the eye or performing eye surgery should have training in how to resuscitate a collapsed patient and should know immediately what to do.

Injection into or through the eyeball

This usually occurs because the needle is directed and advanced incorrectly. It is vital to understand the anatomy. There is not a great deal of space between the floor of the orbit and the eyeball itself. The risk is increased in myopic eyes which are large and have thin sclera. If the injection is into the eye it will become very hard on injection and the cornea may become opaque. This serious complication usually results in blindness, and the operation should be abandoned if it occurs. If the injection is through the eye it may become very soft.

These disasters are best avoided by advancing the needle slowly and not pushing against any resistance once the tip of the needle has passed through the orbital septum. If the needle does meet resistance, in most cases it will be the bone on the floor of the orbit. It should be withdrawn just a fraction and then redirected more upwards. If resistance is still felt it is probably hitting the eyeball, and not the floor of the orbit. In this case it should be very carefully and gently redirected a little more downwards.

Long-term neurological damage

Permanent damage to one of the cranial nerves in the orbit may very rarely occur.

Toxic reaction from excessive anaesthetic

The amounts of local anaesthetic that are given for a facial and retrobulbar block, and for a peribulbar block are quite close to the recommended maximum dose for safety. This is especially true if hyalase is added because it increases the absorption rate of the anaesthetic, and this is why hyalase should not be added to the facial block. By contrast, adding adrenaline slows down the absorption rate. The signs of local anaesthetic toxicity are similar to those from injecting into the blood stream:-cardiac irregularities and collapse.

The peribulbar block

if done carefully and correctly the incidence of serious complications with retrobulbar blocks is extremely low, but the fact that these complications do occur has led to the development of other ways of giving local anaesthesia. One alternative is the peribulbar block (**Figure 5.4**). It avoids some of the possible hazards of retrobulbar injection but requires two injections and takes longer to work. It also tends to cause proptosis because a larger volume of fluid is injected behind the eye. Because the injection is given through the conjunctiva and not the skin it is less painful for the patient.

Principle

Two fairly large volumes of local anaesthetic are given around the eye outside the extraocular muscle cone. These spread slowly into the retrobulbar space as well producing anaesthesia and akinesia of the eye and eyelids.

Method

1. A syringe with 10 ml of local anaesthetic is mounted on a 23G or finer gauge needle. Most surgeons add 1:100,000 adrenaline to prevent rapid absorption and if available 300 units of hyalase to help the injection to spread.
2. The patient is prepared as for a retrobulbar injection. A drop of local anaesthetic is applied to the conjunctiva.
3. The lower lid is pulled down to expose the lower fornix. The needle is inserted through the conjunctiva of the lower fornix lateral to the mid-line. The syringe is held vertically and the needle is advanced backwards and

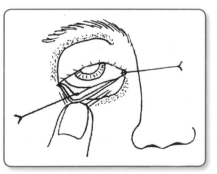

Figure 5.4 Injection sites for the peribulbar block

slightly outwards away from the eye so that it passes to the level of the equator of the eye. It should advance no more than 25 mm. If the patient is asked to move their eye, this will confirm that the tip of the needle is not touching the globe or the extraocular muscles. After withdrawing the plunger slightly to check that the needle has not entered a blood vessel, 5 ml of local anaesthetic is injected and the needle is withdrawn. Gentle pressure is applied for 5 minutes.

4. A second injection is given through the caruncle and passed back and slightly medially towards the nose for 25 mm. The patient should be asked to move their eye and the plunger withdrawn in the same way, and then 4 ml of local anaesthetic is injected. The needle is withdrawn and gentle pressure applied for 10 minutes. The eye is then assessed to ensure an adequate block.

There should be no need for a facial nerve block to be given with a peribulbar block as enough anaesthetic should diffuse out of the orbit to weaken the orbicularis oculi muscle.

The complications of a peribulbar block are the same as for a retrobulbar block. Because larger amounts are given into the orbit the chances of an inadequate block are less. Also there is less risk of injecting into the cerebrospinal fluid or causing permanent neurological damage. However the risks of a retrobulbar haemorrhage, injecting into the eyeball, or into a blood vessel or of toxic absorption are just the same. The same precautions about advancing the needle should be taken as with the retrobulbar injection.

Sub-Tenon's block

Principle
To avoid the risks from using sharp needles, a blunt cannula is advanced into the retrobulbar space to deliver the anaesthetic.

Method
1. The conjunctiva is first anaesthetised with local anaesthetic drops. A small swab soaked in local anaesthetic and left in the lower fornix for a minute is particularly effective. A speculum is inserted to hold open the eyelids.
2. The patient should be told to look upwards and outwards. Using forceps and scissors a tiny incision is made in the conjunctiva in the inferomedial quadrant of the eye about 5 to 6 mm from the limbus and midway between the inferior and medial rectus muscles (**Figure 5.5**). This incision is then deepened very slightly to go through Tenon's capsule. The local anaesthetic drops should prevent any significant pain from this.
3. Specially designed cannulas are made for the sub Tenon's injection, but a blunt lacrimal cannula or blunt bent cannula normally used for viscoelastic is a perfectly satisfactory alternative. It is mounted on a syringe with the same local anaesthetic as for a retrobulbar injection. The cannula tip is then inserted through the small hole in the conjunctiva and Tenon's capsule and passed backwards round the eye with the **tip touching the globe all the way** (**Figure 5.6** and **5.7**). The

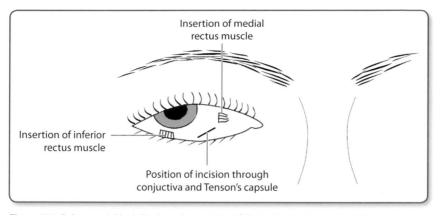

Insertion of medial
rectus muscle

Insertion of inferior
rectus muscle

Position of incision through
conjuctiva and Tenson's capsule

Figure 5.5 Sub-tenon's block. To show the position of the incision in the conjunctiva

patient should continue to look up and out, as this makes it easier to
advance the cannula in the right place next to the globe.
4. After aspirating to check for the absence of cerebro-spinal fluid or
    blood, the injection is then given.
This is an extremely effective and safe way of giving an injection directly into the retrobulbar space. The use of a blunt cannula means there is
minimal risk of damage to the eye, blood vessels, nerves etc. However it
requires more preparation, and sterile instruments are needed to incise
the conjunctiva. It can be done by an assistant wearing sterile gloves or by
the surgeon when he is fully scrubbed up and ready to start the operation.
*It is also a very useful technique if the patient starts having problems in
the middle of the operation, because a sub Tenon's injection can be given
when the eye is open.* During surgery it can be given superiorly in the upper nasal quadrant rather than in the lower nasal quadrant.

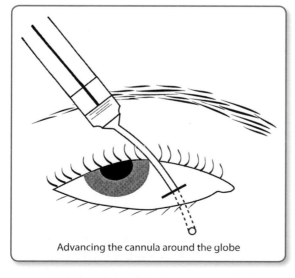

Figure 5.6 Advancing the
cannula around the globe of
the eye

Advancing the cannula around the globe

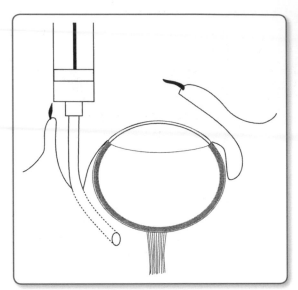

Figure 5.7 To show the final position of the cannula before making the injection

The facial block

if the surgeon plans to give a retrobulbar and a facial block, it is usual to give the facial block first and the retrobulbar block second. The facial block can be given at the neck of the mandible (the O'Brien method), or at the orbital rim (the Van Lint method). In each case 5 ml of 2% lignocaine with adrenaline are used with a 21G or similar needle.

However many surgeons do not use routinely a facial block for most of their patients. As long as the patient is not feeling any pain there is usually no stimulus for them to squeeze their eyes. It is however a useful technique for difficult cases or with anxious patients.

The O'Brien method (Figures 5.8 and 5.9)

Principle

The divisions of the facial nerve are blocked as they pass around the neck of the mandible.

Method

1. The temporo-mandibular joint and the neck of the mandible are palpated while the patient opens and closes his mouth.
2. The needle is inserted perpendicularly through the skin and is pushed down to the neck of the mandible. The tip should touch the bone. This corresponds to a point about 1 cm anterior and 1 cm below the external meatus of the ear.
3. After withdrawing slightly on the plunger to ensure that the needle is not in a blood vessel, up to 5 ml of anaesthetic is slowly injected as close as possible to the bone.
4. The syringe is removed and the site massaged vigorously.

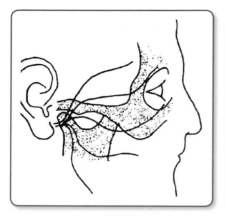 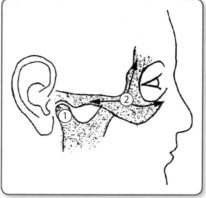

Figure 5.8 To show the course of the facial nerve

Figure 5.9 To show the position of the facial nerve block for the O'Brien method (1) and the Van Lint method (2)

The van Lint method (Figures 5.1 and 5.2)

Principle

Paralysis of the orbicularis oculi muscle by local infiltration around the orbit.

Method

1. The needle is inserted through the skin at the lateral margin of the orbit and pushed down to the bone. There is very little subcutaneous tissue here. Try to avoid blunting the tip of the needle on the bone. A bleb is raised using about
   1 ml of lignocaine.
2. The needle is then advanced to its full extent in three directions. Firstly along the upper orbital margin, then along the lower orbital margin and finally along the zygomatic arch back towards the ear. The needle must be kept close to the bone so as to be under the orbicularis muscle. This is because the motor nerves enter the muscle on its deep side. The lignocaine is injected as the needle is advanced. A total of 4 ml is distributed equally in the 3 directions.
3. On removal of the needle the area is massaged to aid diffusion of the anaesthetic and help its action.

Complications of the facial nerve block

The facial block sometimes causes slight pain as it is being injected because the tissues are quite tense there. The commonest complication is a failure to achieve a satisfactory block. Quite often the block is not complete and the patient can still close the eye with difficulty. A complete block is not necessary but the eyelids should not be able to close forcibly.

If after 5-10 minutes the block has not been effective it should be supplemented by using the other method.

There are also some very rare complications of the O'Brien method. These are:

- Tenderness over the temporo-mandibular joint.
- Permanent weakness of the facial nerve.
- Injection into the branches of the external carotid artery or jugular vein.

General anaesthesia

Safe general anaesthesia requires significant resources:

- Oxygen.
- Uninterruptible power supply.
- Anaesthetic machines.
- Monitoring equipment.
- Air way devices.

Not all of this equipment may be available.

Ketamine is a useful and very safe intravenous general anaesthetic and is particularly valuable for young children who cannot be operated on using L.A.[2] It is ideal for "eye camp" work where full anaesthetic facilities are not available. It can be given by intramuscular or intravenous injection. Alternatively an I.V. infusion can be used for longer periods of anaesthesia. Ketamine provides amnesia, sedation, surgical anaesthesia and analgesia. As various strengths of ketamine are available – 10 mg/ml, 50 mg/ml, or 100 mg/ml it is important to check the strength of the solution before calculating carefully the volume for injection. The recommended dose for intravenous injection is 2 mg/kg body weight, and anaesthesia will start in 30 seconds and last for about 10 minutes. For intramuscular injection the dose is 10 mg/kg body weight, the anaesthesia starts within 3 minutes and lasts for up to 20 minutes. If the effect is wearing off supplementary "top up" injections may be added if necessary, using a slightly smaller dosage.

Clinically, there is a degree of preservation of pharyngeal and laryngeal reflexes after ketamine administration and respiration is usually maintained, however the airway will still have to be managed in order to ensure its patency, and to protect from aspiration. Patients tend to salivate more, so a preoperative intramuscular injection of atropine (an anti-cholinergic drug) should be given. The dose of atropine varies according to the weight of a child, up to a maximum of 0.6 mg (0.1 mg is sufficient for a 10 kg child). Ketamine may cause unpleasant dreams or hallucinations, but these are reduced by giving an oral premedication of diazepam. For a small child 1–2 mg is adequate. Ketamine is a very good analgesic but it does not reduce muscle tone or eye movements. For intraocular surgery it is therefore necessary to supplement the ketamine anaesthesia with a standard retrobulbar block so as to prevent eye movements.

For a child with a small orbit a smaller volume of retrobulbar local anaesthetic should be given – 1.5 ml is usually satisfactory.

Schedule for pre-operative preparation

Day before surgery

- Check blood pressure, urine, heart and lungs
- Check eyelids, lashes and lacrimal system
- Look for septic spots
- Apply antibiotic drops or ointment
- Face and head wash

Morning of operation

- Face wash
- Trim eyelashes (if eyelid drapes are not available)
- Reassure patient

A half to one hour pre-operative

- Give sedation orally, if indicated, but usually not necessary
- Apply antibiotic drops
- Mydriatic drops, if a cataract extraction
- Cyclopentolate (or alternative parasympathetic blocker)
- Phenylephrine 10% (or 2.5% or alternative sympathetic stimulator)
- Prostaglandin inhibitor if available (Ketorolac, Diclofenac or Flurbiprofen)

Immediately pre-operative

- Check the dilatation of the pupil
- Repeat mydriatic drops if not fully dilated
- Instill LA drops
- Give the local anaesthetic blocks and apply pressure to the orbit
- Check that LA block is adequate
- Apply skin preparation
- Drape the eye and insert the speculum
- Irrigate the conjunctival sac

Summary of local anaesthetic blocks, all with 2% lignocaine

Retrobulbar or sub Tenon's block (adrenaline optional)	up to 5 ml without hyalase up to 5 ml with hyalase
Peribulbar block (with adrenaline)	up to 10 ml without hyalase 8 ml with hyalase
Facial block (with adrenaline)	5ml

References

1. Stevens S. How to clean eyelids. Community Eye Health 2011; 24:20.
2. Pun MS, Thakur J, Poudyal G, et al. Ketamine anaesthesia for paediatric ophthalmology surgery. Br J Ophthalmol 2003;87:535-7.

6 Cataract surgery

A cataract is an opacity of the crystalline lens in the eye (see **Figure 6.1**). About 39 million people in the world are blind and just over half of these are blind from cataract.[1] Most patients with cataract are elderly but there are many who are young or middle aged. At present the only treatment for cataract is the surgical removal of the opaque lens. It is not likely that any other treatment or means of preventing cataract will be discovered in the next few years. *Therefore the greatest worldwide challenge for ophthalmology at present is to make cataract surgery available for all.* Some of the issues in providing appropriate cataract surgery have been discussed in general terms in Chapter 1 in the introduction, and the student may find it helpful to think again about these basic principles described on pages 3–13. Not only must cataract surgery be available for all who require it but the standard of surgery and after-care should be satisfactory and especially should **be monitored**, even in rural "eye camps". Regrettably in some areas it is quite common to find patients whose eyes have been spoilt from the complications of poor cataract surgery in the past, or who have never been given corrective spectacles after surgery. For anyone operating on the eye, the most important operation will be a cataract extraction. Cataract surgery is such an important subject that this chapter will describe more than just the technical details of the operation. Each of the following topics will be discussed:

1. The history of cataract surgery.
2. How to restore the focus of the eye once the cataract has been removed.
3. The indications for surgery.
4. The choice of operation.
5. The technical details of the operation both for sutureless extracapsular (SECCE) and conventional ECCE, and how to manage complications during the operation. A brief description of intracapsular cataract extraction (ICCE) will also be given.

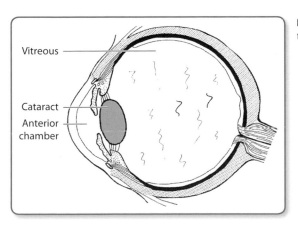

Figure 6.1 A cross section of the eye to show a cataract

Vitreous

Cataract

Anterior chamber

6. The use of intraocular lenses and how to implant them.
7. Routine post-operative care and monitoring of outcomes.
8. Post-operative complications and how to manage them.

The history of cataract surgery

It is not surprising that attempts have been made since the beginning of history to treat a disease as common and disabling as cataract. Surgical treatment of cataract has been described in several ancient cultures, and is thought to have started about 2500 B.C. in India. The aim of this traditional operation was to push the opaque lens downwards and backwards into the vitreous. The operation is usually called *"couching"*. The word is derived from the French word "coucher" – to push down. It has been practised for thousands of years and is still performed today in some parts of the world. The technique is basically as follows:

A needle or similar sharp instrument is inserted into the eye a few millimetres behind the limbus. It is moved around the eye to rupture the suspensory ligament of the lens so that the lens can then be pushed down and back into the vitreous (**Figure 6.2**). At first the patients usually have an improvement in their vision, but there are often late complications and the long-term results are not good. Two particular complications are both common and serious.

- *Infection.* Most people who practise couching are not aware of the nature of bacteria and the importance of sterile techniques. Their instruments are often not sterile and bacteria may enter into the eye during the operation. If an infection occurs in this way the eye is nearly always blinded.
- *Rupture of the Lens.* Often the lens capsule is damaged during couching. Lens protein then leaks out into the vitreous. This usually causes a severe inflammatory reaction in the eye (uveitis) and often raised

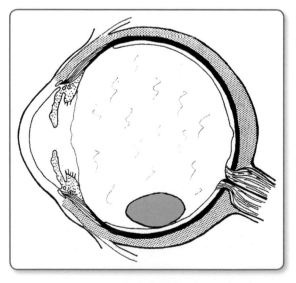

Figure 6.2 The eye after "couching" or dislocation of the cataract into the vitreous

intraocular pressure (glaucoma) By the time this inflammation has subsided and the intra-ocular pressure returned to normal the eye is usually blind or almost blind.

Couching is still practised today in spite of the high rate of complications. Most couchers are not well educated, they usually have little understanding of basic medical science, and travel from village to village practising their art. It is very difficult to trace them and impossible to get any scientific reports about how good or how bad the operation really is. Even with skilled couchers only about 50% of the eyes will recover some useful vision. In most cases the results are much worse. Also most couchers do not give spectacles to their patients after the operation, and so even those who have had successful operations and are free of complications will not recover good vision.

People who are trained in orthodox medicine are often very critical of the activities of these couchers. However they only continue to practise their art because orthodox medicine has not yet completely achieved the goal of making high quality low cost cataract surgery available for all, especially for patients in isolated rural areas.

Is it possible to make couching a safer and more effective operation? The two main complications of couching are intraocular infection and rupture of the lens capsule. With properly sterilised instruments and sterile techniques, the risk of intraocular infection would be reduced. Some people claim that if care is taken, then it is possible to dislocate the lens without rupturing its capsule. However, there have not been enough reliable published reports to recommend it as a procedure, and so it will not be discussed any further in this book.

About 200 years ago attempts were made to remove the cataractous lens from the eye rather than pushing it into the vitreous. The first operation described was an *extracapsular cataract extraction*. This operation removed the lens nucleus and part of the lens cortex but left the lens capsule behind in the eye (see **Figure 6.3**).

The most common complication was that some lens cortex remained in the eye. This caused inflammation in the eye (uveitis) post operatively. Often a thick opaque membrane consisting of the lens capsule and opaque lens cortex and fibrous tissue developed in the pupil. This obscured the vision and required further surgery.

About 100 years ago *intracapsular cataract extraction* was introduced. This removed the whole lens (**Figure 6.4**) and the operation became increasingly popular. The post-operative complications were less than with extracapsular extraction, and until about 25 to 30 years ago intracapsular extraction was the standard operation for senile cataract.

However during the last 30 years the results of extracapsular extraction have greatly improved. There are two reasons for this:
1. With modern surgical techniques, and particularly with the use of operating microscopes, the anterior lens capsule and all the lens cortex can be removed, leaving only the thin transparent posterior lens capsule in the eye.

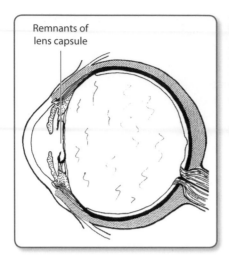

Remnants of
lens capsule

Figure 6.3 The eye after extracapsular extraction

2. Topical steroid treatment postoperatively has greatly reduced postoperative uveitis which was common following extracapsular extraction.

The complication rate of extracapsular extraction is now less than that of the intracapsular method, and it is now the recommended method of cataract surgery. The other great advantage of extracapsular extraction is that intra-ocular lens implants can easily be inserted behind the iris and in front of the posterior lens capsule. This is safest and most secure place for intraocular lens implants to rest within the eye.

Technology continues to advance rapidly. Extracapsular extraction can now be performed using an ultrasonic probe to break up the cataract inside the eye so it is removed through a tiny incision. The operation is called phako-emulsification. Because its results are so good, *phakoemulsification* has now become the standard way of removing most cataracts in developed countries. There are several advantages of phakoemulsification:

The advantages of phakoemulsification

- Because of the smaller incision the wound heals more quickly, and the shape of the eye is not altered so there is very little astigmatism after the operation.
- No suturing of the small wound is required. It means that there are no problems later on from the sutures causing irritation or inflammation.
- The shape and the volume of the eye and the intraocular pressure are maintained throughout the operation. This reduces the trauma to the eye during surgery, and so causes less postoperative uveitis.
- Because of the smaller incision, good local anaesthetic blocks are not so essential. Indeed some expert phakoemulsification surgeons only use topical anaesthetic drops.

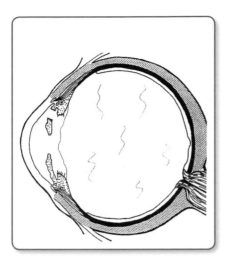

Figure 6.4 The eye after intracapsular extraction

Phakoemulsification is now being introduced in some developing countries and is being enthusiastically promoted. However it is not always an appropriate technique for general use in developing countries for several practical reasons.

The philosophy of this book is to describe technology and methods appropriate for poorer communities. Also phakoemulsification is an operation which is too detailed to be described satisfactorily in this book, and will not be discussed in more detail.

The disadvantages of phakoemulsification

- Cost. The equipment is very expensive and needs expert maintenance. There are additional expenses for disposable items for each case. A top quality microscope with good illumination and focusing controls is also essential, so that the surgeon can see exactly what the "phako" probe is doing inside the lens.
- White, opaque cataracts and advanced cataracts with very dense, brown, hard nuclei are the least suitable cases for phakoemulsification, and these are both very common in developing countries. Phakoemulsification is an ideal procedure for removing cataracts which are in their early stages. As the cataract gets harder and more opaque the risk of serious complications from phakoemulsification also increases, and phakoemulsification is less likely to be successful.(However experts in phakoemulsification using the most expensive modern machines can "phako" nearly all cataracts).
- Training. Phakoemulsification is a difficult technique to learn, and a longer period of training is required. As the consumables for each surgery are also so expensive, this will mean the costs of training are very high.

- Support. On site support from the manufacturers for the set up and maintenance of the machine is often impossible in remote rural settings. Furthermore, the machine itself, as well as the surgeon, will be very sensitive to sudden electricity power cuts and fluctuations, therefore an uninterruptable power supply (UPS) and voltage stabilizer are essential.
- Sustainability. Many phako machines that are available as second hand or donations will be phased out by the suppliers in the next few years, and the consumables needed for them may no longer be available.

There is another rather subtle consequence from recommending phakoemulsification for all cataract surgery worldwide. This concerns the right use of medical resources. Every country, even the richest, has to put some cash limit on the cost of medical care. So-called "developed" countries are already having to face this problem, which will become worse as modern medical care becomes even more complex and expensive. In poor "developing" countries limited medical resources must be used carefully to be of the greatest benefit to the community. A cataract extraction is an extremely cost-effective operation. For quite a small cost it can make a tremendous difference to a patient's life. In fact, cataract surgery is one of the most cost effective of any health intervention in the whole of medicine, in terms of 'disability-adjusted life years'.[2]

Lens implant surgery (see page 94) means that a cataract can be removed at a much earlier stage, and phakoemulsification is such a good operation that cataracts can be removed when the patient is only beginning to have any symptoms. In most developing countries people living in isolated rural areas have the least access to the limited medical care available, and consequently have the highest prevalence of cataract blindness. By introducing phakoemulsification the wealthier patients and those living in the cities may receive more surgery and at an earlier stage. However, this may direct resources away from the rural blind with more advanced cataracts, unless wealthier patients are charged a premium rate to help fund non-phako surgery for those who cannot afford it.

Many developing countries are now in the strange situation that all four methods of cataract extraction may be practised in the same country.

Couching is still performed in some remote rural areas.

Intracapsular cataract extraction is still practised in some areas.

Extracapsular cataract extraction (either sutured or sutureless) has becoming increasingly popular especially as microscopes and good quality, low cost, intraocular lenses have been introduced; and is now the surgery of choice in low and middle income countries

Phakoemulsification is now becoming quite a common procedure in some developing countries especially in the major cities.

The fact that operations using the technology of 2000 years ago are being carried out at the same time as those using the most modern technology shows how great is the need for community based development of surgical treatment, which will help everybody and not just a few.

In recent years extracapsular cataract extraction (ECCE) has improved so that it can now be done very quickly and safely without using any sutures. This operation has been pioneered and developed in low-income countries, while phacoemulsification has developed in high-income countries. The outcomes of sutureless ECCE and phacoemulsification are more or less the same and both very good. However, sutureless ECCE is much faster and cheaper. Therefore high volume high quality cataract surgery is possible without having to rely on very expensive equipment and machinery.[3]

Restoring the focus of the eye after cataract extraction (see Figure 6.5)

An eye that has had the lens removed is called an *aphakic* eye, and the condition is called *aphakia*. The lens helps to focus the light on the retina, and so after a cataract operation without an intraocular lens (IOL) the eye is badly out of focus (**Figure 6.5a**). A strongly positive or convex lens is needed to restore the normal focus of the eye. (The only exception to this is a very myopic patient who will not require such a strongly positive lens after cataract extraction).

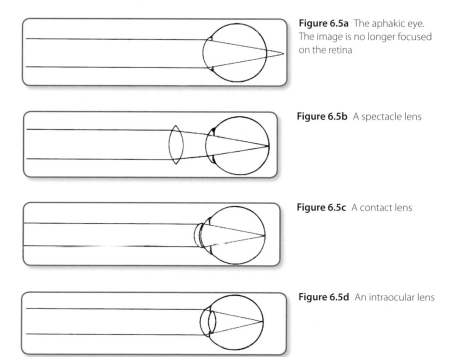

Figure 6.5a The aphakic eye. The image is no longer focused on the retina

Figure 6.5b A spectacle lens

Figure 6.5c A contact lens

Figure 6.5d An intraocular lens

There are three sorts of lens which can be used to restore the focus of the eye: *intraocular lenses, spectacles,* or *contact lenses.*

Intraocular lenses (**Figure 6.5d** and **Figures 6.6–6.9**) IOLs made of high quality non-toxic plastic have been used to correct aphakia for over 50 years. At first there were various problems both with the design of the lens and the materials from which they were made, and in these early years many eyes were damaged or destroyed from the complications of IOLs. Most of these problems have now been overcome, and there is a good understanding of how the IOL behaves inside the eye and what are the best materials and designs. From a patient's point of view a successful IOL implant is by far the best way of correcting aphakia. Virtually normal vision is restored, and there is neither the distortion nor magnification of spectacles, nor the problem of fitting and wearing contact lenses. The IOL is permanent and rests inside the eye where it will neither become scratched nor spoilt. Nowadays in the developed world nearly all patients having cataract extractions receive an IOL.

When the first edition of this book was written over twenty years ago it was difficult to recommend routine use of IOLs because of their cost. At that time nearly all lens implants were manufactured in western countries and would cost about 100 US $, an amount which most poor people, or eyecare programs serving the poor, could not afford. However, high quality lens implants are now manufactured in developing countries and their cost has fallen very rapidly and probably will continue to fall further. At present good quality lens implants can be purchased for about 3 US$ or sometimes even less. Cost alone is no longer a barrier to carrying out lens implant surgery. **An IOL which will last forever is now probably less expensive than a pair of spectacles which will need replacing.**

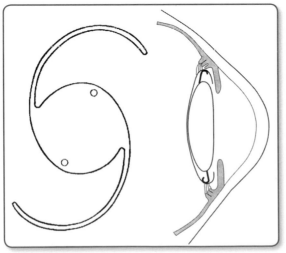

Figure 6.6 A posterior chamber lens implant used with extracapsular extraction (not all posterior chamber lenses have the small dialling holes shown here)

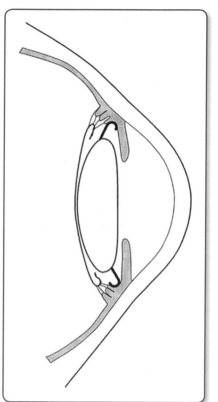

Figure 6.7 A posterior chamber lens with the haptics in the ciliary sulcus. Note how the haptics are in a slightly different position from those in Figure 6.6. The IOL is in the capsular bag

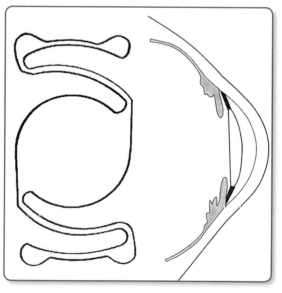

Figure 6.8 An anterior chamber lens implant used with intracapsular cataract extraction

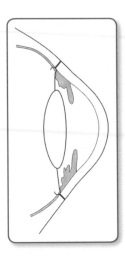

Figure 6.9 A scleral fixated lens. The haptics are secured with sutures which pass through the sclera but the knots must be buried

Several surveys from different countries have shown that a large proportion of patients who have had simple cataract extractions are not wearing their correcting spectacles for one reason or another. The visual acuity in an eye with uncorrected aphakia is less than 6/60. Therefore although these patients can see to get around, they are in some respects classified as still blind. For these reasons intraocular lens implants have now become standard practice during cataract extraction throughout the world.

It is important to remember that intra-ocular lens implants can occasionally cause problems:

- Cataract extraction is not an easy operation and inserting an IOL makes it harder, increases the post-operative complication rate, and requires more careful post-operative management.
- Patients with chronic uveitis or corneal endothelial dystrophy pre-operatively should not be offered lens implants.
- If the operating conditions are not ideal and there is a risk of infection, that risk is much greater if an IOL, which is a foreign body, is left inside the eye.
- If the IOL is badly handled or inserted it will seriously damage the endothelial cells of the cornea, causing bullous keratopathy and permanent loss of sight.
- Cataract surgery without implanting an IOL can be performed without the aid of an operating microscope; but this is very difficult with the best type of intraocular lens implant, a posterior chamber implant.

In surgery it always better to be safe than sorry. Therefore IOLs may not be indicated for any of the reasons listed above.

Lens implant surgery is undoubtedly the best way of treating cataracts, and it is now extremely cost-effective. However, a surgeon who is practising good quality routine cataract surgery without implants, and has a good system for providing low cost spectacles post-operatively, may still be giving a good and valuable service to the community, and should not necessarily be criticised. However in this situation the surgeon would be advised to get training in lens implant techniques. The old proverb "the best is the enemy of the good" is very true when trying to plan a service to eradicate cataract blindness. At present there are still some countries and a few areas where most people get no treatment at all for cataract, and these patients would be grateful for any treatment.

The design of intraocular lenses

All IOLs have two different parts. The central part is called the "optic". This is the lens part which focuses the light on the retina, and has a diameter of 5 to 7 mm. The outer part is called the "haptic" which secures the lens in the eye, so that it does not move or irritate any of the intraocular structures. Most lenses are made of polymethyl-methacrylate (PMMA), which has been used for over 35 years. Nowadays other materials such as silicone and acrylic are also available. The main advantage of silicone and acrylic is that they are softer and so a larger lens can be folded over and inserted through a much smaller incision. These lenses are only used in phakoemulsification surgery, and at present are much more expensive than those made from PMMA which is a solid non-foldable material. Therefore only the use of rigid PMMA lenses will be described in this book.

In most cases the haptics are also made of PMMA, and because the haptics are very thin they are slightly flexible. Ideally the haptics and the optics are made out of one solid piece of PMMA, but it is possible to make the haptics separately and then fix them to the optic in the factory. The haptics can be made from a different material such as polypropylene. (However, a lens made out of one single piece of PMMA is usually the best quality and this is now the standard way of manufacturing lenses.)

There are 4 different places where the IOL can be fixed inside the eye:
1. *In the posterior chamber* in front of the posterior lens capsule and behind the iris (**Figure 6.6**). This is generally considered the **best place** as the lens is fixed very securely, and it is also well away from the sensitive endothelial cells on the posterior corneal surface. These cells can be easily damaged by badly fitting lenses in the anterior chamber. Most posterior chamber lenses now have a fairly standard design. The haptics are angled slightly backwards so that the lens tends to press against the posterior lens capsule, and the optic has a convex curve on its posterior surface which also helps to keep the lens resting tightly against the posterior lens capsule. Many posterior chamber lenses have two small dialling holes at the outer edge of the optic. The purpose of these dialling holes is to make it easier to insert the IOL. There are however two disadvantages in having dialling holes. If the lens becomes decentred slightly, the dialling hole can come into the visual axis and may slightly disturb the vision. Also the dialling hole may become an isolated space where bacteria of low virulence can survive isolated from the body's defences, and these can cause a chronic persistent inflammation in the eye after lens implant surgery. It is fairly easy to insert an IOL without a dialling hole if the haptic loops have the

right amount of flexibility. Therefore dialling holes are becoming less common as IOL design improves, but lenses with dialling holes are easier to insert.

The haptic may be within the lens capsule so that it rests in front of the posterior capsule but behind the rim of the anterior capsule (**Figure 6.6**). This is called *"in the bag"* fixation. Alternatively the haptic may rest in front of the rim of the anterior capsule but behind the iris (**Figure 6.7**) in the ciliary sulcus. This is called 'sulcus' fixation. "In the bag" fixation is generally considered as slightly better than *"sulcus"* fixation, because the lens is more stable and the haptic is protected from touching the rest of the eye by the lens capsule. However in practise there is little difference between the two positions. Sometimes the haptics can be placed very carefully "in the bag", and yet some months later one or both the haptics may have moved spontaneously into the sulcus. Post-operative fibrosis and contracture in the capsule can cause the haptics to move in this way.

2. *In the anterior chamber.* If the patient has had an intracapsular cataract extraction, a posterior chamber lens implant cannot be used because there is no supporting posterior capsule present. The lens implant would just fall back into the vitreous. In most cases the lens is implanted into the anterior chamber (**Figure 6.8**). The haptics of an anterior chamber lens implant are slightly more complicated.

   The most acceptable design for the haptics is shown in **Figure 6.8** so that the haptics touch the anterior chamber angle between the iris and the cornea in four places. (One alternative design has a three point fixation, two in the lower angle and one above.) Therefore anterior chamber lenses must have the correct power of the optic and also the correct diameter of the haptics. If the haptic size is too small then the lens will not fit firmly into the anterior chamber angle. It will therefore be unstable and move around and destroy the endothelial cells of the cornea. These are the most vital cells in the cornea and never regenerate if destroyed. If the lens is too large then it will press too hard in the angle of the anterior chamber and cause pain, discomfort and irritation. Even a perfectly fitting anterior chamber lens will probably cause some very gradual loss of the endothelial cells because the haptics touch the peripheral cornea. There may also be some slight constant rubbing of the lens against the iris causing iritis. (In the early designs of anterior chamber lenses there was a common complication called the 'UGH!' syndrome. This stood for Uveitis, Glaucoma, and Hyphaema.) With modern designs these problems are much less, but the anterior chamber is still not the ideal place for a lens implant. For all these reasons anterior chamber lenses should only be used in elderly patients. They should never be used in patients under 60 and only with caution in patients under 70. Other designs of anterior chamber lenses are available, but these may cause even more damage to the endothelial cells of the cornea.

3. *Iris or pupil fixated lenses.* In the early years of intraocular lens implants it was popular to fix the intraocular lens within the pupil, with two

haptic loops behind the iris and two in front of the iris. This design unfortunately did not stand the test of time, because many of these lenses were found to rub against the endothelial surface of the cornea when the eye moved, causing endothelial cell loss. Sometimes the lens became unstable and fell into the vitreous. There is however one type of iris fixation which has stood the test of time. This is called the "lobster claw" lens which fixes firmly on to the anterior surface of the iris. Although it is probably a good design it is not very popular or widely available and so will not be described any further.

4. *Scleral fixation.* This is a way of inserting a posterior chamber lens behind the iris when there is no posterior capsule to support it. The anterior vitreous is removed with a vitrectomy machine and the haptics of the lens secured through the pars plana to the sclera with non-absorbable, non-irritant sutures (**Figure 6.9**). This is a good way of securing the intraocular lens in young patients who do not have a posterior lens capsule and so cannot have a standard posterior chamber lens. The technique and insertion is a little more difficult, but is described briefly at the end of this chapter on page 192.

Choosing the power of an intraocular lens

Ocular biometry

The best power for an intraocular lens (IOL) is the one that will make the eye very slightly myopic (about minus 0.5 to 1.0 diopter), so that the patient can see fairly well for both distance and near without needing spectacles. Ocular biometry measures the eye so that the correct power of IOL is used. It measures the curvature of the cornea and the axial length of the eye, and with this knowledge the correct power of the lens can be calculated.

There is one other factor which affects the power of an IOL, its position inside the eye. The further forward the IOL rests in the eye, the greater is its effective power. The position that the IOL tends to rest in the eye is measured by a number called the "A" constant. A lens with a high "A" constant rests far back in the eye, and a low "A" constant lens will rest further forward. Posterior chamber lenses have an "A" constant of about 118, and anterior chamber lenses an "A" constant of about 115. In practice this means that a posterior chamber lens must have a power of about 3 diopters more than an anterior chamber lens to have the same effect. When carrying out ocular biometry, the "A" constant for the lens to be inserted is also taken into account.

When choosing the power of the IOL the refraction of the other eye is also important, especially if only one eye is being operated on. For example if the other eye has 6 diopters of myopia what should be the ideal refraction in the operated eye? The most accepted solution is to plan for a refractive error of about half that of the other eye, 3 diopters of myopia in the case described.

Another factor is the occupation of the patient. Someone doing a lot of close work may prefer to be myopic, and someone working outside may prefer to be emmetropic.

"Best guess" for IOL power

If ocular biometry is not available, the surgeon must guess the best strength of IOL. A posterior chamber lens of about 21 diopters should make a normal eye remain emmetropic postoperatively. One extra diopter of IOL power usually changes the refraction of the eye by about 0.5 diopter. Therefore a normal eye with a 22 diopter IOL should have a refraction of minus 0.5 postoperatively. This is a half diopter of myopia which is the ideal. For anterior chamber lenses, 18 diopters should make the normal eye emmetropic, and so a lens of about 19 diopters should be chosen which will result in a refraction of minus 0.5.

The guesswork may be aided by knowing the patient's pre-operative refraction. If the patient was myopic before the operation, a lens of less power will be needed, and a very myopic patient (e.g. minus 20) does not need an IOL at all to become emmetropic postoperatively. (The exception to this is a patient who was myopic preoperatively because of nuclear sclerosis of the lens. This occurs quite frequently, so if you see a patient requiring cataract surgery who is myopic, always ask if they were myopic when they were 30 years old or if they have just become myopic recently). Hypermetropic patients will usually require an IOL of increased power to make them emmetropic. These kind of guesses are not needed if biometry is available. There is one golden rule, if you have to guess the strength of the intraocular lens: "It is always better to leave the patient a little myopic than a little hypermetropic".

Spectacle lenses

Spectacle lenses have been used for many years to restore the focus of the aphakic eye (**Figure 6.5b**). A positive lens of about 10 to 12 dioptres is usually required, and a lens of the correct power will give the patient excellent visual acuity. Spectacle lenses can be easily and cheaply manufactured, but they have certain disadvantages:

- *Distortion*. Some distortion occurs with spectacle lenses of strong powers. Objects appear distorted in shape and many patients feel disorientated, for example a door will tend to change shape as a person approaches it.
- *Magnification*. The image that is produced by a positive spectacle lens of about 10 dioptres is one third larger than the image in a normal eye. This magnification occurs because the lens has been removed from its normal position inside the eye, and has been replaced by a spectacle lens which is at least a centimetre in front of the eye. If the two eyes receive images of unequal size this is called aniseikonia.
- *Prismatic Effects*. When the patient looks through the side of strong spectacles a prismatic effect occurs so that the object looked at is not quite where it appears to be.
- *Discomfort*. Aphakic spectacles are heavy and so may be uncomfortable to wear. They are less heavy if they are made in a special shape but this is usually expensive. Plastic lenses are lighter but will scratch more easily.

For these reasons, patients may take some weeks to adjust to wearing spectacles after a cataract extraction. They have to learn to turn their heads rather than their eyes when looking round, and must get used to the distortion and the magnification which makes judging distances quite difficult at first. However patients who were blind or almost blind before surgery are always delighted to see again, and rarely have real difficulties in getting used to aphakic spectacles. The only patients who do have persistent difficulties are those who have surgery when they can still see quite well, or have had a cataract removed from one eye and have normal vision in the other eye. If a spectacle lens is used to restore the focus in the aphakic eye, then the image in that eye is one third larger than the image in the normal eye. This causes double vision and is very confusing for the patient. It is best not to correct aphakia with a spectacle lens if the other eye is normal. Without spectacles the vision in the aphakic eye will be very blurred and out of focus, but it will not confuse the normal image from the healthy eye.

- "*Wear and tear*". Besides all these optical problems with aphakic spectacles, there is an even more important practical problem, "wear and tear". The glasses easily get lost, broken or scratched. This is especially true for people living in rural areas who do not have anywhere safe to put their glasses, and these are the very people who have difficulty in replacing them. Many surveys have shown that large numbers of patients have either lost or broken their glasses or have never been given any. (In some surveys more than half of all patients after simple cataract surgery were not using any spectacle correction!)

(It is always a good idea for a doctor or surgeon to be able to experience what the patient is experiencing. It will both make the doctor more sympathetic to the patient, and also help them to be able to explain to the patient exactly how they will feel after an operation. It is quite easy for a surgeon to experience what it is like to have a cataract operation and to wear corrective spectacles. If the surgeon has access to contact lenses and someone who fits them, then it is possible to get some soft contact lenses made with a very strong negative correction By wearing these contact lenses, the surgeon will become very hypermetropic, in fact just like a patient who has had cataracts removed but is not wearing glasses. The surgeon can then wear some +10 glasses to correct the refractive error, and in this way experience both what it is like to have had a cataract extraction and have no refractive correction, and also to experience what it is like to have had a cataract extraction and to wear correcting spectacles. The final comparison is to put on a blindfold of thin paper to experience being blind from untreated mature cataract.)

Both contact lenses and intraocular lenses give a much more normal type of vision after cataract extraction than spectacles. A contact lens or an intraocular lens is in almost the same position as the patient's own lens and therefore there is no significant magnification of the image in the operated eye, nor is there any distortion. The lens moves as the eye moves and so gives a much more normal or natural image of the outside world.

Contact lenses (Figure. 6.5c)

Contact lenses have been used for some years, they rest on the surface of the cornea and must be fitted very carefully. The contact lens must be not only the right strength but also the right shape to fit exactly on the patient's cornea. If not the cornea can be damaged.

Contact lenses are made from various materials, and new and improved types of contact lens material are continually being developed. Most are known as either hard or soft lenses. Hard contact lenses are a little smaller than the diameter of the cornea and move freely over the surface of the eye. They are often slightly uncomfortable to wear at first and it takes some time to get used to them. However once the patient's eye has adapted to them they are long lasting, easy to wear and are fairly easy to keep clean.

Soft contact lenses are much more comfortable at first, but need much greater care in cleaning and sterilising and easily become scratched or damaged. Soft contact lenses are a little larger than the diameter of the cornea and do not move over the surface of the eye.

It usually takes some time for contact lenses to be fitted properly and for the patient to get used to wearing them. The patient has to learn how to put them in and take them out of the eye, and to clean and handle them properly.

Some years ago contact lenses were used quite often to correct aphakia, especially for patients who had a cataract extraction in one eye and normal vision in the other eye. However, the increasing use of intraocular lens implants has now meant that contact lenses are hardly ever used as an optical correction for aphakia.

Indications for surgery

At what stage should a cataract be removed? Often this is an easy decision to make. It may be obvious that a particular patient needs a cataract operation, or that another should not have an operation. However, the decision is not always easy and there are several factors to consider.
1. Is an intraocular lens implant planned?
2. How bad is the cataract?
3. What kind of vision does that patient need?
4. Is there evidence of other disease in the same eye?
5. What is the condition of the other eye?
6. What facilities are available?

Is an intraocular lens implant planned?

Nowadays, almost **all** cataract surgeries should be performed using an intra-ocular lens, even if biometry is not available. Cataracts can be removed at an earlier stage if an IOL is planned because this gives much more natural restoration of vision. This is particularly true if a patient has a cataract in one eye and the other eye is fairly normal. Such a patient would gain very little from cataract surgery without a lens implant. By operating on patients at an earlier stage in their disease it means that they are much less handicapped, and no longer must surgeons wait until the cataract is mature. However this policy also means there is much more cataract surgery to be done in the world. The only reasons for not implanting an IOL nowadays, is a patient with chronic persistent uveitis or an extremely myopic patient.

How bad is the cataract?

A brief revision of the anatomy of the lens may be helpful. The lens is enclosed in a membrane called the *capsule*. This is attached to the suspensory ligament at its most peripheral part, the equator. Inside the capsule is a thin layer of fairly soft lens fibres called the lens *cortex*, but most of the bulk of the lens is made up of much harder lens fibres closely packed together and called the lens *nucleus*. In young children all the lens is soft and there is no nucleus. With increasing age the adult nucleus gets harder and bigger, occupying a greater proportion of the lens.

The opacity or cataract may develop in the nucleus which turns brown, and finally black. It may develop in the cortex which turns white and opaque, or it may develop as an opaque layer just in front of the posterior capsule. This is called a posterior subcapsular cataract (PSCC), and it causes a particularly marked loss of vision Often more than one type of cataract may occur in the same lens, and there are other less common types of cataract also.

In the early stages of cataract the patient may see fairly well, and only notice some dazzling or blurring of vision. This is called an immature cataract. Gradually, as the cataract becomes more dense and opaque, the vision deteriorates until the patient is blind, and can only perceive and point out the direction of bright lights. This is called a *mature* cataract.

After this, further degenerative changes may take place in the lens. The lens cortex may become liquid making the lens swell. This is known as an *intumescent cataract*. The lens swelling will make the anterior chamber shallow and may cause secondary angle-closure glaucoma. This is sometimes called 'phakomorphic glaucoma'.

Rarely the lens capsule may rupture spontaneously or leak. The fluid from degenerated lens protein passes into the anterior chamber where it usually causes severe uveitis. This is called *phakolytic uveitis*. The lens protein often blocks up the drainage angle of the anterior chamber causing *phakolytic glaucoma*. Eventually a shrivelled lens capsule and a small nucleus are all that remain, but by this stage the eye has often gone blind from the complications of uveitis or glaucoma.

Most cataracts get worse gradually but the speed with which they do so is variable. The patient may go from having perfect vision to complete blindness in a few months. Usually the process takes a few years, but occasionally cataracts may hardly progress at all or be completely static.

At what stage should the cataract be removed?

- An *intumescent cataract* should be removed as soon as possible, because of the risk of angle closure glaucoma.
- In cases of *phakolytic uveitis* intensive topical steroid treatment should be given and the cataract removed as an emergency.
- A *mature cataract* should also be removed even if the other eye is normal. This will not only restore the sight to the eye but will prevent the risks of future complications developing .
- For *immature cataracts* the decision to operate or not depends very much upon the patient's visual needs and life-style. The use of

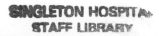

intraocular lens has meant that immature cataracts are now being operated on at a much earlier stage. Without a lens implant there is not much advantage to the patient in having a cataract extraction until the visual acuity has fallen to about 6/60. However with a lens implant many surgeons would recommend a cataract extraction with a visual acuity of 6/18. The exact visual acuity level for an 'operable' cataract will depend on the eye unit, and the burden of blindness in the community. The most modern technique of phakoemulsification can produce such good results that some surgeons are even recommending an operation with a visual acuity of 6/9!! Besides causing a loss of visual acuity the cataract can cause other visual symptoms such as glare in bright light, or "ghost" images which may be quite disturbing. Having these symptoms will also affect how soon the cataract is removed.

What kind of vision does the patient need?

Obviously everyone wants the best vision possible. However a moderate amount of visual loss (e.g. a visual acuity of 6/18) for someone who needs to read fine print or drive a car could mean having to stop work, but for an elderly, illiterate farmer or housewife it would not be a very great handicap. In general, the time for cataract surgery is **when the patient can no longer see well enough to carry out his or her normal activities**.

Is there evidence of other disease in the same eye?

Cataract extraction is most likely to be successful if the rest of the eye is healthy. There are five simple tests to confirm this.

> **Pressure** –check the intraocular pressure.
>
> **Pupil** – check the pupil reaction to bright light.
>
> **Projection** – recognising the direction of a light.
>
> **Posterior part of the eye** – check the retina and the optic nerve.
>
> **Pin-hole** – does the visual acuity improve with a pinhole.

1. *Pressure.* At a routine eye examination the intraocular pressure should be checked. If raised, it indicates glaucoma and it is quite likely that the loss of vision is due to glaucomatous optic atrophy and not to the cataract. Even if it is decided to remove the cataract, the operation may need to be modified to treat the glaucoma at the same time, and the patient counselled that the vision may not improve as much as expected for a cataract alone (i.e. there is a guarded prognosis).

2. *The pupil light response.* A brisk pupil light reaction is excellent confirmation that the eye is otherwise healthy. An absent or poor reaction usually indicates that the retina or optic nerve is diseased especially if the pupil light response is normal in the opposite eye. Sometimes in elderly patients or following iritis or other abnormalities of the iris the pupil reaction may be diminished. Therefore a good pupil reaction is a reliable sign that the rest of the eye is healthy, whereas an absent pupil reaction is very suspicious of retinal or optic nerve disease but does not necessarily confirm it.

However an afferent pupil defect (sometimes called a Marcus–Gunn pupil reaction) in the eye with the cataract indicates that there is other serious disease in the eye as well as cataract. A cataract alone never causes a relative afferent pupil defect. If the pupil reaction is absent, do not operate on the cataract unless there is a very good reason, or you have clearly discussed with the patient that the vision will most likely not improve after surgery.

3. *The projection of light.* When the retina and optic nerve are healthy, a patient with even a dense cataract can still tell the direction from which a bright light is coming when shone into the eye. There are some useful variations of this test. One is to shine two lights held about 15 cms. apart from each other into the eye. A patient with a healthy retina should be able to discern that there are two lights and not one. Another is to shine a bright light into the eye through a special lens called a "Maddox Rod", which is usually a part of a standard trial set of lenses. The patient will see a red line through this lens. If for example the patient has macular degeneration, the central part of this red line will either not be seen at all or will be all broken up and distorted.

4. *The posterior part of the eye (retina and optic nerve).* If the patient has a mature cataract, it is not possible to examine the retina and the optic nerve at all. If the cataract is only partial then the pupil should be dilated with mydriatics to examine the retina and optic nerve with an ophthalmoscope.(In patients with an immature cataract this can be done more easily with an indirect than a direct ophthalmoscope, or with a 90 dioptre lens and a slit lamp.) If there is evidence of another disease and the cataract is only partial, then cataract extraction will probably not benefit the patient very much.

    In doubtful cases the surgeon needs to examine the red reflex from the fundus and compare this with the loss of visual acuity. If the red reflex is only slightly obscured, then the loss of visual acuity should also be fairly slight.

5. *The pin-hole visual acuity test.* This may give helpful information in patients with an early cataract. An early cataract causes the light to be scattered so that there is no clear image on the retina. Looking through a pin-hole cuts down the scattering of the light, and so the visual acuity improves with a pin-hole. This also confirms that the retina is healthy (remember that refractive errors and corneal irregularities will also cause visual loss which improves with a pinhole).

What is the condition of the other eye?

There are 4 basic possible conditions of the other eye, although every case may not fit exactly into one of these groups.

1. The other eye is normal (a unilateral cataract)
2. The other eye also has a cataract (bilateral cataract)
3. The other eye has had a successful cataract extraction (a second eye cataract)
4. The other eye is incurably blind (an only eye cataract)

The other eye is normal (a unilateral cataract). This is a strong indication for an intraocular lens implant, because a cataract extraction without a lens implant will only give very limited improvement to the vision. However it may be worth operating on such an eye even without a lens implant for three reasons:

- The patient's field of vision will improve.
- There is a risk that the cataract may become hypermature or intumescent in the future, and so removing the cataract will prevent the possibility of these complications.
- Cataract will usually develop in the other eye at some time in the future. Very often there may be early signs of this if the other eye is examined closely. In such cases the vision in the other eye is likely to deteriorate and the patient will then see well out of the operated first eye by using aphakic spectacles.

The other eye also has a cataract (bilateral cataract) In this situation cataract extraction should be performed if the patient's sight is bad enough and the cataracts are dense enough. Most people would advise operating on one eye and waiting, at least a day or two, until it was free of immediate post-operative complications before considering an operation on the second eye. However removing both cataracts at the same time is carried out by some surgeons.

The other eye has had a successful cataract extraction (second eye cataract) This is the ideal case for surgery. The patient has already experienced the benefits of one operation, and will be enthusiastic about the second. In any surgical unit which is involved in training, this is the ideal operation for the trainee to perform under supervision.

The other eye is incurably blind (only eye cataract) This is the hardest situation for cataract surgery, because the patient has everything to lose if things go wrong but everything to gain from a successful operation. The level of anxiety is likely to be high both in the patient and the surgeon. These cases should only be operated on by an experienced surgeon unless there are exceptional circumstances. Patients with only one eye will often not consent to cataract surgery until the eye is completely blind. Also, most surgeons are naturally reluctant to operate on an 'only eye'. Always try to discover why the first eye went blind. It may give useful information in planning the operation. For instance, there may be an untreatable retinal detachment in the first eye. This will be a strong indication for doing an extracapsular rather than an intracapsular cataract extraction on the remaining eye.

What facilities are available?

In developing countries good surgical treatment is often not available locally. It may be difficult to decide whether to operate on a blind patient near his home where the facilities are not ideal but the patient is in familiar surroundings, or whether to send the patient many miles to a specialised eye unit. In general, the results of cataract surgery by even relatively inexperienced eye surgeons are fairly good provided that basic surgical principles are followed carefully. However, a young patient who is blind with cataracts or an only eye cataract should be left to an experienced surgeon, with the best possible facilities and support.

Having collected all this information, the surgeon must now decide whether or not to recommend surgery. Usually the decision is straightforward, but some cases are doubtful or uncertain. It is always a good policy to warn patients about the risks of surgery, but especially in uncertain cases where the patient has less to gain and more to lose.

The choice of operation

This is a brief summary of the four different possible ways of removing cataracts and the advantages and disadvantages of each.

Phacoemulsification

Advantages Excellent results and extremely rapid recovery.

Disadvantages Expensive and requires a lot of expensive equipment that needs maintenance, very difficult to perform in patients with hard brown or black nuclei.

Standard extracapsular cataract extraction through a large limbal incision and suturing the wound

Advantages Good results, low cost and requires very little specialist equipment, relatively easy to learn.

Disadvantages The sutures may cause astigmatism or irritation and discomfort, but if the wound is sutured properly these problems should not be very common.

Sutureless small incision extracapsular cataract extraction

Advantages Very good results and very short operating time. Low cost, and requires very little specialist equipment. This is considered the procedure of choice for high volume, high quality, low cost surgery with an experienced surgeon.

Disadvantages It is more difficult to perform than a standard extracapsular cataract operation extraction.

Intracapsular cataract extraction

Advantages Low-cost and can be done without an operating microscope, recommended for patients with subluxated lenses. It is no longer being taught but is still being carried out in some places. It is not in fact a bad operation, especially for elderly patients. It is just that extracapsular cataract extraction. if done properly with an operating microscope is better (in terms of visual outcomes and complications).

Disadvantages More long-term complications, can only really be advised in situations where there is no access to modern microsurgery.

The technology of cataract surgery has been very rapidly progressing and changing as described earlier in this chapter. In developing countries the most modern operation, phacoemulsification, may not always be affordable or available. **The choice of operation for cataract depends on several factors:-**

The equipment available

The most modern treatment for cataracts, phakoemulisification, uses very expensive equipment and the surgeon requires lengthy practical "hands on" training. A more simple sutureless or conventional extracapsular cataract extraction can be performed to a very reasonable standard with fairly basic and simple equipment, as long as an operating microscope with co-axial illumination is available. This method of surgery is now being promoted in most developing countries and by most international agencies concerned with blindness prevention and treatment.[4]

Where a microscope is not available, and it is impossible to send the patient to a properly equipped eye unit an intracapsular extraction is probably a better choice. Intracapsular extraction may also be the surgery of choice if the cataractous lens is dislocated as in Marfan's syndrome, or trauma.), or in some cases during sutureless or conventional ECCE where the zonules are very weak (for example in pseudoexfoliation syndrome) and a very large zonular dialysis occurs.

Is an IOL implant planned?

One of the main advantages of extracapsular extraction is that it is the best type of operation for implanting an IOL. If a lens implant is not planned or not available then the advantages of extracapsular extraction are less, except for young or myopic patients. Extracapsular extraction has a much smaller risk than intracapsular of a retinal detachment and cystoid macular oedema post-operatively. However extracapsular extraction has a greater risk of post-operative uveitis, and thickening of the posterior lens capsule post-operatively is quite common. This is not a problem if YAG lasers are available to treat capsular thickening, but many places do not have a laser. Ideally, an IOL should always be planned.

The age of the patient

Young patients must be treated by extracapsular extraction and in middle-aged patients extracapsular extraction is preferable. A middle-aged patient (40–60 years old) could have a satisfactory intracapsular cataract extraction if absolutely necessary, but anterior chamber lens implants are not generally recommended in this age group. There is also the risk of retinal detachment after intracapsular extraction. (A 50 year-old patient may have 30 years of future life, and so three times the risk of a retinal detachment compared with a person with 10 years of future life). Cataracts in elderly patients can be removed perfectly satisfactorily by either the sutureless or sutured extracapsular technique.

The training and ability of the surgeon

In most training programs, cataract surgeons are initially trained to perform standard sutured ECCE. When they have mastered this technique they would undergo further training in sutureless ECCE.

Surgical technique

Preparing the eye

After the local anaesthetic has been given, the eyelids and conjunctiva cleaned and surgical drapes applied, the eye is ready for operation.

First the eyelids must be retracted. This can be done with eye-lid sutures or a speculum. Most surgeons prefer a speculum. There are many different designs but it is important that the speculum does not press on the eye or get in the way of the operation. The speculum shown in **Figure 3.4**, page 32 is very satisfactory. A slightly heavier speculum in **Figure 3.3**, page 32 can press on the eye. However it can have an advantage if an assistant is available to lift up the speculum gently if required. This tends to create a negative pressure in the eye and can be of help if there is slight pressure on the eye. As the speculum is lifted, the intraocular contents will fall back making more space in the anterior chamber, and lessening the risk of vitreous loss, or posterior capsule rupture.

Before starting the operation check again that the local anaesthetic nerve blocks have worked well:

The patient should not be able to close the eye. If the eyelids can close strongly a facial block may need to be given or to be repeated.

There should be little or no movements of the eye ball on attempting to look in different directions. If there are good ocular movements then the retrobulbar block must be repeated, or a sub-Tenon's block given as well (see page 80).

Slight residual movements in the orbicularis oculi muscle which closes the eye-lids, or in the extraocular muscles moving the eye are acceptable, but the importance of a good local anaesthetic block cannot be emphasised too strongly. The most common cause of complications and difficulties during intraocular surgery is a poor local anaesthetic block. The speculum is inserted to hold open the eye-lids but not to force them apart.

Most surgeons now insert a superior rectus suture, this rotates the eye down and improves access to the upper limbus where the incision is made into the eye. The superior rectus suture should not be used to hold down an eye which is turning up because of an inadequate local anaesthetic block. The technique of superior rectus suture insertion is described on page 33–34. In difficult cases a superior and also an inferior rectus suture can be inserted. These will hold the eye very steady, and also bring it forward a little.

If the palpebral fissure is small, access may be improved with a lateral canthotomy (see page 33). This is more often needed in patients from S.E. Asia who tend to have smaller palpebral fissures.

Extracapsular cataract extraction

In extracapsular cataract extraction the anterior lens capsule, the lens nucleus, and the lens cortex are all removed, leaving the posterior lens capsule and suspensory ligament intact, and using a suture to close the limbal wound. The technique described here is the simplest and easiest way of extracapsular extraction, using a fairly large incision into the eye.

The incision into the eye

The incision into the eye can be made in the sclera, at the limbus where the cornea meets the sclera, or in the cornea.

> **The steps of extracapsular extraction**
> 1 Starting the incision
> 2 The capsulotomy
> 3 Hydrodissection of the lens
> 4 Completing the incision
> 5 Expressing the nucleus
> 6 Irrigation/aspiration of the remaining lens cortex
> 7 Inserting the Intraocular lens
> 8 Wound closure and final irrigation/aspiration

Scleral incisions

Incisions in the sclera will bleed excessively, and some dissection is needed to reach the anterior chamber of the eye. Therefore a limbal incision is usually preferable.

Limbal incisions

Most people recommend that the incision should be at the limbus just under the conjunctiva. Here the sutures become buried under the conjunctiva and do not cause problems or inflammation later on. The surgical anatomy of the limbus is described in detail on page 35–37 and the student may like to revise this.

The incision can be made with a sharp pointed knife called a Graefe knife (**Figure 6.10**). As long as both the point and the blade of the knife are extremely sharp it is a very quick, neat and effective way of making the incision as the wound has a small shelf to it. It also heals well and securely. However, it needs both experience and a very sharp knife to make a successful incision. Bad mistakes can be made if the incision is not done properly and so this technique will not be described in detail.

A slower but safer method is to use a small sharp knife such as a razor blade fragment or a Bard-Parker scalpel (No. 15) to make an incision from the

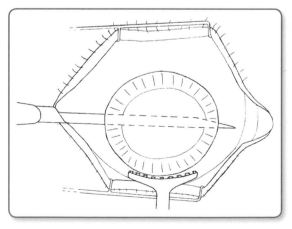

Figure 6.10 A Graefe knife incision

outside of the eye. (N.B. Razor blades made from carbon steel will easily snap obliquely to make sharp knives, but razor blades made from stainless steel will not snap as they are too flexible.) The incision can be started with a knife and completed with scissors, or the entire incision can be performed with a knife. The method is as follows:

1. *Dissecting back the conjunctiva.* A small flap of conjunctiva and Tenon's capsule is dissected back to bare the limbus.
   Either a limbus-based or fornix-based flap may be used (see p.26). Fornix based flaps heal better as they do not interrupt the blood supply to the conjunctiva, so this method will be described. Grasp the conjunctiva gently with non-toothed forceps near the limbus and make a tiny hole in it with sharp scissors. Insert one blade of the scissors through this tiny hole and cut through the conjunctiva keeping as close to the cornea as possible (**Figure 6.11**). Usually and especially in elderly patients, the conjunctiva will retract very easily leaving abouta3mmgap. Ifit will not retract it can be dissected back a little by cutting the attachments between the conjunctiva and Tenon's capsule to the sclera.

2. *Haemostasis.* When the conjunctiva can be retracted about 3 mm back, any bleeding points or large blood vessels in the limbal area should be sealed by applying very light cautery or diathermy (**Figure 6.12**). Do not burn or char the tissues as this prevents wound healing.Take particular care with haemostasis at the two ends of the incision at "2 o'clock" and "10 o'clock" position. There may be numerous small conjunctival blood vessels there, especially if the patient has a small pterygium.

3. *The incision into the eye.* This can now be made where the grey limbal tissue meets the opaque white sclera, which is about 1 mm from the edge of the clear cornea and the attachment of the divided conjunctiva. (Page 35–37 describes in detail the exact anatomy of the limbus.) The size of the incision should be about 140 degrees of the circumference of the eye for an extracapsular extraction, significantly less than half way

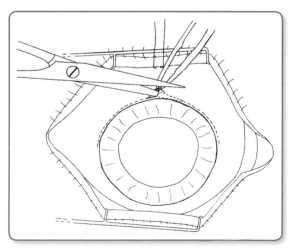

Figure 6.11 The start of a fornix based conjunctival flap and showing the line of the incision

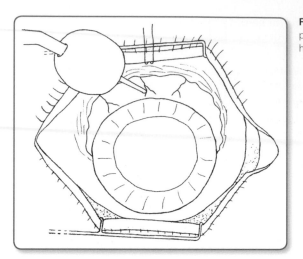

Figure 6.12 Using a "hot point" cautery to achieve haemostasis

round the cornea (**Figure 6.13**). It may need to be larger if the nucleus is very dark and big.

The shape of the incision should be designed so as to make a wound which is as secure as possible and self-sealing. If the incision goes straight through into the eye (**Figure 6.14**) and the eye pressure rises postoperatively the wound can easily leak, but if the incision has a "shelf" (**Figure 6.15**) and the eye pressure rises the wound will tend to seal itself. Another advantage of the wound shown in **Figure 6.15** is that the internal opening into the eye is well away from the trabecular meshwork through which the aqueous drains out of the eye. The shelf also helps prevent the iris prolapsing out from the wound during the operation which can be awkward. One slight problem to guard against with a shelving incision is a stripping of Descemet's membrane from the inside of the cornea (**Figure 6.16**). It occurs if the knife blade is not sharp or if the incision is shelved too much. The Descemet's membrane usually

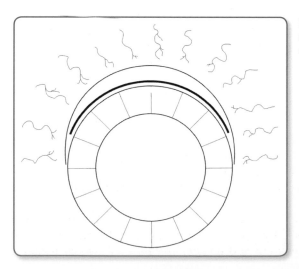

Figure 6.13 To show the size and position of the incision for extracapsular extraction

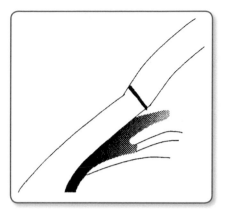

Figure 6.14 An incision straight through into the anterior chamber. An incision shaped like this can easily leak

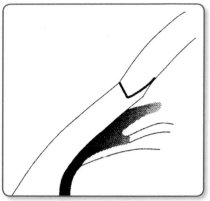

Figure 6.15 An incision with a "shelf". This shape of incision is more watertight

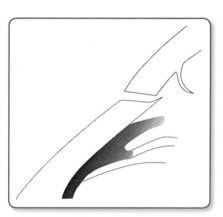

Figure 6.16 Stripping up of Descemet's membrane

sticks back by itself postoperatively, but if some corneal endothelial cells are lost, there may be a localised area of corneal oedema.

The incision starts with a cut that goes about half the depth into the sclera and at 90 degrees (perpendicular) to its surface (**Figure 6.17a**). Here are some hints for a good neat, clean incision:

- Make sure that the knife is sharp.
- Make sure that the eye is grasped firmly with sharp-toothed dissecting forceps.
- Make sure that the blade of the knife is at the correct angle to the eye (**Figures 6.18** and **6.19**).
- Try to cut perpendicular to the surface of the eye (**Figure 6.17a**) and plan to cut half way through the depth of the sclera.
- Try to make one or at the most two firm cuts rather than a lot of small scratches.

If the incision is too deep and enters the anterior chamber at this stage it is not a serious problem. However once the anterior chamber has been opened, aqueous will leak out and the eye becomes soft which makes it

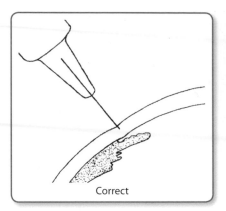

Correct

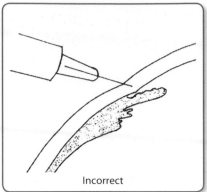

Incorrect

Figure 6.17a The knife blade at the correct angle perpendicular to the surface of the eye

Figure 6.17b The knife blade is not perpendicular to the surface of the eye

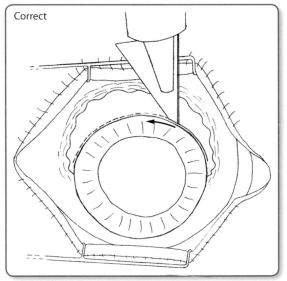

Correct

Figure 6.18 The incision into the eye using a razor blade fragment. Note the cutting edge of the knife is angled towards the direction in which the blade is moving

more difficult to continue to incise the eye from outside using the knife. Also if the incision goes right through into the anterior chamber it means that the shape of the incision is not ideal for producing a shelved secure wound.

Once a half thickness groove has been made into the sclera the incision is deepened to enter the eye. The angle of the knife to the surface of the eye should be changed to point obliquely into the eye (**Figure 6.20**) in order to make a secure shelved wound. Alternatively the incision can be completed with a small angled keratome (**Figure 6.53c**). These are now readily available because they are used for phakoemulsification incisions.

Another way of constructing a secure wound is to make the first part of the incision halfway through the depth of the sclera. Then advance the incision

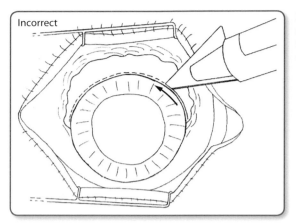

Figure 6.19 The cutting edge of the knife is angled away from the eye and so will not cut effectively

into the cornea and make the second half of the incision straight down into the anterior chamber (**Figure 6.21**).

Once a small entry site has been made into the anterior chamber, it is usual to carry out the anterior capsulotomy and the hydrodissection of the lens. These are the first two steps of an extracapsular cataract extraction, and they can be performed more easily through a small incision so that the anterior chamber stays formed. This also protects the cornea. Then the wound is fully opened up (see page 121) and the rest of the cataract extraction performed. Alternatively the capsulotomy needle can be mounted on a 2 ml syringe with irrigating fluid, and pushed through the groove of the incision before the eye is opened. In this way the capsulotomy can be done through a watertight incision.

Corneal incisions

Incisions further forward in the cornea are quick and bloodless, which is an advantage. However they do not heal so well and they will tend to cause more post-operative astigmatism because the incision is nearer the optic axis of the eye. In particular there may be problems from sutures

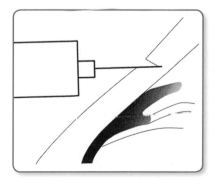

Figure 6.20 The angle of the knife to complete the incision into the eye

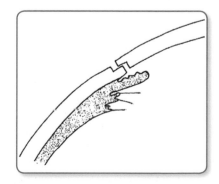

Figure 6.21 An incision with a "shelf"

with corneal incisions. If there are knots or suture ends left on the surface of the cornea these will cause considerable irritation and inflammation. Monofilament suture material such as 10-0 nylon or polyester will not cause any irritation as long as the knots are buried in the tissue, because the suture material becomes covered by corneal epithelium and does not irritate. However, the sutures may become loose, and after about nine months nylon sutures will begin to soften and then break. The broken ends will then cause considerable irritation. There are three rules for the suturing of corneal incisions:

1. Always use fine monofilament suture material(10-0 nylon or polyester.)
2. Always bury the knot.
3. Always remove the suture after 4 to 6 months. This last rule can be ignored for polyester sutures, because they do not weaken and break up even after many years.

If a particular suture is very tight and is causing excessive astigmatism, it can be removed sooner, after about 6 to 8 weeks. Loose sutures should be removed immediately. A lose nylon suture can be recognised very easily. It will stain green with fluorescein because it is not covered by the corneal epithelium. (The suturing of corneal incisions is also described in chapter 3.)

Corneal incisions are specifically recommended if the patient has had a previous glaucoma operation as this avoids damaging the drainage bleb. Corneal incisions are also advisable if the patient has a high risk of developing glaucoma later, because a limbal incision will cause scarring of the conjunctiva, which reduces the chance of success of a glaucoma operation later. For all other patients a limbal incision is better.

A corneal incision is made in the same way as a limbal incision. The incision can have the same shape as a limbal incision to provide a watertight wound, but care must be taken not to cut into the central part of the cornea, as this would affect the vision. Remember that a corneal incision will need to extend further round the eye than a limbal incision to have the same size opening into the eye.

The capsulotomy

Incising the anterior lens capsule – the capsulotomy

Several different methods have been recommended for this. The aim is to remove the anterior capsule, but to keep intact the posterior capsule and the capsule at the equator of the lens where it is attached to the suspensory ligament. Nearly all methods use a small, specially shaped hypodermic needle called an irrigating cystotome. This can be made from a hypodermic needle simply by bending it into the right shape (**Figure 6.22** and **6.23**). It is very important at all times to protect the delicate endothelial cells on the back of the cornea and not to damage them either chemically or mechanically. The best way to ensure this protection is to use visco-elastic fluid, which is injected into the eye before doing the capsulotomy. (Various visco-elastic fluids are available. Some are very expensive, but hypromellose is quite cheap. It *must* be manufactured specially for intraocular use, and it *must* be

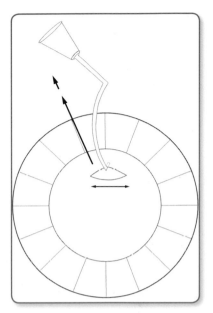

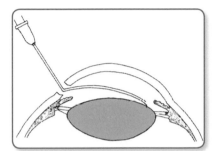

Figure 6.22 The position of the irrigating cystitome in the eye

Figure 6.23 To show how the capsule usually tears into the opposite direction to the movement of the cystitome

completely pure and non-toxic.) If visco-elastic fluid is not available, then the cornea can be protected by injecting a bubble of air into the eye or alternatively by connecting the cystotome to the irrigating fluid. The constant flow of irrigating fluid will maintain the anterior chamber and protect the cornea throughout the procedure. It will also wash away any debris from the lens which may be released during the capsulotomy.

There are 3 commonly accepted ways of cutting and removing the anterior capsule. The first is called the "endocapsular" or "envelope" method, the second is called the "can opener" method, and the third is called the "continuous circular capsulo-rexis" method.

It is important to understand the way the lens capsule tears when it is punctured by the cystotome. The capsule is a thin elastic membrane. When the sharp point of the cystotome needle is pushed into the lens, it punctures the capsule and makes a small tear in it. If the tip of the cystotome is then moved over the surface of the lens this tear then becomes bigger rather like tearing a thin piece of paper. If the cystotome is moved in one direction the capsule usually tears in the opposite direction, at 90 degrees to the movement of the cystotome (see **Figure 6.23**). However it may tear in the same direction as the cystotome is moved.

The endocapsular method

This is probably the safest and easiest way of performing the capsulotomy. A horizontal opening is made in the upper part of the lens capsule (**Figure 6.24**), but none of the capsule is removed at this stage. The nucleus and the cortex are removed through this opening. The intraocular lens is then inserted into the "envelope" between the anterior and posterior lens capsule, and finally

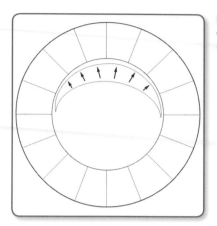

Figure 6.24 Anterior capsulotomy by the endocapsular method. The arrows show the movements of the tip of the cystotome

the bulk of the anterior capsule is removed with intra-ocular scissors. The advantages of the endocapsular method are:

- the intact anterior capsule helps to protect the corneal endothelium during the operation.
- it ensures that the intraocular lens is placed correctly inside the lens capsule.
- if the posterior capsule ruptures during the operation, the intact anterior capsule may still provide enough support for a posterior chamber IOL. However the haptics will be in the ciliary sulcus and not in the capsular bag.

The main disadvantage of the endocapsular method is that it is sometimes difficult to remove the anterior capsule at the end of the operation without the use of visco-elastic fluids and fine intra-ocular scissors.

In the endocapsular method the cystotome punctures the lens capsule and short vertical movements are made across the upper part of the capsule. In this way a horizontal tear is made across the upper part of the capsule (**Figure 6.24**). Finally the tip of the cystotome is moved across the surface of the lens from left to right to make sure that the tear is complete.

The "can opener" anterior capsulotomy

The aim of this is to tear the anterior capsule round its periphery and to leave a large hole in the centre. In the "can opener" technique the point of the cystotome is first pushed into the lens at the pupil margin at the 6 o'clock position at the bottom of the eye (**Figure 6.25**). The cystotome is then pushed about 1–2 mm downwards making a small tear in the capsule. The cystotome tip is then lifted out of the lens and pushed into it again at the 5 o'clock position and again moved 1–2 mm peripherally in order to enlarge the tear in the lens capsule. Altogether about 10 short radial cuts are made, first at the bottom of the lens, then at the sides and finally at the top, each cut pierces the lens towards the edge of the pupil and pushes outwards by 1–2 mm. In this way these radial cuts should produce a large round tear of the lens capsule (**Figure 6.25**). It is sometimes helpful to end by passing the cystotome right round in a circular direction to make sure that the cut is complete.

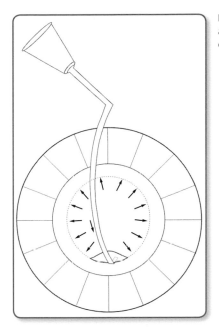

Figure 6.25 The "can opener" capsulotomy. The arrows show the movements of the tip of the cystitome

The advantage of the can-opener method is that no more manipulation in the eye is needed to remove the anterior capsule. This helps if visco-elastic fluids or fine intraocular scissors are not available. The disadvantages are:

- The capsule does not always tear in the way that is planned.
- The intraocular lens cannot always be placed reliably in the capsular bag.
- The lens nucleus may rub against and damage the corneal endothelium during expression of the nucleus.

Continuous circular capsulo-rexis

This is in theory the best way of incising and removing the anterior lens capsule, as it is torn without any jagged or irregular edges. There is therefore almost no risk of any small tear in the capsule extending backwards round the equator of the lens capsule into the posterior capsule. It also ensures that the intraocular lens is placed very safely and securely inside the lens capsule. Continuous circular capsulo-rexis is the only safe way of performing the anterior capsulotomy with a phakoemulsification operation. The method is to start with a small U shaped tear in the capsule, to fold this over with the tip of the needle, and then tear it right round in a circle in the same way as a thin piece of paper might be torn (**Figure 6.26**). There are however two problems with the technique. Firstly, it is very difficult to do in patients with dense opaque white cataracts, because the surgeon needs to see the edge of the capsule. Secondly, it is difficult to manoeuvre a large lens nucleus through the capsulo-rexis opening and into the anterior chamber and so out of the eye. For these two reasons it is difficult to recommend capsulo-rexis for surgery without phakoemulsification.

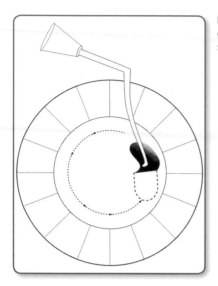

Figure 6.26 Continuous circular capsulorexis capsulotomy. The folded over piece of capsule is shown as black.

Difficulties during capsulotomy

These may occur especially if the cataract is very dense or hypermature. The capsule may not tear in the planned direction, and as soon as the capsule is punctured, fluid white lens matter may leak out into the anterior chamber. This obscures the view and has to be washed away with irrigating fluid.

On rare occasions the capsule may be thick and calcified, and will not tear at all with the cystotome. In these patients the capsule may have to be cut using fine intra-ocular scissors, or the surgeon may have to do an intracapsular extraction instead.

Hydro-dissection

This separates the nucleus and the layer around it called the epinucleus from the capsule of the lens, and in this way it makes it easier to express the nucleus from the eye. It is done using a blunt cannula placed just under the capsule and injecting some infusion fluid which will help form a plane of cleavage between the nucleus and capsule.

Completing the incision

The incision into the eye must now be enlarged and completed. The *knife* or *keratome* can be used for this, but if the eye is soft it is very difficult to use the knife to cut into a soft eye. Visco-elastic fluid can be injected into the anterior chamber to keep the eye firm, so the incision can be completed with a knife or keratome making a shelf as already described. If the eye is soft or it is difficult to complete the incision with a knife, corneal scissors should be used. The opening made by the knife must be big enough to get one blade of the *corneal scissors* into the anterior chamber. Make sure that this blade does not catch or go through the iris. Use the scissors to complete the incision taking several small snips (**Figure 6.28**). If the scissors are sharp and held at the correct angle the incision can usually be completed easily. If there is any pressure on the eye the iris will bulge out through the incision.

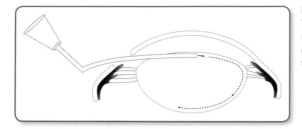

Figure 6.27 Hydro-dissection. The fluid separates the lens nucleus from the cortex and can also separate the cortex from the capsule

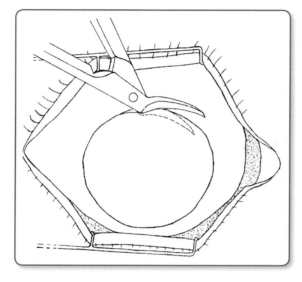

Figure 6.28 Using corneal scissors to complete the incision

The iris will then catch on the tip of the scissors, and it is then very easy to make the mistake of cutting through the iris as well as cornea with the scissors. **Figure 6.29** shows the profile of the completed incision using a knife to start with, and scissors to complete the incision.

Expressing the nucleus of the lens

The nucleus of the lens can now be expressed out of the eye, through the hole in the anterior capsule and out through the wound. The usual way to do this is with a lens expressor and a lens loop. These are shown in **Figure 6.67** on page 156. In young patients the nucleus is fairly soft and fairly small having the consistency of paste, but with increasing age the nucleus becomes larger and harder and fills most of the lens. Sometimes in intumescent cataracts the nucleus begins to shrink again, although it remains hard.

During the expression of the lens nucleus it is very important to prevent it from rubbing against the corneal endothelium. If it does, the vital endothelial cells will be damaged and will never be replaced. The more the nucleus rubs against the corneal endothelial cells, the more likely these cells are to be damaged or destroyed. The best way to protect the corneal endothelium is to use visco-elastic fluid. This may have been washed out during the hydro-dissection and more may need to be inserted into the anterior chamber. If visco-elastic fluid is not available, air costs nothing and is perfectly satisfactory.

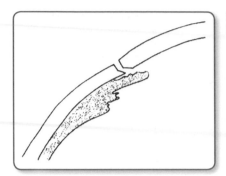

Figure 6.29 The profile of the wound using a knife to start the incision and scissors to finish it

During the expression of the nucleus try to keep a small air bubble in the anterior chamber to act as a cushion between the corneal endothelium and the lens.

The endocapsular method also helps to protect the corneal endothelium, because the intact anterior capsule prevents the nucleus from rubbing against the cornea. The capsule has a smooth surface and will not damage the endothelium so easily.

The technique of expressing the nucleus is as follows:

1. Fill the anterior chamber with visco-elastic fluid or a small air bubble (**Figure 6.30**).
2. Place a lens expressor at the lower limbus (**Figures 6.30 and 31**).
3. Put counter-pressure usually with a lens loop well above the upper limbus about 3 mm on the scleral side of the incision (**Figures 6.30 and 31**).
4. Press gently but firmly with the lens expressor and the lower pole of the nucleus will tilt back so that the upper pole of the nucleus tilts forwards. Gentle pressure with the lens loop on the posterior lip of the wound will now open up the incision and push the upper pole of the nucleus forward into the incision. The black arrows in **Figure 6.30** show where the expressor and the lens loop press into the eye. If the lens loop is too near the edge of the incision, then pressure with it will press the upper pole of the nucleus backwards and so stop it coming out of the eye. It is very important to have both the lens loop and the expressor in the right place to slide the nucleus out of the eye. The pressure with expressor at A should be a little more than that with the loop at B. The upper pole of the nucleus should now appear between the lips of the incision. By moving the lens expressor upwards a little over the lower part of the cornea and continuing with gentle pressure from the lens loop, the nucleus will be pushed further out of the eye. Do not let the expressor come right up over the central cornea as it will press the cornea against the lens and damage the endothelium.

Difficulties during the expression of the nucleus

If the nucleus is reluctant to emerge from the eye it may be held up in 3 possible places:

1. The incision may be too small so the nucleus is trapped inside the anterior chamber. *This is the usual reason why the nucleus will not come out.*

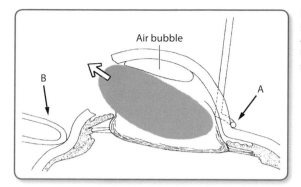

Figure 6.30 and 6.31 To show the position and action of the lens expressor and lens loop when expressing the nucleus

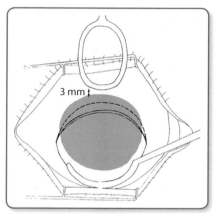

- Make the incision larger. But, before doing this, inject some visco-elastic into the anterior chamber to push back the nucleus and protect the endothelium. It is important to remember with the shelved incision that its internal size is smaller than its external size, because of the shelf. Therefore a very shelved incision may need to be enlarged.
2. The iris sphincter may be too small so the nucleus is trapped behind the pupil. There are various ways of trying to deal with this situation .
   - The pupil may be stretched using two small hooks such as the diallers for an intraocular lens.
   - Alternatively, you can grasp the upper part of the iris with forceps and place it behind the upper pole of the lens
   - If neither of these work or possible you can do a sphincterotomy of the iris to enlarge it. To do this a vertical cut is made in the upper part of the iris starting at the pupil margin. The iris can be resutured after the IOL has been inserted using 10-0 polyester suture, but that is not essential.
3. The capsulotomy may be too small so the nucleus is still trapped inside the lens capsule
   - Enlarge the capsulotomy with radial incisions at 10 and 2 o'clock.
4. Sometimes the lens nucleus may be particularly large and hard. This is found especially in "black" nuclear cataracts.

Once the nucleus is half out of the eye it can be wheeled out using a lens loop, or the tip of a needle (**Figure 6.32**). It can be squeezed right out of the eye using the expressor but this tends to rub the endothelial cells of the cornea against the lens.

There are other ways of removing the nucleus from the eye. Some surgeons place an irrigating lens loop(sometimes called an irrigating Vectis) inside the eye, behind the nucleus but in front of the posterior capsule (see page 144 and **Figure 6.54**).This is connected to a syringe or the infusion bottle and hydrostatic pressure will then force the nucleus out of the eye. Great care must be taken to avoid scooping the nucleus upwards against the corneal endothelium, and thus damaging it.

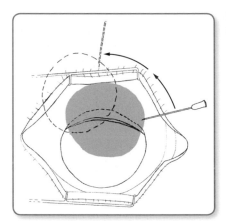

Figure 6.32 Using a needle tip to "wheel" a nucleus out of the incision

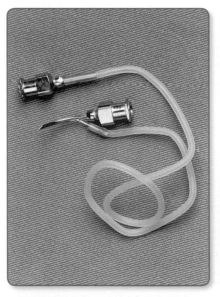
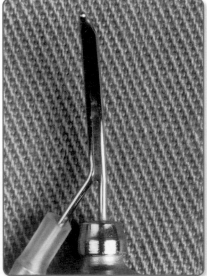

Figure 6.33 A two-way irrigating/aspirating cannula

Removing the lens cortex by irrigation and aspiration

This may be easy or difficult depending mainly on the consistency and transparency of the lens cortex. If the cataract is almost intumescent, the cortex is white and opaque and semi-fluid. It breaks up easily and therefore it is both easy to see and to remove. If the lens cortex is fairly transparent, as it is in most nuclear cataracts or in less mature cataracts, it can be difficult both to see and remove. It is difficult to see because it is transparent, and difficult to remove because it will not break up and sticks to the capsule. For these cases an operating microscope with co-axial illumination makes all the difference. The almost transparent cortical lens matter and the edge of the lens capsule can only be seen against the red fundus reflex with co-axial illumination (see plate 1 and plate 2).

The standard way of removing the cortical lens matter is with a two-way cannula (sometimes called a Simcoe cannula) which will both irrigate and aspirate (**Figure 6.33**). The irrigation is attached to an infusion line so that there is a constant gentle flow of fluid which keeps the anterior chamber formed. The aspiration is attached to a 5 ml syringe. Make sure that the cannula is connected the right way round as shown in **Figure 6.34**.

The epinucleus

Most cataracts have a layer of lens cells around the nucleus called the epinucleus. This is softer than the nucleus but harder than the cortex. The epinucleus may come out with the expression of the nucleus or it may remain in the eye. It can be removed by irrigation and aspiration but this can be very time consuming. It is more easily removed by injecting irrigating fluid through a blunt cannula into the anterior chamber which will wash it out of the eye in one piece. This is sometimes called hydro-expression.

The technique of irrigation and aspiration

Removing the cortical lens matter without damaging the posterior capsule is

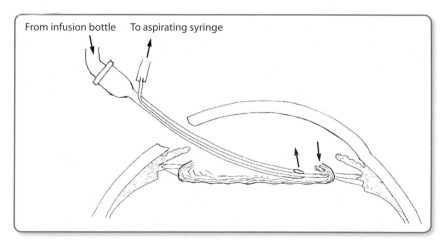

From infusion bottle   To aspirating syringe

Figure 6.34 To show the lens cortex being aspirated whilst maintaining the anterior chamber with irrigation

probably the hardest part of an extracapsular cataract extraction. It is made easier by a good hydrodissection (see p.115), which helps to separate the cortex from the capsule. Here is a list of helpful tips to assist this delicate part of the operation.

- Before starting the aspiration, it is often a good plan to just wash out the anterior chamber with irrigating fluid in a 10 ml syringe and a cannula. This will wash away any large fragments of lens cortex and any epinucleus, and the last pieces can be removed with irrigation and aspiration.
- Maintain a constant, gentle continuous flow of irrigating fluid. Keep watching the tip of the cannula. The aspirating port hole at the tip of the cannula should be facing forwards (**Figure 6.34**). It may be necessary to turn it so the hole is facing side-ways to remove lens cortex which is caught under the iris or stuck to the posterior lens capsule. It should never face backwards or it will suck in the posterior capsule and rupture it. If the two-way cannula has been sterilised by chemical methods or by boiling, make sure that all the chemical and the water has been very thoroughly washed out of it so that only pure irrigating fluid enters the eye.
- Keep the tip of the cannula in the plane of the pupil or just behind it. Do not press on to the posterior capsule or it may rupture. Place the cannula so that the tip is close to the lens cortex to be removed.
- Now apply gentle suction on the syringe, and the lens cortex should be sucked into the tip of the cannula and strip away from the lens capsule. As a general rule do not move the tip of the cannula in the eye while applying suction with the syringe. However, if the lens cortex is firmly attached to the lens capsule, it may help to move the cannula tip very slowly whilst aspirating to help strip the lens cortex from the capsule. When doing this always move the cannula tip from the edge of the pupil towards the centre–not the other way. Try to peel away all the lens cortex starting at the bottom of the eye at 6 o'clock, then at the sides and finally from the top.
- As well as watching the position of the tip of the cannula, also watch where the cannula enters the eye through the lips of the wound. If the shaft of the cannula is not resting gently between the wound edges but is either pressing upwards or downwards it will keep the wound open so the anterior chamber will not remain full of fluid. This makes the aspiration more difficult and the cannula is more likely to damage the corneal endothelium or rupture the posterior lens capsule.
- A technique called "suck and spit" is quite helpful to remove little pieces of cortex that are reluctant to come out of the eye. The cannula is left in one place and with the syringe, fluid is alternately aspirated and injected into the eye.

Difficulties during irrigation and aspiration of the lens cortex

1. ***Failure to remove all the lens cortex*** It is important to remove as much lens cortex as possible. However if there are a few pieces still attached to the capsule which are reluctant to emerge, it is best to leave them as long as the centre of the pupil is clear of lens cortex, and continue

with the operation. Once the IOL is in place and the wound closed with sutures, a further irrigation/aspiration should be performed by passing the two way cannula between two sutures. The anterior chamber will then deepen when the irrigating cannula is placed in the eye because the wound is almost closed. The IOL will act as a splint holding the posterior capsule in place, and the haptics will help dislodge some of the peripheral pieces of lens cortex, and these last few pieces will then be aspirated out of the eye more easily.

Lens cortex at the 12 o'clock position under the upper iris may be particularly difficult to remove because the tip of the cannula cannot easily reach there.

2. *A poorly dilated pupil* If the pupil is not well dilated, it is difficult to aspirate cortical lens matter which is hidden behind the iris. A poorly dilated pupil is best avoided by taking all the steps described on pages 71–72 to make sure that the pupil is well dilated. If the pupil is not well dilated the tip of the cannula must be passed behind the iris and suction applied without being able to see the tip. If it is obvious that the iris has become caught in the aspirating port hole, then release the suction and move the point of the cannula very slightly. Once it seems that the tip of the cannula has engaged cortical lens matter then maintain gentle suction with the syringe and very gently withdraw the cannula to the centre of the pupil. Usually the lens cortex will strip away from the lens capsule. One helpful tip with a constricted pupil is to pass the tip of the cannula behind the iris, and then use the syringe to squirt a small amount of irrigating fluid under the iris which may dislodge pieces of lens cortex that cannot be seen.

3. *The tight eye or the eye under pressure* If the eye is tight or under pressure it becomes very difficult to maintain the depth of the anterior chamber, and the posterior capsule appears to be pushing forwards the whole time. In this situation it is very likely that the tip of the irrigating cannula will rupture the posterior lens capsule, and vitreous loss will then occur. The other signs of a tight eye are that the wound may gape a little or there may be a small horizontal fold across the centre of the cornea (**Figure 6.35**). A tight eye and forward pressure on the open eye may have four basic causes (see **Figure 6.36**):

  a. *An incomplete facial block.* This is the most common cause and the eye-lids will tend to squeeze shut. The speculum may also be pressing slightly on the eye. Ask the assistant to lift the speculum gently, and bring the two limbs of the speculum together a little, and usually the signs of pressure on the eye will disappear and the anterior chamber will become more deep. The operation can proceed, but the assistant will need to hold the speculum up until the wound has been closed with sutures.

  b. *An incomplete retrobulbar block.* This will cause pressure on the open eye because the extraocular muscles are still contracting. This should have been identified before reaching this stage. If this is causing a serious problem and the operation has already started, a sub Tenon's

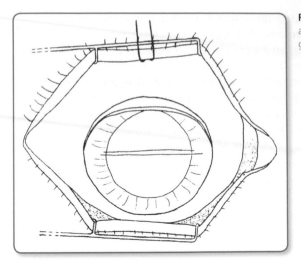

Figure 6.35 A horizontal fold across the cornea with slight gaping of the wound

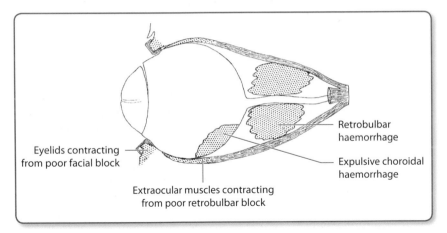

Eyelids contracting from poor facial block

Extraocular muscles contracting from poor retrobulbar block

Retrobulbar haemorrhage

Expulsive choroidal haemorrhage

Figure 6.36 The causes of a tense or tight eye

block using a blunt curved cannula can be safely given, as this has very little risk of rupturing or damaging a blood vessel behind the eye (see page 80).

c. *A retrobulbar haemorrhage.* This is a complication of the retrobulbar block and causes pressure on the open eye. A severe retrobulbar haemorrhage should have been identified before the operation begins, but a small or delayed retrobulbar haemorrhage may not be noted until this stage.

d. *An expulsive haemorrhage.* This is an extremely rare but disastrous complication causing forward pressure of the lens and the posterior capsule. This is caused by a ruptured choroidal artery causing bleeding into the choroid and forcing all the intraocular contents out of the eye. With a severe haemorrhage first the lens, then the vitreous and finally the choroid and retina will be progressively extruded from the eye. This very rarely happens. With less severe choroidal haemorrhage the eye will just appear very tight for no obvious reason.

Treatment The best treatment for a choroidal haemorrhage is to sew up the eye as quickly and securely as possible. This restores the intraocular pressure and acts as a tamponade stopping the haemorrhage and in this way the eye may be saved. After a few weeks, the haemorrhage will absorb and any further surgery can be safely performed.

The management of a tight eye and a shallow anterior chamber

If the anterior chamber if still rather shallow despite lifting up the speculum, the surgeon will rightly be worried about rupturing the posterior lens capsule with the irrigating cannula when trying to remove the last pieces of lens cortex. The best thing to do is to try to insert the IOL with the help of visco-elastic fluid and sew up the wound. With a closed wound the anterior chamber will deepen with irrigation/aspiration, and the last pieces of lens cortex can be removed much more easily. With a very tight eye it may not be possible to insert an IOL at all.

Posterior capsule rupture and vitreous loss

The most common complication of extracapsular extraction is that the posterior capsule ruptures and vitreous starts to emerge from the wound. It can happen for various reasons. The eye may be tight, or there may be external pressure on the eye so the anterior chamber is very shallow. Sometimes there may not be sufficient care taken during irrigation and aspiration of the lens cortex, and the two-way cannula may catch and rupture the posterior lens capsule. Most cases of posterior capsular rupture cause a loss of vitreous through the wound as well, but in some cases no vitreous loss occurs. Even the best surgeons experience vitreous loss, but with care and foresight it should not happen frequently.

A vitreous loss rate of 5% or less is acceptable. The complication rate will depend both on the ability of the surgeon and whether the cases are straightforward or not.

Vitreous loss can cause serious complications, but they are not common if managed correctly. The vitreous is a gelatinous substance containing protein fibrils and tends to stick to anything solid that it touches. Therefore if the vitreous prolapses through the wound it will stick to the wound edges. This may prevent the wound healing well, and it may cause the iris and pupil to be drawn up into the wound post operatively. The posterior surface of the vitreous is attached to the retina, especially to the peripheral retina. If the anterior part of the vitreous becomes trapped in the wound, there is traction on the posterior part of the vitreous. This will pull on the peripheral retina and may cause a retinal detachment. Severe cystoid macular oedema is also much more common after vitreous loss. The five main complications of vitreous loss are therefore (**Figure 6. 37**):

- *a retinal detachment*
- *cystoid macular oedema*

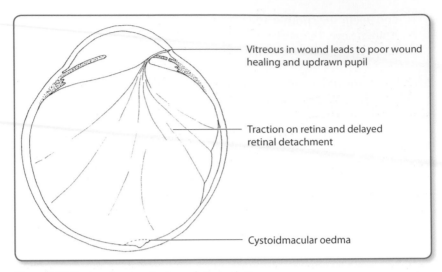

Vitreous in wound leads to poor wound healing and updrawn pupil

Traction on retina and delayed retinal detachment

Cystoidmacular oedma

Figure 6.37 To show the complications of vitreous loss

- *poor wound healing*
- *an updrawn pupil*
- *infection; a vitreous strand to the wound will act as a direct route for infection to enter the eye*

Management of vitreous loss

The correct management of vitreous loss is to cut and clear all the vitreous from the wound and the anterior chamber. In all cases no vitreous should be left touching the wound, and ideally none left in the anterior chamber. Removing the vitreous in this way is called an *anterior vitrectomy*. The best way of performing this is with a vitrectomy machine, which slowly aspirates the vitreous while chopping and dividing it. If a vitrectomy machine is not available the recommended method is to use a small cellulose sponge and a pair of iris scissors, "the sponge and scissors vitrectomy" (**Figure 6.38**). A small dry cellulose sponge is inserted into the wound edge where it will adhere to the vitreous, and as the sponge is gently lifted from the wound scissors are used to cut the attached vitreous. The surgeon will need to put the sponge repeatedly into the lips of the wound, lift it up and cut the vitreous to which it is attached. If the assistant lifts the speculum at the same time this may help to reduce any pressure on the eye, and help the vitreous to fall back from the wound. A "sponge and scissors" vitrectomy should continue until there is no formed vitreous left in the anterior chamber or in front of the pupil (**Figure 6.39**). If vitreous is still present in the anterior chamber, each time the sponge is inserted into the wound edge and gently withdrawn it will be seen to have gelatinous strands of vitreous attached to it. A "pupil tug" will also be noticed so that as the sponge is withdrawn slightly the vitreous pulls on the pupil margin and slightly distorts it. When there is no "pupil tug" and no strands of vitreous attached to the cellulose sponge, then the anterior chamber is clear of vitreous and this can be confirmed by inserting a small air bubble into the anterior chamber. If vitreous is still present the air bubble will be distorted.

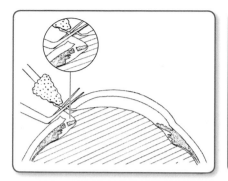

Figure 6.38 The technique of sponge vitrectomy

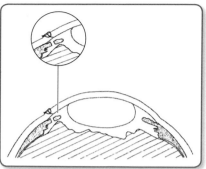

Figure 6.39 The end result of sponge vitrectomy with an air bubble in the anterior chamber

Do not suck the vitreous out of the eye with a syringe as this risks pulling on the posterior vitreous and causing a retinal detachment. There is always a temptation when vitreous loss occurs not to clear away all the vitreous from the wound and anterior chamber. *However it is much better to remove too much vitreous rather than leave it trapped in the wound.* Sometimes the vitreous is fluid and degenerate and it may keep coming forward into the anterior chamber as fast as it is excised. This type of fluid vitreous is less likely to stick to the wound edges or the iris and so cause significant traction on the retina. Therefore the complications of leaving degenerate fluid vitreous in the anterior chamber are much less. Remember that a rapid, continuous and unexplained loss of vitreous could be caused by an expulsive haemorrhage, but fortunately this is very rare.

When vitreous loss has occurred the surgeon must decide whether to implant a posterior chamber lens, an anterior chamber lens or no IOL at all. If there is only a very small rupture in the posterior capsule, it is reasonable to implant a posterior chamber lens but to position the haptic loops where the posterior capsule is intact.

If the cataract extraction has been done by the endocapsular method so that the anterior capsule is still present, it may be best to insert the lens in front of both the anterior and the posterior capsule rather than into the capsular bag.

If the posterior capsule has ruptured extensively and it does not seem possible to insert a posterior chamber lens, then an anterior chamber lens may be inserted (see page 165–166). In that case the capsule remnants are not serving any useful function and it may sometimes be better to remove them. If the surgeon decides to convert from a posterior chamber lens to an anterior chamber lens implant, then a peripheral iridectomy must be performed as well to prevent any risk of blocking the flow of aqueous (see page 151).

Inserting a posterior chamber intraocular lens

It is very much easier to insert the intraocular lens if the anterior chamber is deep. Visco-elastic fluid should be used to fill up the anterior chamber, and also the capsule bag. If this is not available irrigating fluid or an air bubble must be used, and it may be helpful to put 2 interrupted sutures at each edge of the wound just leaving a 7mm gap through which the intraocular lens can be inserted. This will help to maintain the air bubble or irrigating fluid in the anterior chamber and prevent it collapsing. Make sure that the orientation of the intraocular lens is correct (see **Figure 6.41**).The tip of the lower haptic should be pointing towards the left. Also make sure that as the intraocular lens goes into the eye it does not brush against the eyelids or eyelashes and so risk becoming contaminated with skin bacteria. If the "can-opener" anterior capsulotomy technique was used, then insert the lower haptic so that it goes behind the pupil. If the endocapsular anterior capsulotomy technique was used, insert the lower haptic so that it goes behind the anterior capsule and into the capsular bag. (This may be a little bit difficult if an air bubble is being used to maintain the anterior chamber depth, as the air bubble will tend to press the anterior capsule back onto the posterior capsule.) Once the first haptic is in place and the optic of the lens is in the anterior chamber, the second haptic must be inserted into the eye. This is done by rotating or "dialling" the lens through 90 degrees so that the haptics lie transversely in the eye at 3 and 9 o'clock. There are three methods for doing this:

1. *Using the lens dialler with a pointed tip and the dialling holes at the edge of the optic of the IOL* (see **Figure 6.40** and **6.41**). The tip of the dialler engages the upper dialling hole and moves down and to the left. This pushes the intraocular lens into the centre of the eye and also rotates it at the same time. As it rotates the upper haptic should naturally pass into the capsular bag in the case of the "endocapsular technique", or behind the iris into the ciliary sulcus in the case of the "can opener" technique.

2. *Using the dialler with a groove at the tip at the junction of the optic and upper haptic* (**Figure 6.42** and **6.43**). Some lenses do not have dialling holes. With this type of lens the dialler can be placed where the upper haptic is attached to the optic and in the same way the lens can be "dialled" or rotated into the eye.

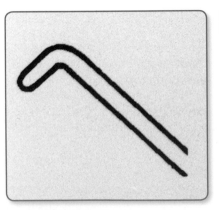

Figure 6.40 Enlarged view of the tip of the Dialler for use with lenses with dialling holes

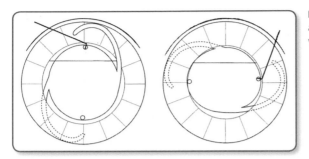

Figure 6.41 To show the action of the Dialler for IOLs with dialling holes

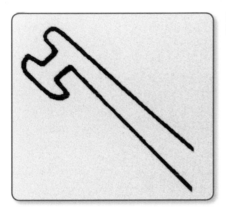

Figure 6.42 Enlarged view of the tip of the Dialler used for lenses without dialling holes

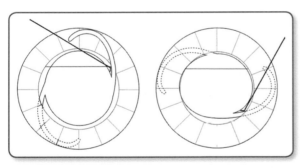

Figure 6.43 To show the action of the Dialler for IOLs without dialling holes

3. *Using the fine intra-ocular Kelman-McPherson capsule forceps* (**Figure 6.44**) gently grasp the upper haptic and flex it towards the centre of the eye downwards and to the right (**Figure 6.45**). The grip on the upper haptic is then released so that it springs back into place behind the iris or in the capsular bag.

Once the IOL is in place, the anterior capsule is removed if the endo-capsular technique was used. With the anterior chamber full of viscoelastic fluid, the capsular scissors (**Figure 6.46**) are used to make two vertical cuts at either side of the anterior capsule (**Figure 6.47**) The central flap is then grasped with the Kelman-McPherson capsular forceps shown in **Figure 6.44** and torn off at its base (**Figure 6.48**) Alternatively the central

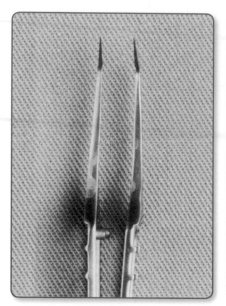

Figure 6.44 Kelman-McPherson capsular forceps

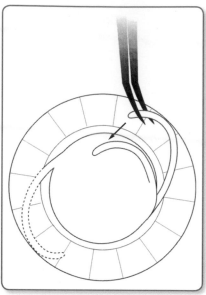

Figure 6.45 To show the action of the Dialler for IOLs without dialling holes

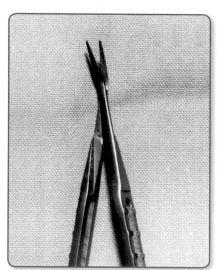

Figure 6.46 Capsular scissors

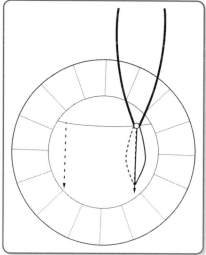

Figure 6.47 Making two vertical cuts in the anterior capsule with capsulotomy scissors

flap can be left in the eye until the wound is sutured and closed, and then grasped and torn off with the two way cannula during the final irrigation/aspiration.

Difficulties in inserting the IOL

Sometimes if the eye is rather tight or the anterior chamber is shallow, it may be difficult to get the IOL into the eye. In some cases the second haptic

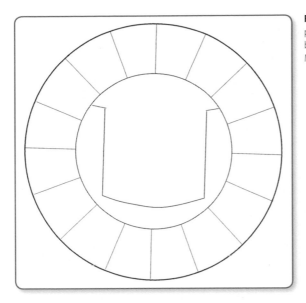

Figure 6.48 The central piece of anterior capsule has been removed with Kelman-McPherson capsular forceps

will not go behind the iris, but in really difficult cases it may be difficult to get the second haptic even to stay in the anterior chamber, and it keeps coming out of the eye. In this situation it is best just to leave the IOL where it is, either in the anterior chamber or with the second haptic of the IOL outside the eye, and sew up the wound completely and tightly. The anterior chamber is then filled with fluid, preferably visco-elastic but failing that with irrigating fluid. This will deepen the anterior chamber and create downward pressure on the posterior capsule and the IOL. This makes it very much easier to dial the IOL into place by inserting the dialler between two sutures.

Wound closure

The methods of wound closure have already been described on pages 42–49. The basic rules are:
- Place the suture at the right depth (**Figure 6.49**); too shallow causes poor wound healing and too deep causes a "wick" from the anterior chamber to the outside, and a possible route of infection into the eye.
- Have the suture at the right tension; too tight causes astigmatism, and too loose causes poor wound healing and astigmatism in the opposite direction.
- With virgin silk or absorbable suture material, 4 to 5 interrupted sutures should be used. The knots should be placed at the scleral end of the wound where they will be covered by conjunctiva (**Figure 6.50**).
- With monofilament nylon (9-0 or 10-0) or polyester(10-0 or 11-0) it is much better to bury the knots (see pages 43–4). For sutures on the cornea the knots **must** be buried.
- A continuous "bootlace" nylon or polyester suture with a single buried knot at one end gives a very quick, secure and neat wound closure (see page 44).
- Make sure the knots are properly tied (see pages 47–48)

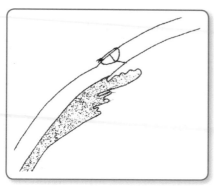

Figure 6.49 The closed wound

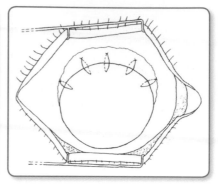

Figure 6.50 The position of the knots when closing the wound

- Make sure that the iris is neither adherent to the wound nor trapped in it. This is done by gently inserting an iris repositor between the lips of the wound in between the sutures. If the iris has actually prolapsed from the wound it is better to use the side of the iris repositor to stroke it back into the eye (see **Figure 6.51**) rather than the tip to poke it back in.

When the wound has been closed or almost closed there should a final irrigation of the anterior chamber, using the two-way cannula. The cannula can be inserted into the eye between two of the sutures. If a continuous suture is used for wound closure, then the first half hitch of the knot can be tied, the cannula placed between the sutures, and when the cannula is finally removed the suture can be tightened and the second half of the knot completed.

This final irrigation and aspiration of the anterior chamber will wash out all the viscoelastic fluid and also any last pieces of lens cortex which may have been dislodged by the IOL. *It is a very important step and will help to prevent post-operative uveitis.* The IOL acts as a splint keeping the posterior capsule in place, and the sutured wound means that the anterior chamber stays very deep. Therefore this final irrigation and aspiration can be more easy and effective.

It is not essential to suture the conjunctiva if a fornix based conjunctival flap has been used, but some surgeons like to place a "purse-string" suture to tighten the conjunctiva and bring it down to cover the wound giving extra protection. (see **Figure 6.52**). This suture can either be placed at the 12 o'clock position or at one or other end of the conjunctival incision. If a nylon suture is used for this, again make sure that the knot gets buried under the conjunctiva and is not on the surface.

Sutureless extracapsular cataract extraction

Sutureless extra-capsular cataract surgery (SECCE), is also known as small incision cataract surgery (SICS), or manual small-incision cataract surgery (MSICS), the incision is not all that small although it is smaller than for a conventional extracapsular cataract extraction.

Most people think that SICS is the best and most appropriate operation where the aim is to provide good quality, high volume, low cost surgery. It is

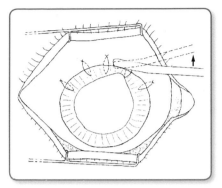 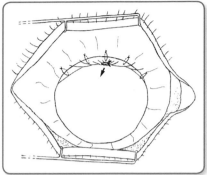

Figure 6.51 The use of the iris repositor to replace the iris and free it from the lips of the wound

Figure 6.52 A small suture (arrowed) to bring down the conjunctiva incision

however significantly harder to learn than the large incision sutured extracapsular extraction.

The idea of sutureless extra-capsular cataract surgery has developed from phakoemulsification, and has been pioneered in developing countries. Cataracts can be removed without phakoemulsification through an incision which is self-sealing and therefore sutureless. Because no suturing is needed, this saves both time and money, and because the incision is watertight the eye is more stable during the operation. The main disadvantage is that the operation is harder to perform than a standard operation particularly if the nucleus is fairly large. Small incision cataract surgery requires 3 separate steps, each one must be completed successfully to enable the next one to be performed.

- The incision needs to be self-sealing and yet large enough to allow the entire lens nucleus to be removed in one piece. This can be achieved with a tunnel shaped incision.
- The nucleus is then mobilised inside the eye, and inside the lens, to enable it to be removed.
- The nucleus is then removed without damaging either the cornea or the posterior lens capsule.

These stages of sutureless ECCE can be further broken down into to following:
- Preparation
- Superior rectus suture
- The incision:
    - Conjunctical peritomy & cautery
    - Scleral fixation & incision
    - Paracentesis/'side port'
    - Scleral tunnel
- Capsulotomy
- Hydrodissection & nucleus mobilisation
- Nucleus extraction
- Soft lens matter removal
- IOL implantation
- Irrigation/aspiration

Preparation, superior rectus suture

This is covered in the previous paragraph, and in more details in Chapter 3, and thorough cleaning of the skin around the eye, eyelashes (with Povidone Iodine 10%) and a drop of 5% Povidone iodine into the eye at least 5-10 minutes before surgery is essential; as is careful draping to hold the lashes out of the way.

The incision

Until the surgeon has gained plenty of experience, this is quite difficult to construct. It is easier if the eye is fairly firm and so we would recommend making a small side port incision first, to fill the eye with viscoelastic fluid. This also has advantages later on in the operation when removing the lens cortex. For a right-handed surgeon this will be made in the eight o'clock position in the clear cornea, and should be shelving and just big enough to fit the Simcoe irrigating and aspirating cannula. After the side port incision has been made the anterior chamber is filled with viscoelastic fluid so the eye is firm but not hard. This side port incision, also known as the paracentesis, can be made with any sharp blade.

There are three parts to the incision. The opening into the sclera, the tunnel and the opening into the cornea.

The opening into the sclera (see Figure 6.53a)

A superior rectus suture is inserted and a fornix based conjunctival flap dissected. The incision into the sclera is about 8 mm long and usually shaped like a "frown". It can be slightly smaller (6–7 mm), especially if the nucleus is small or the surgeon is very skilled. It can be even larger. The incision goes halfway through the sclera and can be made with any sharp knife or razor blade fragment. Because it is a little way from the limbus, it is quite vascularised and the blood vessels will need **gentle** cautery or diathermy first. At its closest point, it should be at least 2 mm from the clear cornea. The incision can be made straight across rather than frown-shaped but the frown incision produces less post-operative astigmatism.

The incision doesn't need suturing because the large distance of at least 4mm between the internal and external opening (see **Figure 6.53d**) makes the wound self-sealing as the intraocular pressure rises. Therefore the width of the incision from side to side does not really matter. The post-operative astigmatism is usually about 1 dioptre. It will be greater if the incision is nearer to the limbus or if it is larger. However larger incisions make the operation easier, and the astigmatism can always be reduced by a single suture in the middle of the wound.

Making the tunnel (Figure 6.53b)

This is the most critical part of the incision, and for it a standard crescent knife is used. Since the coming of phakoemulsification, these knives are readily available and usually "disposable". However, with care between cases and sterilising the blade in spirit based povidone-iodine solution or autoclaving at a lower temperature (115° C.), one knife and handle may remain sharp for a whole operating list or more.

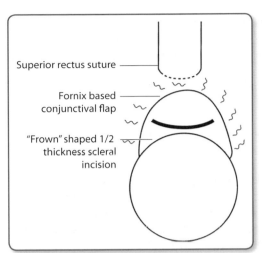

Figure 6.53a The Incision

Superior rectus suture

Fornix based conjunctival flap

"Frown" shaped 1/2 thickness scleral incision

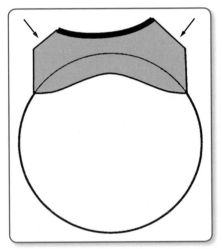

Figure 6.53b The Tunnel (shaded), note its shape and size

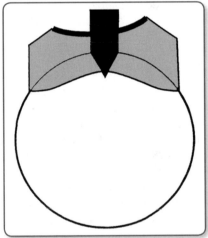

Figure 6.53c Completing the incision into the eye

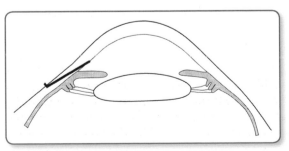

Figure 6.53d To show the profile of the scleral tunnel

First establish a plane of cleavage about half the thickness of the sclera. With experience, you will be able to judge how deep this is. If you can't really see the metal of the Crescent knife, you are probably too deep; and if you can see it very clearly you're probably too shallow. It is possible to go deeper by pointing the tip of the Crescent knife down, or alternatively by pressing it down. It is possible to go less deep by pointing it up or by lifting it up. Then enlarge by making sweeping movements with the crescent knife, both downwards 2 mm into clear cornea, and then sideways at the edge of the incision, to make a tunnel which stretches from limbus to limbus at the ten o'clock to two o'clock position (see **Figure 6.53b**). The knife will cut much better if you sweep it from side to side rather than trying to push it. Remember to keep the heel of the Crescent knife resting on the eye all the time so that the plane of the knife is the same as the plane of the sclera The tunnel must be *long* and enter the eye well into clear cornea in order to be self-sealing and free of the risk of iris prolapse. It must be *wide* in order to accommodate the entire nucleus. Make sure that the incision is wide enough throughout the length of the tunnel, especially in its outer part as shown by the arrows in **Figure 6.53b**. While making the initial scleral incision, and making the tunnel with the crescent blade, use a toothed scleral fixation forceps to gently but firmly grip the sclera and immobilize the eye. For a right-handed surgeon this is done with the left-hand, and make sure that the fixation forceps is neither **pushing** down on the eye, nor **pulling** up on the eye but just **grasping** it.

Completing the incision into the anterior chamber (Figure 6.53c)

This is done with a sharp pointed keratome knife which can be re-sterilised in the same way as the crescent knife. Advance the tip of the keratome to the centre end of the tunnel. Make sure it doesn't go through the back of the tunnel but once its tip has reached the end of the tunnel, then point it sharply backwards so that it will enter the cornea.

It is usually easier to make the cut with the sharp side-edge of the keratome as it goes into the eye rather than as it comes out of the eye. Having a firm eye also lessens the risk of creating a rip of the corneal endothelium or Descemet's membrane, which is a possible complication of cutting obliquely through the cornea. In particular, the internal opening into the anterior chamber must be wide, reaching all the way to the limbus at each end of the incision. The tip of the keratome should disappear beyond the margin of the clear cornea at each end of the internal opening. If the keratome is getting blunt, it may fail to cut the full width of the incision. The profile of the completed incision is shown in **Figure 6.53d**.

The capsulotomy

This can be done by the endo-capsular, can-opener, or capsulorrhexis method (see page 116–120) Once the internal opening is complete, many surgeons use the same keratome knife to make an incision at the top of the lens capsule, known as the endocapsular or "envelope" technique, or 'linear capsulotomy' (see **Figure 6.24**). This can alternatively be done with a cystotome, but the incision in the lens capsule must be from pupil margin to pupil margin and big enough to allow the nucleus to come out easily. Some surgeons prefer a complete 360° "can opener" capsulotomy (see **Figure 6.25**). This makes it easier to mobilise the nucleus into the anterior chamber, but it risks damaging the corneal endothelium from the nucleus rubbing against it. The endocapsular method is probably safer.

Difficulties during scleral tunnel construction

The two most common difficulties while making the scleral tunnel are when using the crescent blade making the tunnel too shallow (and causing a "button-hole") or making the tunnel too deep (and causing premature entry).

- Button hole. If the crescent blade is too shallow and comes out of the sclera, a button hole will appear. It will be necessary to start a new scleral tunnel, starting again at a part as far away from the button hole. Very careful tunneling will now aim to 'undermine' the button hole.
- Premature entry. If the blade is too deep, it will enter the anterior chamber too soon. If this occurs, carefully complete the tunnel trying not to enter the eye too soon at other parts of the tunnel. If during the rest of the operation the iris is prolapsing, and especially if there is any iris prolapse at the end, it will be necessary to place a suture in the scleral tunnel at the end of the operation.

The mobilisation of the nucleus

The nucleus must first be separated from the capsule. This is done by hydrodissection. It is then mobilised by rotating it. Once fully mobile an instrument can be passed behind the nucleus without any risk of rupturing the posterior capsule. *A well dilated pupil is absolutely essential for a satisfactory mobilisation of the nucleus*. It enables the surgeon to see what he or she is doing, and allows the mobilised nucleus to come forwards either wholly or partly into the anterior chamber. The best way to ensure that the pupil is well dilated is described on page 71–2. Sometimes before starting hydrodissection the nucleus can be mobilised partially using the cystotome. After the capsulotomy has been done by whatever method the tip of the cystotome is put into the nucleus and used as a lever to rotate it or to lift up one edge.

Hydro-dissection

Hydro-dissection helps to separate the lens nucleus from the capsule and the lens cortex and so makes it easier to express the nucleus. A 5 or 10ml syringe is filled with the irrigating fluid and mounted on a fine blunt cannula. This cannula is then inserted just under the capsule and irrigating fluid injected fairly vigorously just under the capsule (**Figure 6.27**). This helps to separate the lens nucleus and cortex from the capsule. A good hydro-dissection makes the expression of the nucleus easier. It also helps to separate the lens cortex from the capsule, so that the cortex can be stripped away from the capsule more easily.

The hydrodissection fluid should pass around the nucleus both behind and in front of it. Some surgeons like to hydrodissect in two planes, one just under the capsule and the other deeper into the lens between the nucleus and the epinucleus. This is to make the nucleus as small as possible so it will come out of the tunnel more easily. However this second hydrodissection is not really necessary. When the nucleus passes out through the tunnel, the epinucleus strips itself off and stays behind in the anterior chamber.

Once the nucleus has been separated from the capsule by hydrodissection, it must be mobilised by rotation. The blunt cannula tip is used as a lever to spin it round. For this the cannula is placed at the side of the nucleus. Once it has rotated through 180 degrees it is well mobilised. If it is difficult to rotate, the sharp tip of an irrigating cystotome can be placed in the nucleus and will give better leverage. In order to remove the nucleus from the eye it must be brought from behind the iris, into the anterior chamber. This often happens by itself with the hydrodissection, but if it doesn't you can use the tip of the hydrodissection cannula like a tyre lever to manoeuvre it into the anterior chamber. If it will not come one useful tip is to press gently on the outside of the eye at the limbus at three o'clock, which will tilt the nucleus so that the part at nine o'clock tends to come up a little, and the hydrodissection cannula can then be used to tyre lever it into the anterior chamber.

Very mature cataracts with fluffy white cortex are usually fairly easy cases. The fluffy cortex can easily be washed out of the eye during hydrodissection, and there is often a fairly small nucleus and no obvious epinucleus. First wash out the cortex in front of the nucleus, then at the side of the nucleus. Sometimes this loose cortex can be removed from behind the nucleus as well, but always maintain a flow of fluid in the cannula, especially if the tip is behind the nucleus, as this protects the posterior capsule. Also press the shaft of the cannula very gently backwards on to the posterior side of the wound, as this keeps the wound open and helps the cortex come out.

The removal of the nucleus

This is the hardest and most critical part of the operation but there should be no problem if:

1. The incision has been properly constructed,
2. The pupil is well dilated,
3. The lens nucleus has been fully mobilised into the anterior chamber (if an irrigating vectis is used)
4. The nucleus is not excessively large.

Various instruments have been described for removing the nucleus. The easiest is probably the irrigating lens loop, or vectis.

- First inject some visco-elastic fluid, both between the nucleus and the corneal endothelium to help preserve the corneal endothelium, and also just behind the upper tip of the nucleus to help insert the lens loop behind the nucleus without damaging the posterior lens capsule. *The cannula should be used at the same time to check the two sides of the tunnel to make sure that the whole length of the tunnel is wide enough.*
- The irrigating loop *must* be at the correct angle to open the tunnel by pressing *backwards* on the posterior lip of the incision (see **Figure 6.54b**). This can be helped in different ways:
  i.   strong traction is applied to the superior rectus suture which will rotate the eye down.
  ii. Alternatively the eye may be grasped at the lower limbus and forcibly turned down.
  iii. If the patient has a rather sunken socket it also helps to have a backward curve on the shaft of the irrigating loop, so that the shaft is pressing backwards on the posterior lip of the tunnel.

iv. A slightly different way of putting backward pressure on the posterior lip of the wound is to do the entire operation at the side of the eye rather than at the top. This is called a temporal approach. From this direction it is very easy to put backward pressure on the wound. The main disadvantage is that the wound is not covered by the upper lid at the end of the operation.

- The lens loop, mounted on a 5ml syringe, is now inserted through the incision into the eye. The loop is advanced so its tip is just under the upper pole of the nucleus (this is why the previous injection of visco-elastic is helpful), and it is then slowly advanced further into the eye just behind the lens nucleus. It helps at this stage to inject fluid very gently through the loop as this keeps the posterior capsule well clear of the loop. Once the tip of the loop has reached the lower pole of the lens nucleus, then the nucleus can be extracted (**Figure 6.54a**).

- It is particularly important to have both the *shaft* and the *tip* of the lens loop in the correct position. The shaft should be pressing downwards (**Figure 6.54b**) on the posterior lip of the incision (as shown by the arrows A). This opens up the tunnel. However the tip of the loop should be resting just behind the nucleus. It should not press downwards or it might rupture the posterior capsule, nor should it press upwards or it might rub the nucleus against the endothelium

- There is always a great temptation to lift the tip of the loop forwards towards the cornea to "scoop" the nucleus out of the eye. This temptation must be resisted. It will rub the nucleus against the corneal endothelium and permanently damage the endothelium. It will also close off the tunnel instead of opening it. Instead, the nucleus comes slowly out of the eye because of the hydrostatic pressure created by more forceful pressure on the plunger of the syringe (see B in **Figure 6.54b**). This raises the pressure in the anterior chamber, and this pushes the nucleus into the tunnel (see arrow C).

- Once the nucleus has started to enter the tunnel, then the lens loop is gently withdrawn whilst maintaining the hydrostatic pressure of the injection (B in **Figure 6.54b**) and also maintaining the downward pressure on the posterior part of the wound (A in **Figure 6.54b**). As the loop is gently withdrawn it will help to drag the nucleus through the tunnel and out of the eye.

- Once the nucleus is properly in the tunnel and no longer in the anterior chamber, the lens loop can, of course, be used as a kind of scoop because upward pressure now can no longer damage the corneal endothelium and the nucleus itself will keep the tunnel open. Once the nucleus is almost out of the eye, the pressure on the syringe should be released.

Removing the nucleus using a specifically bent 30G needle as a 'fish-hook'

It is important that the nucleus is mobile after hydro-dissection, as described above.

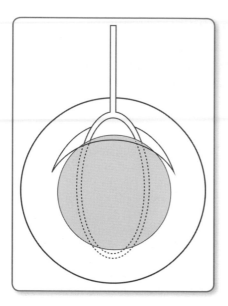

Figure 6.54a An irrigating lens loop is inserted behind the nucleus

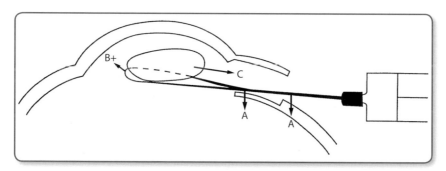

Figure 6.54b Removing the nucleus to show the position of the lens loop

Some visco-elastic is injected into the anterior chamber to protect the endothelium, and then the cannula is laid flat on the scleral tunnel, and pressed gently backwards towards but above the upper equator of the nucleus so as then to tip the top of the nuclued forwards. If the cannula is too close to the centre, the nucleus will simply move backwards. Stop and try again a little further above the nucleus until the top of the nucleus tips forward, and then inject some visco-elastic behind the nucleus to push back the posterior capsule while at the same time moving the cannula downwards and forwards to move the top of the nucleus into the anterior chamber. Then inject a bit more visco-elastic behind the nucleus. Advance the bent 30G needle/fish-hook behind the nucleus towards the lower equator, turn, engage the nucleus and remove it through the sclearal tunnel. It may be helpful to push back on the tunnel while you remove the nucleus, and also pull on the superior rectus suture: both of which help to open the scleral tunnel.

Difficulties and complications

The most common problems encountered are:[5]

1. The nucleus enters the tunnel but will not come out through the external opening. There are several possible solutions to this.

   - The keratome can be used to widen the external opening of the tunnel.
   - There is a simple manoeuvre which may help to remove a nucleus which has definitely entered the tunnel but has become stuck in it. A lens dialler can be passed along the tunnel in front of the nucleus and the pointed tip of the dialler then turned down into the front of the nucleus. This with the lens loop which is behind the nucleus will act as a "sandwich" enabling the nucleus to be pulled out through the tunnel.
   - The lens loop can be pressed forward into the upper pole of the nucleus to chip off its upper part. If the nucleus is a then pushed back into the anterior chamber, and then rotated round through 90 degrees using a cannula with visco-elastic, the nucleus diameter will be less and it should now come out through the tunnel.
   - In all cases, it is helpful to inject some visco-elastic into the anterior chamber above the nucleus to protect the endothelium, and behind to push back the posterior capsule; before enlarging the tunnel or trying to extract the nucleus.

2. The iris keeps prolapsing through the wound. The reason for this is either that the tunnel does not go far enough into the clear cornea, or else the pupil is not well enough dilated.

3. The nucleus may remain posterior to the iris or it may not be possible to mobilise it at all into the anterior chamber. The usual reason is that the pupil is too constricted or possibly the capsulotomy hole is not large enough. You should not even attempt to remove the nucleus until it is in the anterior chamber.

4. If the nucleus is particularly large and hard it will not enter the tunnel at all.

The best solution to problems 2, 3, is to convert to a standard sutured extracapsular extraction. The incision in the sclera is extended right along the edge of the shaded area in **Figure 6.53** and the incision can be further enlarged around the limbus with corneal scissors or a blade. For problem 4: The incision can be converted in this way, or it is possible to widen the incision and still keep it as a tunnel.

There are some skilled surgeons who use techniques and instruments to divide a particularly large nucleus into two or more fragments inside the eye, and in this way can still remove a large nucleus using a sutureless tunnelled incision.

5. Bleeding from the incision may occur especially if the tunnel is very wide. If the bleeding is into the eye, patience is usually the best treatment and it should stop. The blood can then be washed out. The side port incision will enable the anterior chamber to be filled with irrigating fluid under slight pressure, and this should prevent any further bleeding by compressing the bleeding point (tamponnade).

For the expert, sutureless cataract surgery is an extremely quick and effective operation which can be performed in almost every patient. For the beginner, it is definitely harder than the standard extracapsular technique. Apart from obtaining some "hands on" training, it is best to wait until one feels entirely confident with routine extracapsular surgery, and to choose easier cases. These are younger patients, those with posterior subcapsular cataracts and mature cataracts with white, fluffy cortex. Hard cases are those with dense nuclear sclerosis and those with partially dilated pupils. It is also essential to have a really sharp crescent knife and keratome to make the incision, and a well-manufactured lens loop – preferably one with more than one irrigation hole at the tip. Grooves in the front surface of the loop will also help it to pull the nucleus through the tunnel.

Alternative methods

There are various alternatives ways of removing the nucleus.

The technique pioneered by Professor Blumenthal from Israel uses an anterior chamber maintainer (see **Figure 6.55**). This is inserted at the lower part of the cornea to maintain the hydrostatic pressure throughout the operation. A plastic lens glide (see **Figure 6.81**) is used to open the tunnel and remove the nucleus.

The technique developed by Dr Ruit and Dr Tabin, also in Nepal uses a triangular capsulotomy, and a lens expression using either hydroexpression with a simcoe canula, or an irrigating vectis.[6, 7]

Videos describing the techniques are also available (see end of chapter for details).

Cataracts and glaucoma

Sometimes patients may require treatment for both cataract and glaucoma. When both cataract and glaucoma are present in the same eye it may be difficult to decide the best plan for the treatment. It is important to assess how much of the visual loss is from the cataract, and how much from glaucoma. In each case a very careful clinical examination is absolutely essential

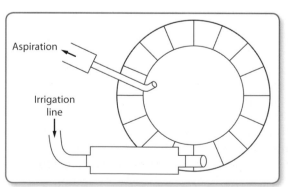

Aspiration

Irrigation line

Figure 6.55 An anterior chamber maintainer inserted through the lower part of the cornea. There is also an aspiration cannula inserted into the anterior chamber

to avoid performing an unnecessary or harmful operation. As well as a careful examination of the eye, helpful clues may come from the history, from examining the other eye, from gonioscopy etc.

Both cataract and glaucoma cause loss of vision. Cataract causes a loss of visual acuity, and the vision will be restored after successful surgery. Glaucoma causes a loss of the visual field and the sight that is lost will not be restored even with successful surgery.

The pupil reaction is normal in cataract but patients with glaucoma have an afferent pupil defect. The most valuable clinical sign of glaucoma is the appearance of the optic disc, but this may be difficult or impossible to see in an eye with cataract.

Sometimes an eye with an advanced cataract may develop secondary glaucoma as a complication. This may be *phakomorphic glaucoma* when the lens enlarges and causes secondary angle closure glaucoma, or it may be *phakolytic glaucoma* when fluid lens protein leaks out and obstructs the trabecular meshwork.

Sometimes patients who have had successful glaucoma surgery may subsequently develop a cataract in the eye.

The following are some general principles in helping to decide how to treat a patient with both cataract and glaucoma:

1. In all cases of cataract with glaucoma extracapsular extraction is preferable to an intracapsular extraction. Glaucoma surgery has a much higher rate of failure after intracapsular extraction, because there is no physical barrier to stop the vitreous becoming incarcerated in the glaucoma drainage operation.
2. Always try to reduce the intraocular pressure to normal before the start of the operation. Operating on an eye with raised intraocular pressure risks causing an expulsive choroidal haemorrhage.
3. In certain cases it may be best to operate only on the cataract and leave the glaucoma untreated:
    *   If there is a risk of angle closure glaucoma this is prevented by cataract extraction.
    *   If there is open angle glaucoma but it is only mild, the intraocular pressure may often fall just from removing the cataract.
4. If a cataract extraction is performed on a patient who may later need a trabeculectomy operation for glaucoma, a clear corneal temporal sutured is best. This leaves the conjunctiva unscarred, which makes any subsequent glaucoma operation more likely to succeed. If a cataract extraction is performed in an eye which has previously had a successful glaucoma operation, the incision should be through the cornea, so not to disturb the successful glaucoma drainage procedure. One way of avoiding the glaucoma bleb is by performing the cataract extraction through a teuporal approach.
5. In some cases the surgeon may decide to operate on the glaucoma and the cataract at the same time. This has obvious practical advantages for the patient by avoiding two operations, and in most cases the results are good.

Cataract extraction combined with trabeculectomy

This may be planned in several different ways.

1. A standard trabeculectomy may be performed (see page 208). On completing the operation the cataract is then extracted through a corneal incision in front of the trabeculectomy and without disturbing it. This is probably the simplest method.
2. A standard extracapsular cataract extraction may be performed but with an alteration to the shape of the incision in the sclera (**Figure 6.56**). A partial thickness flap of sclera is made, the anterior chamber entered in the usual way, and the cataract removed and the IOL inserted. Then a peripheral iridectomy is performed, and a small piece of deep corneo-scleral tissue excised just as for a trabeculectomy. The incision in the sclera is then sutured, and then the conjunctiva is sutured very tightly. Finally the test described on page 216 should be done to confirm that the aqueous is draining satisfactorily.
3. The technique of sutureless cataract surgery can be very easily modified to function as trabeculectomy as well. The tunnel is constructed, but a small horizontal slit is made into the posterior wall at the limbus, before opening the tunnel into the anterior chamber. After the lens has been removed and the IOL inserted, this slit is enlarged to remove a piece of trabecular tissue. Through this hole an iridectomy is done. The scleral incision and the conjunctiva should be sutured just as for a trabeculectomy.

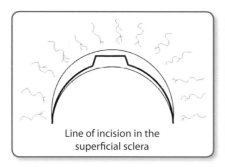

Line of incision in the superficial sclera

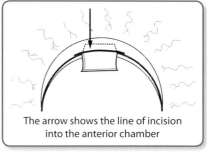

The arrow shows the line of incision into the anterior chamber

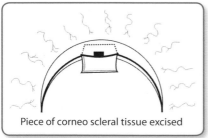

Piece of corneo scleral tissue excised

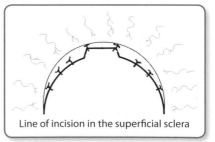

Line of incision in the superficial sclera

Figure 6.56 The incision for combined cataract extraction and trabeculectomy

4. An alternative method is to place the incision for sutureless cataract extraction in one part of the eye, and the incision for the trabeculectomy in another part.

For all combined cataract and trabeculectomy procedures the conjunctiva must be tightly sutured down to make sure that the aqueous does not leak out of the subconjunctival space. Testing that the trabeculectomy is draining and the conjunctival flap is watertight as described on page 216 and **Figure 6.18** is also very helpful.

Intracapsular cataract extraction (ICCE)

There are a few cases which have subluxated lenses or calcified capsules where intracapsular extraction is best. Occasionally during a complicated ECCE where the capsule is not stable, conversion to ICCE with and anterior chamber IOL is necessary. Finally, although ICCE is not being taught anywhere, there are many places where it is still being performed, and it does not require an operating microscope. Visual outcome results comparing ECCE and ICCE can be similar when done well.[8]

With an intracapsular extraction, the entire lens is removed by rupturing the attachment of the lens capsule to the suspensory ligament.

The incision

The principles of the incision are basically the same as for extracapsular extraction but the incision needs to be larger because a larger space is needed to remove the entire lens within its capsule. The size of the incision needs to be just less than half way round the limbus, about 170 degrees in all (see **Figure 6.57**).

Pre-placed sutures

Once the incision has been completed most surgeons place one or more sutures in the wound at this stage, but of course these sutures are not tied.

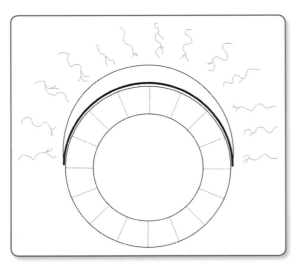

Figure 6.57 To show the size and position of the incision for intracapsular extraction

The reason for inserting sutures at this stage is that the eye is more stable with the lens in place. Once the lens has been removed, manipulations on the wound edge while inserting the sutures may press on the eye and force some vitreous into the wound or even out of the eye. If one or more sutures are in place before the lens is extracted these sutures can be tied immediately after the lens has been removed. This secures the wound, allowing further sutures to be inserted without disturbing the wound edge very much. The only problem caused by placing sutures before removing the lens is that these sutures may get in the way when trying to remove the lens. Therefore only one or at most two pre-placed sutures should be used. The sutures should be inserted to about half the depth of the cornea and once inserted they should be looped out so that they do not get in the way when the cornea is lifted (**Figure 6.58**).

A pre-placed suture has another advantage. The assistant can use fine forceps to hold the loop of the suture which goes through the cornea, and in this way open up the eye for the surgeon. Otherwise the assistant has to grasp the

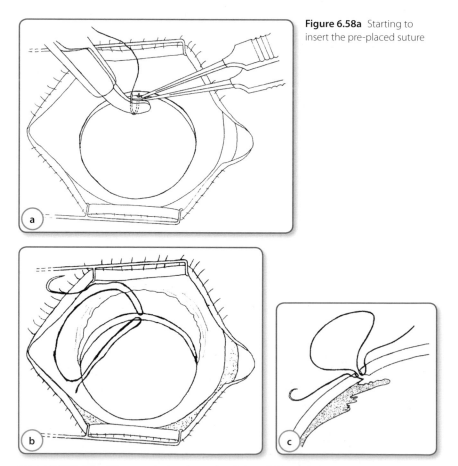

Figure 6.58a Starting to insert the pre-placed suture

Figure 6.58b and c The suture is then looped well clear of the wound cornea itself with forceps which is harder to do and may damage the corneal endothelium.

The iridectomy

There are two reasons for doing an iridectomy:

1 *To prevent pupil block glaucoma.* After an intracapsular extraction the vitreous face may rest against the pupil and stick to the pupil margin. This can stop aqueous circulating into the anterior chamber and cause a condition known as pupil block glaucoma (**Figure 6.59**). This can be prevented by making a small hole in the iris. This may be a peripheral iridotomy when a small slit is made in the iris, or a peripheral iridectomy (**Figure 6.60**) when a small hole is made in the iris.

2 *To make the cataract extraction easier.* The iris is a sphincter lying in front of the lens. If this sphincter is divided the lens will come out more easily. A full or broad iridectomy divides the iris sphincter (**Figure 6.61**). This makes removing the cataract easier especially if the pupil is not well dilated. After a full iridectomy, grasping the lens with the cryoprobe or the capsule forceps is easier. Therefore a full iridectomy is recommended for intracapsular extraction if the pupil will not dilate well or the surgeon is very inexperienced.

Always perform an iridectomy if you plan to implant an anterior chamber lens.

There are however three advantages of a peripheral iridotomy or iridectomy over a full iridectomy:

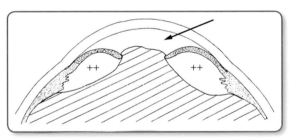

Figure 6.59 Pupil block glaucoma. A knuckle of vitreous (see arrow) blocks the pupil and prevents circulation of the aqueous

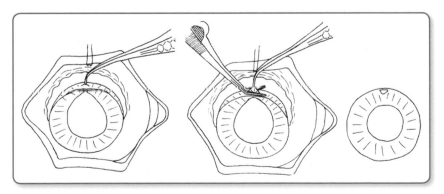

Figure 6.60 A peripheral iridectomy

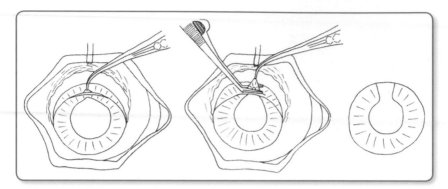

Figure 6.61 A full or broad iridectomy

- With a peripheral iridectomy the iris sphincter is intact. An intact iris sphincter means that the pupil will constrict in bright light and on accommodation. This improves the visual acuity and depth of focus of the eye and prevents glare. However in most cases patients do not seem to have any problems with their vision after a full iridectomy, as the iridectomy is usually hidden by the upper eye-lid.
- An intact iris helps to prevent vitreous loss by holding the vitreous back.
- If an IOL is planned, then a full iridectomy makes IOL fixation very difficult.

Technique of iridectomy

1. The assistant gently lifts the cornea at 12 o'clock preferably by traction on the pre-placed corneal suture (**Figure 6.62**).
2. For a peripheral iridectomy, grasp the iris fairly near its root with fine iris forceps. Lift it very gently and gradually, then using deWecker's scissors excise the small portion of iris tissue held in the iris forceps (**Figure 6.60** and **6.62**).
3. For a peripheral iridotomy, the scissors cut into the iris without excising any tissue.
4. For a full iridectomy, the iris is grasped about half way between its root and pupil margin and a slightly larger segment of iris including the pupil margin is excised with de Wecker's scissors (**Figure 6.61**).
5. Take great care not to touch the lens capsule with the iris forceps (**Figure 6.63**).

Bleeding into the anterior chamber

Sometimes the view of the lens is obscured by bleeding into the anterior chamber. This may come from the incision into the eye or from the iridectomy. Blood usually clots quite quickly in the anterior chamber. A few tiny blood clots on the surface of the iris do not matter. However if they obscure the view of the lens they should be removed. This is best done with a cellulose sponge or with gentle irrigation using balanced salt solution or normal saline. All is now ready to remove the lens.

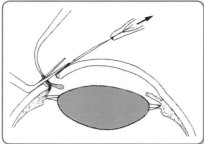

Figure 6.62 Performing the iridectomy

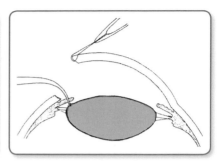

Figure 6.63 Damage to the lens capsule from the iris forcep

The extraction of the lens

First check the eye is suitable to proceed with an intracapsular extraction. For this there should be no evidence of pressure on the open eye. The lens should be resting, without forward pressure, slightly behind and clear of the cornea. If the lens is coming forwards and pressing against the cornea, and especially if the wound is gaping a little or there is a small horizontal fold across the centre of the cornea (**Figure 6.35**), it is likely that something is pressing on the open eye. Therefore the vitreous is likely to prolapse out of the eye when the lens has been removed.

The causes of pressure on the eye and how to manage it have already been described on page 127–8. The assistant should lift up the speculum and if there is still pressure on the open eye despite lifting up the speculum, it is best to change plans from an intracapsular to an extracapsular cataract extraction. If you are satisfied that you can proceed with an intracapsular extraction, then lift the edge of the cornea to check that the incision is both complete and big enough to allow the lens to be removed.

Methods of intracapsular extraction

There are several different instruments used for intracapsular extraction. Three of these will be described here: the cryoprobe, capsule forceps and the lens loop (sometimes called the "Vectis" loop). The cryoprobe is considered the best method, but in case a cryoprobe is not available or not functioning, the other methods will be described.

The cryoprobe

This is a small probe which can be cooled so that it forms an ice-ball at its tip which adheres to whatever the tip of the probe is touching. If it is in contact with the lens it will adhere to it and so it can be lifted out of the eye. The most sophisticated cryoprobes work off nitrous oxide or carbon dioxide gas. The gas is released under some pressure through a very fine jet at the probe tip and this cools the temperature of the tip down to -50 C. This then forms an adherent ice-ball in the tissues on which it is resting (**Figure 6.64**). The main

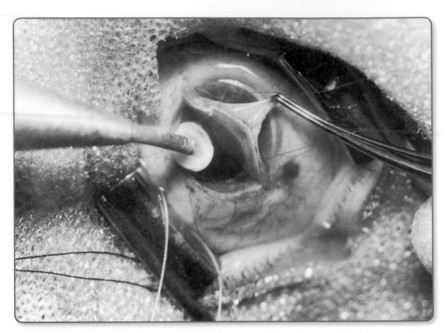

Figure 6.64 A photograph of cryo-extraction of the lens with a carbon dioxide probe

disadvantage of the cryoprobe is that it will stick very firmly to whatever it touches. It can cause serious intraocular damage if it sticks to the iris or the endothelial cells lining the inside of the cornea. Most cryoprobes therefore have a rewarming circuit so that the tip can be rapidly rewarmed to melt the ice-ball if it is sticking to the wrong tissue. The greatest advantage of this type of cryoprobe which gets very cold is that the ice-ball forms inside the lens capsule in the substance of the lens and so sticks to it very firmly and securely. The disadvantages are that the machine is expensive and the probe is difficult to sterilise. The recommended method of sterilisation is a formalin cupboard or careful autoclaving. The probe can be disinfected by immersing the tip in methylated spirits, acetone or a similar disinfecting solution which will evaporate. Unfortunately these fluids do not kill all micro-organisms and the cryoprobe tip must be thoroughly rinsed before use inside the eye.

A more simple cryoprobe is formed by a plastic cylinder with a silver rod at it tip (**Figures 6.65, 6.68** and **6.69**). Freon gas from a small pressurised container is injected under pressure into the cylinder and the gas liquefies. This liquid rapidly evaporates and as it does so becomes cold. The plastic cylinder is held with the tip down, so that the low temperature of the boiling freon is transmitted along the silver rod and forms an ice-ball at its tip. The sides of the silver rod are insulated with plastic so that only the tip gets cold. This type of cryoprobe is cheap and easily portable and can be boiled or carefully autoclaved, but has some disadvantages. It does not get as cold as a cryoprobe which works off carbon dioxide or nitrous oxide gas, and so the ice-ball is not as adherent. There is no rewarming apparatus, so if the probe sticks to the iris or cornea, the only way of separating it is to irrigate the eye with balanced salt solution or normal saline to melt the ice-ball.

Capsule forceps

Capsule forceps (**Figures 6.66** and **6.71–6.74**) are delicate forceps with smooth rounded cups which can grasp the lens capsule. In this way the lens can be pulled out of the eye. There are 2 different methods of doing this. The lens may be grasped at its lower end and somersaulted or "tumbled" out of the eye. Alternatively the lens may be grasped at its upper pole and lifted or "slid" out of the eye. The sliding technique is generally considered easier to learn than the tumbling one so will be described.

There are several disadvantages of capsule forceps:

- The grip on the lens capsule is a delicate one, so the capsule can easily tear. Some capsules are relatively tough while others are very fragile.
- If the cataract is intumescent the lens capsule is swollen and tense, and it is then very difficult or impossible to grasp the lens capsule with forceps at all.
- Because forceps do not grip the lens as securely as a cryoprobe, the lens has to be pushed out of the eye with the help of the lens expressor as well as being pulled by the capsule forceps. This increases the risk of vitreous loss.
- The technique of extraction with capsule forceps is harder to learn than the cryoprobe.

For all these reasons the use of capsule forceps has declined since the introduction of cryoprobes. However capsule forceps have certain advantages. They can be easily and effectively sterilised. They are not expensive, do not require expendable gases, nor is there any equipment that can go wrong at the vital moment. Also the part played by the assistant is not so critical. It is however very important that the forceps are in good condition. The ends should meet along their length and they must not be damaged. Damaged forceps are more likely to rupture the capsule.

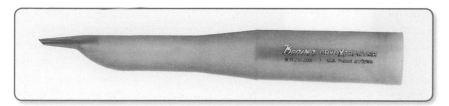

Figure 6.65 A hand held cryoprobe which uses freon gas

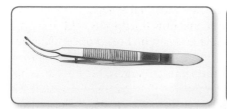 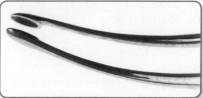

Figure 6.66 Capsule forceps for intracapsular extraction

The lens loop (Figures 6.67 and 6.75–6.79)

This is a small metal loop, which is used to "tumble" or somersault the lens out of the eye. It can also be used to scoop out the lens if it has dislocated downwards into the vitreous.

The expressor (Fiugres 6.67)

With all three methods of extraction a lens expressor is held in the other hand, and placed near the lower limbus. In this way the lens is both "pushed" and "pulled" out of the eye at the same time. Careful use of the expressor is absolutely essential when using the forceps or the loop to extract the lens. It is not so essential with the cryoprobe.

Alpha-chymotrypsin

Alpha-chymotrypsin (Zonulysin) is an enzyme which dissolves the suspensory ligament of the lens. It does not seem to harm any of the other intra-ocular structures but it may cause a slight rise in intraocular pressure for 1–2 days post operatively. It is irrigated into the eye under the iris usually with a lacrimal cannula placed in the iridectomy. Only about 0.5 cc of appropriate solution is required. After about 3 minutes the suspensory ligament of the lens should be dissolved. Some people like to irrigate the eye with balanced salt solution or saline after the chymotrypsin has worked, but many surgeons think this is unnecessary. Alphachymotrypsin makes intracapsular cataract extraction easier by dissolving the suspensory ligament so that the lens can just be lifted out of the eye. It is not essential. It is especially helpful for an inexperienced surgeon using forceps, or in a middle-aged patient whose suspensory ligament may be quite tough. There is much less of a commercial market for it now because intracapsular extraction is so rarely performed in the Western world, and it is not so easy to obtain.

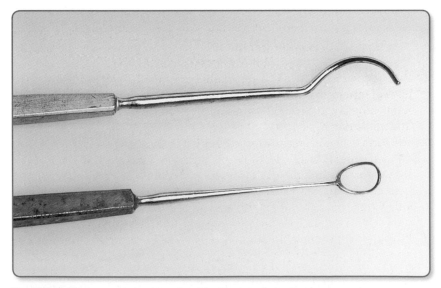

Figure 6.67 The lens expressor (above) and the lens loop (below)

The general principles of intracapsular extraction

The aim of the operation is to remove the entire lens intact in its capsule from the eye. Obviously the suspensory ligament of the lens must either be broken mechanically or dissolved with alpha-chymotrypsin. Using the cryoprobe or capsule forceps, there are three manoeuvres which will help to break the supensory ligament:

1. Pulling on the lens with the cryoprobe or the capsule forceps. The main complication of excess pulling is that the lens capsule may rupture before the suspensory ligament does.
2. Pushing the lens out of the eye with the lens expressor. The main complication of excess pushing is that the suspensory ligament will break and the vitreous will be pushed out of the eye rather than the lens.
3. Rotating the lens. This provides a shearing force on the suspensory ligament and in this way helps to rupture it.

Using the capsule forceps, it is usually necessary to carry out all three manoeuvres at the same time, pulling, pushing and rotating. Using the cryoprobe a much firmer grip on the lens is achieved. Therefore the lens can be pulled from the eye with much less rotation or pushing.

If alpha-chymotryspin is used, the suspensory ligament is weakened to such a degree that the lens can be simply lifted from the eye with minimal pulling and little or no pushing or rotation. The main disadvantage of alpha-chymotrypsin is the risk of chemical or bacterial contamination when it is injected into the eye. It is also quite expensive, and may not be easily available now that intracapsular extraction is not performed in the developed world.

For an intracapsular extraction using the lens loop, the principle is slightly different, because the lens is "tumbled" or somersaulted out of the eye so that the lower pole of the lens comes out first.

The technique of intracapsular extraction using the cryoprobe

1. The assistant must lift the edge of the cornea preferably by gentle traction on the pre-placed suture at 12 o'clock (**Figures 6.68** and **6.69**). Lifting the cornea the right way is very important. Do not allow the assistant to touch the corneal endothelium with the forceps. Lift up the edge of the cornea enough to insert the cyroprobe into the eye without it touching the back of the cornea or iris. The cornea must only be lifted and not folded right over.
2. The surface of the lens must next be dried by mopping away any aqueous from it. If it is wet the ice-ball will not form easily at the tip of the cryoprobe, and instead it will spread to the iris and cornea causing damage. The aqueous is mopped away using small cellulose sponges which also should not touch the back of the cornea. If the assistant has a spare hand he can carry out this drying, but if his other hand is holding the speculum to stop any pressure on the eye, then the surgeon himself will have to dry the eye. If the pupil has contracted down a little or a peripheral iridectomy has been done, it may be necessary to retract the iris in order to make enough room to apply the cryoprobe to

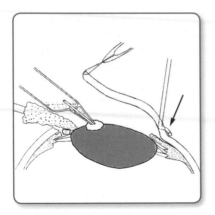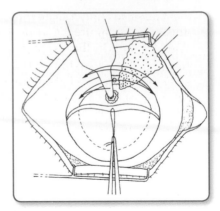

Figure 6.68 and 6.69 Intracapsular extraction with a freon gas cryoprobe. The assistant is retracting the cornea

the surface of the lens. This can be done by retracting the iris at the 12 o'clock position with the same small cellulose sponge or using a metal iris retractor. If a full iridectomy has been done or the pupil is well dilated there is no need for iris retraction.

3. Now rest the cryoprobe on the surface of the lens half-way between its centre and upper equator (**Figure 6.68**), and wait for a few seconds so that it is frozen not just to the surface of the lens, but also causes an ice-ball to form inside the lens. This will happen very quickly with a cryoprobe that runs off carbon dioxide or nitrous oxide. It may take 10 seconds or more with a cryoprobe which uses freon gas.

4. Sometimes it is easier to apply the cryoprobe to the cataract if a lens expressor is placed at the lower limbus and pressed very gently on the eye (**Figure 6.68**). This presses the lower pole of the lens back and so pushes the upper pole of the lens forward. This makes it easier to apply the cryoprobe and to get it to stick to the lens. However the surgeon may not have a spare hand free to use a lens expressor in this way. Pressure with a lens expressor is not often needed to help extract the lens when a sophisticated cryoprobe is used, because the cryoprobe gets such a good grip of the lens. The small cryoprobe which uses freon gas does not become so cold and so does not adhere so well to the lens. Therefore some expression of the lens is often required as well.
   Note:
   i.   the position of the sponge swab to retract the iris as well as drying the lens.
   ii. the use of the expressor at the lower limbus in **Figure 6.68** to tilt the upper part of the lens forward.
   iii. rocking the cryoprobe from side to side to help rupture the suspensory ligament (zonules).

5. Once the cryoprobe has adhered firmly to the lens, start lifting it very gently out through the wound, while at the same time rocking it from

side to side to apply a slight rotational force to the lens (**Figure 6.69**). This helps to rupture the suspensory ligament. As the upper pole is lifted forwards by the cryoprobe, the iris retractor or cellulose sponge being used to retract the iris can be removed. The lens should peel away from the suspensory ligament and can be lifted completely out of the eye. If the suspensory ligament is particularly tough or if a cryoprobe using freon gas is being used, then gentle pressure at the lower limbus with the lens expressor may help to extract the lens.

6. As soon as the lens starts coming out of the eye and the tip of the cryoprobe is clear of the wound, the assistant should release the traction which is holding open the corneal edge of the wound.

The most common complication of cryo-extraction is that the probe adheres to the iris or the back of the cornea (**Figure 6.70**). If this happens the probe should be rewarmed as quickly as possible if it has a re-warming device, if not the eye must be irrigated with balanced salt solution or saline to melt the ice-ball. The lens should then be dried and the cryoprobe reapplied in the correct position.

The other two possible complications of extraction with a cryoprobe are capsule rupture described on page 164 and loss of vitreous described on page 129–131.

The technique of intracapsular extraction with the capsule forceps

This requires a more delicate touch from the surgeon, especially if alpha-chymotrypsin is not being used. However there is less need of skilled assistance because it is not necessary to dry the eye, and the forceps are less likely to damage the cornea or the iris. Indeed it is possible to do a forceps lens extraction without any assistance at all. There are 3 secrets to success when using capsule forceps and the sliding method:

*   The lens capsule must be grasped correctly. This should be done with the forceps "side on" or transversely rather than "end on" or vertically (**Figure 6.71**). The forceps should take a large bite of lens capsule rather than a small one, and the lens should be grasped as near to the equator as possible rather than at the anterior pole where the capsule is thinner (**Figure 6.72**).

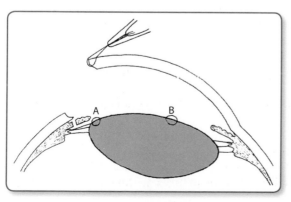

Figure 6.70 Wrong positions to apply the cryoprobe, at "A" it is likely to stick to the iris, at "B" it is likely to stick to the back of the cornea. Compare with Figure 6. 68

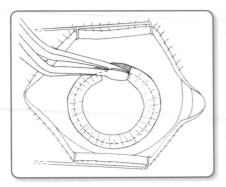

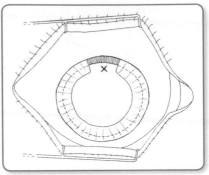

Figure 6.71 The correct way to apply the capsule forceps.Try to take a large "bite" of capsule

Figure 6.72 Applying a rotation movement to the lens with capsule forceps

- For a successful forceps extraction there must be a balance between pulling the lens out of the eye with the forceps and pushing the lens out of the eye with the expressor. If it is all "pulling" and no "pushing" the capsule is likely to rupture. On the other hand if there is excessive pushing then the vitreous may prolapse before the lens.
- Applying a rotatory force to the lens helps to rupture the suspensory ligament (**Figure 6.73**).This may be more effective than trying to pull or push the lens out of the eye.

If alpha chymotrypsin has been used the lens can be virtually lifted out of the eye with only very slight rotation and expression.

A right-handed surgeon usually prefers to hold the capsule forceps in his right hand and the lens expressor in his left, but some people prefer the other way round.

1. The assistant should first lift the edge of the cornea a little.
2. The surgeon should then press gently at the lower limbus with the lens expressor. This will push the lower part of the lens slightly backward and so tilt the upper part of the lens slightly forward (**Figure 6.74**).

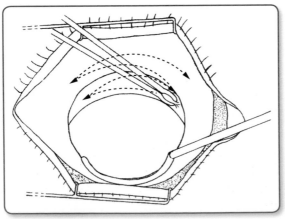

Figure 6.73 Applying a rotation movement to the lens with capsule forceps.

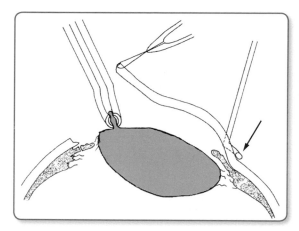

Figure 6.74 Pressure with the expressor at the lower limbus tilts the lower pole of the lens backwards and the upper pole of the lens forwards. This helps the capsule forceps to grasp the lens more securely

3. The forceps should now be applied at the top of the lens near the equator. A broad iridectomy or a very well dilated pupil both help to get a good grasp of the lens in the correct place. It is quite a common mistake to catch the iris as well as the lens capsule in the forceps especially if the pupil is not very well dilated. The surgeon must make sure he has a good view of exactly what the forceps is grasping. The assistant can help by retracting the iris with a small cellulose sponge. Once a good grip has been secured the forceps should be rotated first towards the 10 o'clock position and then towards the 2 o'clock position (**Figure 6.73**). The gentle pressure should be maintained all the time at the lower limbus of the eye with the lens expressor. Some people like to keep the pressure point on the lower limbus exactly opposite the forceps so that when the forceps are rotated to 10 o'clock the tip of the expressor is at 4 o'clock. When the forceps are rotated to 2 o'clock the expressor is at 8 o'clock.

4. As the suspensory ligament begins to rupture, the lens can be lifted very slowly out of the eye. All the time the capsule forceps should be slowly rotated from the 2 o'clock position to the 10 o'clock position and back again. Gentle pressure should be maintained on the lower limbus with the lens expressor.

Some surgeons use even more rotation to break the suspensory ligament. Using this technique the capsule forceps are applied at the 2 o'clock position rather than at the 12 o'clock position and they are then rotated to the 10 o'clock position. Whilst maintaining very gentle pressure with the lens expressor, the forceps are opened to let go of the lens which is grasped again at 2 o'clock and rotated once more to 10 o'clock. In this way the lens is "wheeled" out of the eye.

The technique of intracapsular extraction with the lens loop

When using the lens loop much firmer pressure must be applied with the lens expressor. Instead of being placed at the lower limbus it is placed about 3 mm below the lower limbus.

For intumescent cataracts The lens loop can be used for intracapsular extraction of intumescent cataracts if a cryoprobe is not available. (Obviously capsule forceps will not grip the capsule of an intumescent cataract.) The technique is as follows:

1. Place the lens loop on the posterior scleral lip of the incision and press very gently back in to the eye (**Figure 6.75**). This has two effects: it slightly opens up the lip of the wound. It also presses back the upper pole of the lens. Now rest the lens expressor 3 mm below the lower limbus (not at the limbus) and apply gentle pressure and massage to it. This pressure which is behind the lens will tend to push the lower pole of the lens forwards.

An intumescent cataract contains fluid and so the shape of the lens will be moulded by this pressure. The lower (inferior) fibres of the suspensory ligament will be stretched and will rupture, and the lens will "somersault" or "tumble" out of the eye (**Figure 6.76**).

If an extraction with the lens loop is planned the iridectomy should not be done until after the lens has been extracted. For this technique it is vital that the lower (inferior) fibres of the suspensory ligament rupture before the upper (superior) fibres so that the lens somersaults out of the eye. An intact iris helps to keep the upper pole of the lens and the upper fibres of the suspensory ligament intact.

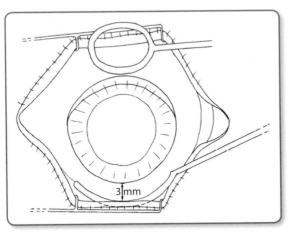

Figure 6.75 To show the position of the lens loop and the lens expressor for expressing an intumescent cataract

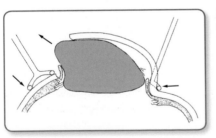

Figure 6.76 Gentle pressure with the lens loop and pressure and massage with the expressor

For other cataracts This same technique of using the lens loop and the expressor to "somersault" the lens out of the eye can be used for intracapsular extraction of any cataract and not just an intumescent cataract. However solid cataracts will not mould as easily as intumescent ones, so the lower fibres of the suspensory ligament will not be stretched or ruptured so easily. The lens expressor is placed in just the same place, but the lens loop must be placed actually in the eye and pressing down on the upper pole of the lens (**Figures 6.77** and **6.78**). Quite a lot of pressure may be necessary and the suspensory ligament may suddenly rupture causing vitreous loss or dislocation of the lens backwards into the vitreous. With skill and training it can become a very effective technique where only basic facilities are available.

For a dislocated lens If the lens has dislocated into the vitreous, the loop is used to get right under the lens so that it can be scooped out of the eye (**Figure 6.79**). Inevitably some vitreous will be lost. Sometimes the lens is only partially dislocated or sub-luxated. This means that some but not all of the suspensory ligament fibres have ruptured. Always insert the loop where the fibres of the suspensory ligament have ruptured and make sure that the loop gets right under the lens before scooping it out of the eye. With a partially dislocated lens a cryo-extraction is a possible alternative to the loop.

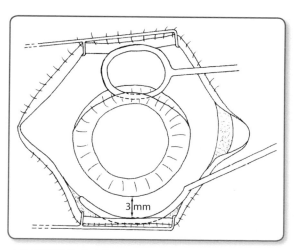

Figure 6.77 and 6.78 To show the position of the lens loop and lens expressor for expressing a solid cataract. Note that the lens loop is actually inside the eye and is in a different position from Figures 6.75 and 6.76

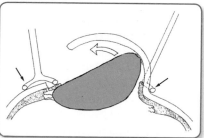

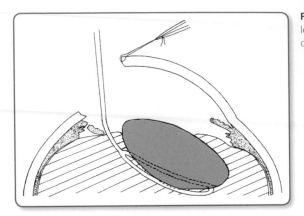

Figure 6.79 The use of the lens loop for a subluxated or dislocated lens

Complications of intracapsular extraction

The two main complications of intracapsular extraction are rupture of the lens capsule and vitreous loss.

Rupture of the lens capsule

This is more common using capsule forceps than the cryoprobe, because the cryoprobe gets a much better grip on the lens. Capsule rupture may occur for several reasons:

- The lens capsule is sometimes very weak.
- The capsule forceps may be applied incorrectly or may be in poor condition.
- The surgeon may try to pull the lens from the eye before the suspensory ligament has ruptured.
- If using a cryoprobe, it usually occurs because the probe has only frozen to the capsule and not formed an ice-ball inside the lens.
- If the incision is too small, there may not be enough room for the intact lens to be removed from the eye.

If the capsule rupture is small, it may be possible to reapply the cryoprobe or the capsule forceps and to get another grip of the lens so that an intracapsular extraction can be completed. However, often this is not possible because the rupture is too large.

If the capsule breaks when the suspensory ligament is still intact, the best way to proceed is as follows:

1. Express the nucleus of the lens from the eye in the same way as for an extracapsular extraction (see page 121–4).
2. The surgeon may then choose to convert to an extracapsular cataract extraction by irrigating and aspirating the remaining cortical lens material from the eye, and just leaving the posterior capsule intact.
3. Alternatively the intracapsular extraction may be completed by removing the rest of the capsule and cortical lens remnants. The assistant should lift the corneal flap to allow a good view of the anterior chamber. Then grasp the edge of the ruptured capsule with capsule forceps and gently pull the capsule containing the remaining pieces of lens cortex out of the eye (**Figure 6.80**). It is best to do this with a capsule forceps in each

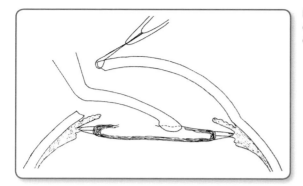

Figure 6.80 The use of the capsule forceps to remove capsule remnants

hand. Use the first capsule forceps to grasp the edge of the ruptured capsule, and then the other capsule forceps to get a more secure grip of the capsule. In this way the ruptured capsule containing cortical lens remnants can be very gradually pulled out of the eye "hand over hand". Occasionally the capsule ruptures after the suspensory ligament has been broken, and then the surgeon is faced with a difficult situation as to how best to remove the lens. If the lens is almost out of the eye it may be possible to express the lens nucleus from the eye and then using the capsule forceps pick out of the eye any fragments of capsule and lens cortex that remain. If both the capsule and the suspensory ligament have ruptured and the lens is still in the eye do not try to express the lens or the nucleus. Almost certainly vitreous will come out through the wound and the lens or its nucleus may well be pushed down deeply into the vitreous. If any lens matter ends up deep in the vitreous it will set up a chronic and persistent inflammatory reaction in the eye. Instead use the lens loop, identify where the suspensory ligament has broken and place the lens loop through the gap in the ligament so that it lies behind the lens. Then scoop the lens out of the eye.

Vitreous loss

There are usually two reasons for vitreous loss during intracapsular extraction:

- From some external pressure on the eye (page 127–9). Either the assistant should have lifted the speculum to overcome this pressure or the surgeon should have planned an extracapsular and not an intracapsular extraction.
- From too much pressure on the lens expressor by the surgeon during the extraction, which pushes the vitreous out of the eye.

The management of vitreous loss has already been described on page 129–31.

Insertion of anterior chamber intraocular lenses

When inserting an anterior chamber intraocular lens the haptics need to be the right size (diameter), as well as the optic power of the lens being correct. The standard lens is designed so that it has a four point contact in angle of the anterior chamber between the back of the cornea and the front of the iris (see **Figure 6.8**, page 95). If the size is too small the lens will move in the anterior chamber. This will cause chronic uveitis and in particular it will damage the endothelial cells of the cornea causing corneal oedema. If the size of the haptics is too large, they will cause pressure in the anterior chamber angle and this causes persistent tenderness and pain in the eye. The normal way of sizing the intraocular lens is to measure the horizontal corneal diameter (white sclera to white sclera) and add 1 mm to give the correct size (diameter) for the haptics. Recently an anterior chamber lens has been introduced with three point contact in the angle which is more flexible so that there is only one size of haptic. It has two point contact inferiorly and only one superiorly. The anterior chamber depth must be maintained with either viscoelastic fluid, air or irrigating fluid. When using air or irrigating fluid, it is very helpful to partly close the incision with two interrupted sutures leaving a gap of 7mm through which to insert the intraocular lens.

Inserting an IOL in the anterior chamber is made much easier if a small sheet of plastic called a "lens glide" is first inserted into the anterior chamber right down to the bottom of the anterior chamber angle between the iris and the cornea (**Figure 6.81**). The intraocular lens can then slide down the front surface of the lens glide, so that the lower haptics of the lens rest nicely in the lower part of the anterior chamber angle. Without a lens glide, the lower haptics may catch against the lower iris rather than sliding into the anterior chamber angle. Once the lower haptics are well placed in the angle, the lens glide is removed and the superior haptics are tucked under the scleral lip of the incision so as to lie in the upper part of the anterior chamber angle. At this stage the pupil should be round and central, confirming that the

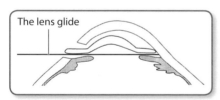

The lens glide

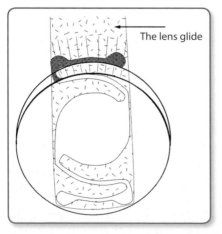

The lens glide

Figure 6.81 Inserting an anterior chamber intraocular lens. To show the position of the lens glide and how the IOL slides on the surface of it

haptics of the lens have not got caught in the iris. Care must be taken that the intraocular lens does not touch the eyelashes or skin and so become contaminated with skin bacteria, and also that it does not touch the posterior surface of the cornea and cause damage to the corneal endothelium. It is often quite difficult to prevent the haptics from catching on the iris and so causing a distorted pupil, especially if the anterior chamber is shallow. Many surgeons like to constrict the pupil at this stage with pilocarpine or acetyl choline (Miochol), because it makes the insertion of the IOL easier. Any drop used when the eye is open must be sterile and non toxic to the corneal endothelium, and free of preservatives. The use of these miotic drops is not essential. When using an anterior chamber lens the surgeon must check that the iridectomy or iridotomy is patent.

Wound closure

Once the lens is in place then the wound can be sutured. The preplaced sutures should now be tied, unless this has already happened.

Usually a total of five interrupted sutures is enough to secure the wound. Wound closure has already been described on pages 42–29. If viscoelastic fluids have been used, they should be washed out of the eye once the wound has been closed.

Post-operative care

The routine post-operative care for all different types of cataract surgery is essentially the same. Modern cataract surgery is both safe and effective. Serious post operative complications are not common but may occur even with the very best of care. Different surgeons have different ideas about post operative care and management, and the care that is given will depend upon the circumstances and treatments available. Therefore basic principles will be discussed here rather than rigid rules.

Routine post operative examination of the eye

The eye must be examined from time to time to make sure that there are no complications. Ideally it should be examined on the first and second post-operative days, then after one week and finally about one month after the operation. However all this may not be possible.

It is important to check the visual acuity post-operatively, with and without pinhole; and to record this along with any reasons for a 'poor outcomce'. See Table 2.1 on page 17.

Mobilising the patient

Early mobilisation is probably the biggest change in recent years in the post operative care of eye patients. Some years ago patients were kept in bed and carefully rested after an eye operation. Nowadays most patients are mobilised immediately after the operation, which can be done as an out patient. The main reason for this change is improved suture techniques. The wound is now closed securely so it is no longer necessary to immobilise the patient's head and eye waiting for the wound to heal. Early mobilisation has many advantages. It lessens the risk of post operative venous thrombosis, urinary retention, chest infection and constipation. It is much more pleasant for the patients themselves, they can be discharged from hospital sooner, and nursing care is easier. Indeed many surgeons are quite happy to operate on patients as outpatients and allow them to walk off the operating table and go straight home. This may not be practical in rural situations or where the patient's understanding is poor.

Protecting the eye

Although the wound is closed securely, the eye must still be protected from the patient rubbing it or from something or someone else knocking or hitting it. It is therefore routine practice to apply a shield to the eye immediately after the operation. Applying a sterile pad also helps the corneal and conjunctival epithelium to heal by preventing movements of the eyelid against the eye. The pad also keeps flies off the eye.

The main disadvantage of a pad is that bacteria multiply more rapidly in the conjunctival sac when the eye is padded. Most surgeons would not keep the eye padded for more than one, or at most two days post operatively. If some protection is still required this can be given by placing a shield across the eye but leaving it unpadded.

Prevention of infection

Post operative infection in the eye is a disaster. Sometimes with prompt and energetic treatment some or all the sight may be saved, but frequently the eye is lost. *The only way to avoid post operative infections is by keeping strictly to the rules of good theatre procedures and by good surgical technique. Nearly all infections enter the eye at the time of surgery*. Hygiene and cleanliness in the post operative environment is much less important. Giving lots of antibiotics pre-and post operatively is no way to cover up for bad theatre procedures or surgical techniques. They do not usually prevent post operative infections in any case. In spite of this fact nearly all surgeons do use topical antibiotics routinely after intraocular operations.

Antibiotic ointment is applied at the end of the operation, and then either drops or ointment are given 2 or 3 times a day for another 2 to 4 weeks post operatively. Chloramphenicol is the most widely used topical antibiotic but others such Neomycin, Gentamicin or Tetracycline may be used.

If there is any concern about contamination of the eye during the operation, then the best way of preventing post operative infection is to give a subconjunctival antibiotic injection at the end of the operation. Subconjunctival antibiotics give a high level of antibiotic in the aqueous and conjunctiva for about 24 hours and are more effective than systemic antibiotics. The most popular subconjunctival antibiotics are Cefuroxime 100 mg or Gentamicin 20 mg (If there is a very severe risk of contamination it may be appropriate to inject both antibiotics at different sites, but do not give Cefuroxime to patients with penicillin allergy.) Most surgeons routinely give subconjunctival antibiotics post operatively to every case.

Some surgeons recommend adding antibiotic to the infusion bottle during extra capsular extraction, however the benefit of this is uncertain and there is a great risk of damaging the eye if the wrong concentration is given.

Intracameral cefuroxime

There is good evidence that an injection into the anterior chamber (an intra-cameral injection) of Cefuroxime antibiotic is an excellent way of preventing endophthalmitis. If you have Cefuroxime available then this is a good choice, however it is of **critical importance that the correct dose is injected.** *An incorrect dose or conentration can damage the corneal endothelium and lead to vision loss.*

Cefuroxime – for intra-cameral injection[9]

Dilution to 1mg in 0.1ml solution
Items needed:
- Cefuroxime powder 750mg vial
- 1ml syringe (insulin syringe)
- 10ml syringe
- 20ml syringe
- Sterile 'water for injection' 30ml vial

In sterile conditions (using sterile syringes, tray, and gloves):
1. Draw 15ml sterile water for injection into a 20ml syringe
2. Inject the 15ml of water for injection into a 750mg vial of Cefuroxime (= 50mg per ml)
3. Shake Cefuroxime vial with water in it
4. Draw 2ml from Cefuroxime solution into a 10ml syringe
5. Add a further 8ml of 'water for injection' into 10ml syringe, making a total of 10ml. (= 10mg per ml; or 1mg per 0.1ml)
6. Finally draw 0.1ml from the 10ml syringe into a 1ml syringe; ready for use
7. Repeat step 6 for each patient on the operating list for that day

Suppressing inflammation in the eye

There is always some inflammation in the eye after an intraocular operation. In particular this inflammation will occur in the iris and ciliary body which are the most vascular structures in the eye, causing an irido-cyclitis. There will also be some inflammation in and around the wound at the corneo-scleral junction. This inflammation will be slight if the eye is otherwise healthy and the operation has been performed neatly and with minimal intraocular manipulation. Poor surgical technique or excessive intraocular manipulation will obviously increase the severity of iridocyclitis.

Iridocyclitis is more common after extracapsular than intracapsular extraction. Firstly, there is more manipulation inside the eye, and secondly, any lens cortex left in the eye will slowly dissolve in the aqueous causing an inflammatory reaction. The use of intraocular lenses will also cause some inflammation in the eye, although with good technique and a good quality lens this should only be slight. The Afro-Caribbean eye may be more susceptible to post-operative inflammation.

The standard way to reduce inflammation in the eye is to use mydriatics and corticosteroids.

Mydriatics As modern surgical techniques are improving, many surgeons no longer routinely use mydriatics postoperatively. However if there is significant inflammation, mydriatics should be given post operatively for a few days. Mydriatics paralyse the iris sphincter muscle and the ciliary muscle. In this way the inflammation in the iris and ciliary body is suppressed and the pupil is kept dilated. This also lessens the risk of adhesions developing between the pupil margin and the IOL or the posterior lens capsule in an extracapsular extraction, or the anterior vitreous face in an intra capsular extraction.

Atropine 1% drops or ointment given daily is the most effective mydriatic. Occasionally it causes an allergic reaction, or it can be absorbed and cause a dry mouth, tachycardia and even mental confusion in elderly patients. Homatropine, Tropicamide and Cyclopentolate 1% are alternative mydriatics which have fewer side-effects, but are less powerful and should be given twice daily.

Corticosteroids Corticosteroids are the standard drug used to suppress post-operative inflammation, and most surgeons use them routinely after any intraocular operation. They can be given as drops, ointments or by subconjunctival injection. They suppress iridocyclitis and also suppress inflammatory reaction in the wound, cornea and conjunctiva caused by surgical trauma. There are many different steroid preparations; Hydrocortisone (the weakest), Prednisolone, Betamethasone or Dexamethasone (the strongest). Topical steroids are often combined with an antibiotic so that the 2 medications can be given at the same time. In an uncomplicated case it is usual to give steroid drops or ointment 3 times a day for about a month post operatively. If there is severe inflammation the drops or ointment should be given more frequently (up to every hour) and for longer.

A subconjunctival injection will deliver high levels of drug to the eye, and most surgeons routinely give a subconjunctival steroid injection (about 10 mg of prednisolone) following extracapsular extraction and especially with a lens implant. This is usually given together with the sub-conjunctival antibiotic.

Complications of steroid use

Steroids are very effective drugs but they may cause side-effects in the eye. They can also cause systemic side-effects, but the dose given topically to the eye is too small for this. The local side-effects in the eye are:

- *Delay in wound healing.* Steroids suppress the inflammatory reaction of the body to injury, so wound healing is delayed. In practice if the wound has been carefully sutured this does not create any significant problems.
- *Increased risk of infection.* Steroids suppress the reactions of the immune system to infection. There is an increased risk of post operative infection occurring in an eye if steroids are used. Such post operative infections are fortunately rare. If the organism is a virulent one the infection is so severe that stopping local steroids will not make much difference (see page 176). However much less virulent organisms which are usually only slightly pathogenic, for example fungi or commensal skin bacteria, may enter the eye. The steroids may encourage the growth of these organisms by suppressing the natural defences of the body, and so produce a chronic but mild

endophthalmitis. These infections are also rare but they are difficult to both diagnose and treat. It may be necessary to identify the organism by taking a culture of the vitreous.

- *Steroid-induced glaucoma.* In a few patients steroids can cause the intraocular pressure to rise. Exactly why this happens is not understood. However if a steroid sensitive patient is given prolonged local steroid treatment, loss of vision from steroid-induced glaucoma can occur. There is neither pain nor discomfort and the patients may not be aware that their vision is gradually fading. Usually steroids are only given for a few weeks post operatively and so steroid induced glaucoma is not a significant problem. However the intraocular pressure should be checked routinely before final discharge at one month.
- *Steroid-induced cataract.* Excessive and prolonged use of topical steroids can also cause cataract. This obviously does not matter after cataract extraction, but it can be important after other intraocular operations which do not involve removal of the lens.

Many surgeons use a combination (antibiotic and steroid in the same bottle) eye drop for patients post-operatively. This is often easier for the patient who would then have only one rather than a number of different bottles of eye drops to use.

Prescribing spectacles

- The great majority of patients after lens implants should not need glasses except perhaps for driving or reading small print.
- It is best to wait for 4-6 weeks before giving glasses as the curvature of the cornea may alter a little as the wound heals.
- If the wound has been sutured too tightly there will be astigmatism with the plus axis at 90º. This can be corrected by removing tight sutures about three months post operatively.
- If the sutures are too loose there will be astigmatism with the plus axis at 180º. Either the patient must accept this or the wound must be resutured
- If the patient has not had a lens implant (i.e they are aphakic and not pseudoaphakic) a strong level of about +10 diopters will be required. However this should not be prescribed if the sight in the other eye is still good

Instructions to the patient

It always helps if the patient and their attendant understand the importance of postoperative treatment and exactly how to apply drops or ointment to the eye. Compliance is the word used to describe whether the patient takes the treatment correctly. Compliance is always much better if the nursing staff spend a little time helping the patient and the attendant to apply medication correctly.

Post operative complications

Post operative complications can be divided into two groups:
1. Early complications presenting during the first few days after the operation.

2. Late complications presenting at least a month or even years after the operation.

Serious complications should be rare, but anyone responsible for the care of eye patients should know how to recognise and treat them. Most early complications can be seen with a good light and magnifying spectacles, a slit lamp is helpful but not essential. For delayed complications which involve the retina, ophthalmoscopic examination is also needed. The table on page 189 lists what to look for at a post operative eye examination and what each abnormal finding might signify.

Early complications

Poor wound closure

If the wound is not properly closed 2 possible complications may develop, either a leak of aqueous from the wound or an iris prolapse through the wound.

Aqueous leakage (see plate 3 and 4 and 18–21)

Symptoms and signs

This is usually apparent on the first post operative day. The anterior chamber will be flat or, in less severe cases, very shallow. The iris will appear to be resting up against the cornea or very close to it. A useful way of detecting a small aqueous leak is to apply fluorescein drops to the conjunctiva. The aqueous will be seen diluting the fluorescein dye and so the site of the leak is detected. This is called Seidel's test. If a blue light is used, the leak is much more obvious. A flat anterior chamber due to wound leakage must be distinguished from a flat anterior chamber due to pupil block or malignant glaucoma (see the table on page 188).

Treatment

Unless there is a very obvious gape in the wound, apply a firm pad and bandage for 24 hours and then examine the eye again. In many cases the wound leak will seal off and the anterior chamber will reform. If after a day the anterior chamber is still completely flat then the leak should be identified and the wound re-sutured.

Iris prolapse

Symptoms and signs

This is usually fairly obvious. The pupil will be distorted and the iris will be seen coming out through the wound edge (see plate 5). In mild cases the iris may be trapped or incarcerated in the wound edges but not actually prolapsed out of the eye. The anterior chamber may be flat as well if the aqueous is also leaking out, but the iris tissue may plug the hole so the anterior chamber may be formed.

Treatment

Nearly every case of iris prolapse should be treated surgically. However if a small prolapse of the iris is covered by the conjunctiva this is not absolutely necessary. The wound will eventually heal and the iris will be protected by the conjunctiva. However, if the iris is not covered by conjunctiva, it must be treated surgically.

Early complications
   Poor wound closure
   Aqueous leakage
   Iris prolapse
   Striate keratopathy
   Hyphaema
   Infection
   Iridocyclitis
   Pupil block and malignant glaucoma

Late complications
   Retinal detachment
   Cystoid macular oedema
   Corneal oedema and bullous keratopathy
   Thickening of the posterior lens capsule
   Glaucoma
   Chronic uveitis
   Infection

Post-operative complications can often lead to total or partial loss of sight. Often this can be prevented by the right treatment given promptly. Nearly all the colour plates are to show what these complications look like, so as to help identify the problem.

The aims of surgical treatment for an aqueous leak or an iris prolapse are essentially the same:-to close the wound properly.

Local anaesthetic is sometimes difficult in these cases. Most people do not recommend retrobulbar anaesthesia in the early post operative period. If a retrobulbar haemorrhage occurs it may have disastrous consequences on a recently operated eye. If the patient is co-operative, surface anaesthesia with drops and some local anaesthetic injected into the surrounding conjunctiva will be adequate. A facial block to stop the patient squeezing is helpful. However a full nerve block may be necessary for an unco-operative patient if general anaesthesia is not available. The best way to give this is by a "subTenon's" injection (see page 80). This uses a **blunt** needle and so there is less risk of causing a retrobulbar haemorrhage.

If there is an iris prolapse it can be either excised or replaced in the eye. If seen within 24 hours and in a clean eye replacement is better, but if there is any suspicion of infection excision is safer. The iris will often have stuck to the wound edges and must first be mobilised. This is done by holding the lips of the wound and gently sweeping an iris repositor between the wound edge and the iris. Once mobilised the prolapsed iris can either be excised or replaced.

Excision Grasp the prolapsed iris with forceps and cut it off with de Wecker's scissors flush with the surface of the eye.

Replacement Use an iris repositor to replace the iris gently back into the eye. The aqueous will usually drain from the anterior chamber whilst this is being done. The gap in the corneo-scleral wound should be repaired securely with sutures. It may be helpful if a small flap of conjunctiva is mobilised and used as an extra covering for the wound. Because of the risk of infection it is usual to give a sub-conjunctival antibiotic injection.

Striate keratopathy

This is the name given to the appearance of the cornea post operatively if the endothelial cells have been damaged by physical or chemical injury during the operation. **Figure 6.82** shows some of the different ways this can happen.

Signs and symptoms

Irregular white opaque lines and folds appear in the deeper corneal layers and in Descemet's membrane (see plates 6 and 11). The cornea will appear hazy particularly near the incision. Striate keratopathy is always caused by damage to the corneal endothelial cells and is evidence of excessive trauma to the eye or poor surgical technique.

Treatment

There is no specific treatment, although steroids may help it to clear. Damaged or destroyed endothelial cells do not regenerate but in most cases the

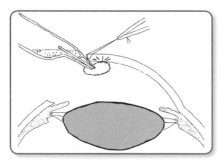

Figure 6.82a Touching it with an instrument. The cryoprobe is particularly dangerous because it can damage the corneal endothelium cells by freezing as well as by touch

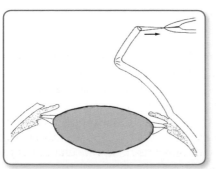

Figure 6.82b Deforming the cornea

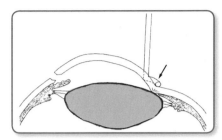

Figure 6.82c Rubbing the lens against the cornea with external pressure

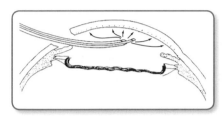

Figure 6.82d Damage from faulty irrigation fluid. This is the most serious damage because it will affect the entire endothelium

undamaged endothelial cells compensate, and after 1–2 weeks the cornea gradually becomes clear. In severe cases striate keratopathy progresses to irreversible corneal oedema (see below, page 185).

Hyphaema

This means blood is present in the anterior chamber (see plates 3, 8 and 11). There may be a small amount of bleeding in the anterior chamber from the wound or the iridectomy at the time of the operation. This blood will be absorbed in a few days and does not usually cause any complications.

Rarely there may be fresh bleeding into the anterior chamber post operatively. This nearly always occurs because of poor wound closure. Delicate capillaries bridge the gap in the wound. If the sutures are not secure and the eye is rubbed or knocked, these fragile blood vessels rupture and bleed into the anterior chamber.

Signs and symptoms

Recent slight bleeding will cause the anterior chamber to appear cloudy. Soon the red blood cells settle with gravity to form a layer of blood (plate 3). In severe hyphaema the whole anterior chamber becomes filled with dark blood so no iris details are visible (plate 8).

Treatment

Hyphaemas will absorb in time and usually no treatment is necessary, but with a total hyphaema, the intraocular pressure may rise. It is then best to milk out the blood clot and reform the anterior chamber with saline or air. Otherwise there is a risk of developing secondary glaucoma, or the cornea becoming stained with blood pigments. It is very difficult to decide when to intervene surgically with a postoperative hyphaema. If there is both a complete hyphaema so the iris cannot be seen and a rise in intraocular pressure then surgery is essential, for most other cases it is best to wait.

Method

Apply local anaesthetic blocks as described for iris prolapse or wound repair. Use an iris repositor to open up a space in the wound between 2 sutures. The thick, treacle-like fluid blood should be massaged or irrigated out of the eye, and visco-elastic fluid may help. It may be necessary to remove a corneo-scleral suture to do this. Do not try with forceps to remove formed solid blood clot which is stuck in the anterior chamber as it will probably make the bleeding start again.

Infection

This is the most serious post operative complication and is known as acute endophthalmitis. The severity of the infection may vary according to the virulence of the organism and the number of infecting micro-organisms. Mild infections may be difficult to recognise and may not appear till some time after the operation, but a severe infection will completely destroy an eye in 24 hours. Most infections will cause blindness if left untreated, and must therefore be treated extremely seriously. Almost always the infection enters the eye at the time of surgery. Any of the pyogenic bacteria can cause endophthalmitis. Staphylococcus, Streptococcus and Pseudomonas are probably the most common species. The bacteria multiply very rapidly in the vitreous and aqueous and their toxins will quickly destroy the delicate intraocular structures. Only very rapid and very specific treatment can save the eye from total destruction and blindness.

In good eye units the incidence of endophthalmitis is about one case in a thousand. If infections are occurring much more frequently than this, the entire surgical arrangements should be carefully examined.

Obviously medical science has tried hard to think of ways of preventing postoperative infection. These include giving antibiotics prophylactically before, during or after the operation in the hopes that this will kill any bacteria.

Preoperative antibiotics are usually given as topical drops or ointment. At the time of operation antibiotics are usually given by sub-conjunctival injection. Both these methods probably help a little. There is not much evidence that giving postoperative antibiotics either topically or systemically makes much difference. Excess use of antibiotics can even be harmful by encouraging resistant bacteria to grow. Antibiotics applied topically can cause allergies and may be toxic to the conjunctiva and cornea. Systemic antibiotics can have all sorts of side effects, both minor and life-threatening.

It cannot be emphasised too much that the only effective way to prevent postoperative infection is reliable sterilisation, excellent surgical technique and careful skin and eyelid preparation.

Signs and symptoms

The signs of infection develop rapidly (see plates 9 and 10). They are sometimes present on the first post operative day and are usually obvious by the second day. Rarely the infecting micro-organisms may be less virulent and then the signs of infection appear very gradually after a week or two. The following are the typical features of an eye with acute endophthalmitis:

1. There is pain, tenderness and often photophobia.
2. The vision is usually affected, and can become very blurred in a matter of hours.
3. The eyelids are often swollen.
4. There is vasodilation of the ciliary vessels around the cornea especially in the area of the incision, and the conjunctiva is often swollen (chemosis).
5. There may be mucopurulent conjunctival secretions/discharges.
6. The cornea is often hazy.
7. The anterior chamber is turbid and cloudy, containing protein exudate and circulating white cells. Later these cells settle with gravity to form a hypopyon.
8. There is sometimes a collection of pus around the incision, or one of the sutures.
9. The intra-ocular pressure may be raised.
10. An afferent pupil defect is a sign of retinal and optic nerve damage and that the vision will not recover to normal.
11. The fundus may be very difficult to visualize, and there may be a poor "red-reflex".
12. There are inflammatory cells in the vitrous.

Treatment

Intensive and urgent antibiotic treatment is necessary to save the eye but even with the most vigorous treatment the eye is often lost.

The antibiotics can be given in 4 different ways:

1. By injection into the vitreous.
2. Systemically.
3. Topically.
4. By sub conjunctival injection.

Intravitreous injection of antibiotics

There is now no doubt that an intravitreous injection of antibiotic is by far the best way of saving an eye with suspected or confirmed endophthalmitis, and it is much more effective than all the other routes. Without an intravitreous antibiotic the eye is very likely to become blind. However the injections **must** be given **exactly** the right way and with **exactly** the right amount and concentration. Even when properly given there is a slight risk of toxicity or damage to the eye, and so they should only be given if there is little doubt that the eye is infected. At the same time as the injection is given, there is an opportunity to remove a very small sample of vitreous for Gram stain and culture to try to identify the bacteria. It usually takes 48 hours to get a result but the injection can be repeated then, and there may then be some bacteriological information to help decide which antibiotic to give if a second injection is necessary.

Choice of antibiotics

It is usual to give *both* an antibiotic which is effective against Gram positive bacteria *and* an antibiotic which is effective against Gram negative bacteria.

Choosing which antibiotics to give may be difficult, and will also depend on what is available locally.

Vancomycin is thought to be the best choice for Gram positive infections. (Teicoplanin or the earlier cephalosporin antibiotics such as Cephazolin or Cefuroxime are alternatives.)

The choice for Gram negative infections is a little more complicated. Until recently the aminoglycoside antibiotics Gentamicin or Amikacin were thought to be the best. However there have been several reports that Gentamicin can be toxic to the retina, and possibly this is true of Amikacin as well. If available, the newer cephalosporin Ceftazidime has a good spectrum of action against Gram negative bacteria. Therefore the choice at present is either *Amikacin* or *Ceftazidime*, but if neither are available, Gentamicin

New forth generation fluoroquinolones such as Moxifloxacin are becoming available for intravitreal, topical, and intra-cameral use in the treatment and prevention of endophthalmitis.

Preparation of the injection

Note that the volume of each injection is 0.1 ml and the antibiotic must be diluted with preservative free normal saline. If possible the dried antibiotic powder or solution should be free of preservative as well. The solution is prepared so that 10 times the amount to be given is dissolved in a one ml syringe. 0.9 ml of this is discarded, leaving just 0.1 ml to be injected.

Here are some examples of how to prepare the injections:

Vancomycin (or Cefuroxime or Cephazolin if Vancomycin is not available) – Dose: 1.0 mg in 0.1 ml. Therefore 10 mg must be prepared in one ml and 9/10 of it discarded.
1. Reconstitute a 500 mg vial with 8 ml of normal saline.
2. Withdraw entire contents and make up to 10 ml with normal saline = 50 mg/ml.
3. Inject 1 ml back into vial and add 4 ml of normal saline = 10 mg/ml.
4. 0.1 ml of this solution = 1.0 mg.

Amikacin – Dose: 0.4 mg in 0.1 ml Therefore 4 mg must be prepared in one ml and 9/10 of it discarded.
1. Take 2.0 ml from a vial of amikacin at 250 mg/ml (contains sodium citrate and bisulphite).
2. Make up to 10 ml with normal saline = 50 mg/ml.
3. Discard 9 ml and make up remaining 1 ml to 12.5 ml with normal saline = 4 mg/ml.
4. 0.1 ml of this solution = 0.4 mg.

Ceftazidime – Dose: 2.0 mg in 0.1ml. Therefore 20 mg must be prepared in one ml and 9/10 of it discarded.
1. Reconstitute a 500 mg vial with 10 ml of saline (beware some vials may contain 250 mg or some 1.0 gm) to make 50 mg /ml and then withdraw entire contents of the vial.

2. Inject 2 ml back into the vial and add 3 ml of normal saline =20 mg/ml.
3. 0.1 ml of this solution=2mg.

Gentamicin (Only give gentamicin if amikacin and ceftazidime are un-available) – Dose: 0.1mg in 0.1ml. Therefore 1.0 mg must be prepared in 1.0 ml and 9/10 discarded.
1. Take 0.5ml from an vial of gentamicin containing 40mg/ml = 20 mg.
2. Make up to 20 ml with normal saline in a syringe = 1.0 mg/ml.
3. 0.1ml of this solution = 0.1mg.
The two injections should be given through the same needle using different syringes.

Technique of intravitreous injection

The smallest and the sharpest needle available should be used. It should be inserted directly into the centre of the vitreous through the pars plana, 4 mm posterior to the limbus in the infero-temporal quadrant. The needle is inserted up to 1 cm into the eye. Alternatively after intracapsular extraction, the needle can be inserted directly through the incision. With these very small amounts for injection, try to avoid having any air making a "dead space" in the base of the needle. It may help to have the bevel of the needle pointing forward, and to inject slowly so that the antibiotics aren't pushed back on to the retina. A small swab soaked in topical anaesthetic drops will help to anaesthetise the area, and a subconjunctival injection of local anaesthetic will also help. Even then the injection will be somewhat painful. Intravitreous injections can be repeated after 48 hours. If laboratory facilities are available, and if the vitreous will come out through a small needle, aspirate 0.2mls of vitreous to send to microbiology in a separate empty small syringe before then injecting the antibiotics.

Identifying the organism

In acute cases the priority is to get some antibiotics into the eye and not worry too much about identifying the organism. So the first injection will be given without knowing the cause of the infection.

If a reliable bacteriological service is available, a Gram stain or culture may be very helpful for chronic cases or cases which have not responded to treatment. The laboratory must be used to handling tiny specimens from the eye. However it needs a good microbiologist to grow bacteria from the very small sample that is available, and in most cases the services of a skilled microbiologist will not be available.

If a vitrectomy kit is available a tiny amount of vitreous can be obtained before giving the injection. Some surgeons try to aspirate a tiny bit of vitreous just by using the same needle to inject the antibiotic. Alternatively there may be some pus from the wound to examine and culture.

It is best for a hospital to be prepared, so that some vials of antibiotic powder are always available with detailed instructions of how to dilute the solution so that the right amount is given (see chart on page 181). Patients with endophthalmitis have a habit of arriving in the evening or at weekends when nobody is prepared, the antibiotics cannot be found and the correct dose is not known.

We advise you to photocopy the table and place it in a prominent place in the operating theatre. This will save time and stress if a case of post-operative endophthalmitis needs urgent treatment.

1	VANCOMYCIN	2mg in 0.1ml	Kills coagulase -ve and +ve Cocci (incl. MRSA)
		and	
2	CEFTAZIDIME	2mg in 0.1ml	Kills most Gram +ve organisms (incl. *Pseudomonas aeruginosa*)
		or	
	AMIKACIN	0.5mg in 0.1ml	Use in patients allergic to PENICILLIN (NB risk of retinal toxicity)

VANCOMYCIN

From 500mg vial: Add 10ml water for injections to vial Remove 4ml of vial contents into 10ml syringe Add further 6ml water for injections to make up 10mls in syringe Remove 1ml of this solution into a 1ml insulin syringe Inject 0.1ml of this solution = 2mg total	Total in 1ml syringe is now 20mg

CEFTAZIDIME

From 1g vial: Add 10ml water for injections to vial Remove 2ml of vial contents into 10ml syringe Add further 8ml of water for injections to syringe to make up 10mls total Remove 1ml of this solution into a 1ml insulin syringe **Inject 0.1ml of this solution into vitreous = 2mg total**	Makes 100mg/ml = 200mg = 20mg/ml Total in 1ml syringe is now 20mg

25 G needle 4 mm from limbus, 1 cm into vitreous, bevel facing forward, avoid air. Use same needle for both injections and vitreous tap. Remove 0.2 ml vitreous before injection, if sample to be sent for microbiology.

Systemic

Systemic antibiotics should also be given, but they are not nearly as effective as intravitreal. They should be started by injection and then by mouth. Ciprofloxacin and the Cephalosporins have good tissue penetration and a good spectrum of activity. Ampicillin and Flucloxacillin (sometimes called Co-fluampicil or Magnapen) combined are a good alternative.

Postoperative infection is an emergency. Prompt and effective treatment can save the eye, but delay of even a few hours or ineffective treatment may result in blindness. It is useful to have an 'endophthalmitis protocol' printed and ready, together with the required equipment, In case of an emergency.

Topical

Topical antibiotics probably help a little but are not really effective for infections inside the eye. Chloramphenicol drops have a good spectrum and penetrate a little into the eye. Alternatively a combination of Gentamicin and a Cephalosporin can be given. Gentamicin has a good range of action against Gram negative organisms and the Cephalosporins such as Cephazolin or Cefuroxime have a good range of action against Gram positive organisms. Topical drops should be given every hour.

Sub-conjunctival injection

This produces good levels of antibiotic in the anterior chamber, but is less effective for the vitreous. It is recommended as the best alternative if an intravitreous injection cannot be given. Gentamicin together with a Cephalosporin again make a good broad spectrum combination and are probably the treatment of choice.

The table below shows the doses of subconjunctival antibiotics as well as other drugs which can be given subconjunctivally.

Sub-conjunctival injections

Antibiotics

These are usually made up to 0.5 ml with water for injection. A small injection of lignocaine should first be given if the injection is painful. Antibiotics which are particularly painful by subconjunctival injection are indicated with an asterisk.

Ampicillin	125–250 mg
Benzylpenicillin*	500,000 units with 0.5 ml lignocaine
Carbenicillin	100 mg
Cefuroxime	100 mg
Cephazolin	125 mg
Chloramphenicol*	100 mg with 0.5 ml lignocaine
Cloxacillin	100 mg
Gentamicin	20 mg
Methicillin	125–500 mg
Streptomycin*	100–250 mg with 0.5 ml lignocaine
Vancomycin*	25 mg with 0.5 ml lignocaine

Anti-inflammatory

Betamethasone	2–4 mg
Cortisone	20 mg
Hydrocortisone	20 mg
Depomedrone	20–40 mg

Mydriatic

Atropine	0.6 mg

Anti-fungal

Amphotericin*	0.15–0.3 mg with 0.5 ml lignocaine

Technique of sub-conjunctival injection

The injection is fairly easy and if done carefully should not cause excessive pain.

- Anaesthetise the conjunctiva. A small swab should be soaked in a topical anaesthetic drop, and left in the lower fornix for 2–3 minutes.
- The lower lid is then pulled down and a fine needle inserted through the conjunctiva and advanced for 2-3 mm under the conjunctiva.
- The injection is then given slowly. Multiple injections can be given through the same needle with a change of syringe.

Steroids

As well as antibiotics most people also recommend intensive steroid treatment for acute endophthalmitis. As a general rule steroids should never be used for treating infections, however they are used in the treatment of endophthalmitis. The damage to the eye from an acute infection is caused by bacterial toxins, which produce an inflammatory reaction in the delicate intraocular tissues. Even if the bacteria are all destroyed the inflammation caused by the toxins can still blind the eye. Therefore this inflammation must be suppressed as well as destroying the bacteria with antibiotics. Steroids are usually given as hourly topical drops and most surgeons would give a short course of systemic steroid treatment as well, starting with a high dose (60 mgm of prednisolone daily) and tapering this off very rapidly over the next few days according to response.

Mydriatics

These should also be given to all cases of endophthalmitis.

Acute iridocyclitis

Sometimes there may be an acute inflammatory reaction in the eye which is not caused by an infection, particularly after extracapsular extraction. Pieces of lens cortex may dissolve in the aqueous and cause iridocyclitis, or alternatively there may be chemical impurities in one of the solutions used to irrigate the eye.

Signs and symptoms

A non-infective iridocyclitis is often very hard to distinguish from endophthalmitis caused by infection. In non-infective iridocyclitis pain is usually less, and the eyelids and conjunctiva are much less inflamed. However there may be many inflammatory cells in the anterior chamber. The pupil is often constricted and irregular. An inflammatory reaction from cortical lens material usually occurs a few days later than acute infective endophthalmitis.

Treatment

The basic treatment is steroids and mydriatics. If there is uncertainty about infection, antibiotics may be given as well. For mild cases topical steroid drops (e.g. Prednisolone drops 2 hourly) are appropriate, more severe cases should be given subconjunctival injections and/or systemic treatment. Mydriatic drops should also be given.

Pupil block and malignant glaucoma

Both of these are fortunately very rare complications, especially malignant glaucoma. They usually develop within a week or two of operation but may come on later. The intraocular pressure rises because the aqueous fails to circulate from the ciliary processes where it is produced, to the trabecular meshwork where it is absorbed. In pupil block glaucoma following intracapsular extraction the anterior face of the vitreous becomes adherent to the pupil, in this way blocking the aqueous circulation. This is the main reason for doing an iridectomy in an intracapsular extraction. For pupil block glaucoma to develop, the iridectomy must have closed off for some reason (see **Figure 6.59** and page 151). It may also occur following extracapsular extraction if the pupil adheres to the lens capsule.

In malignant (or ciliary block) glaucoma the aqueous passes backwards into the vitreous, forcing the vitreous forwards against the iris, so that the aqueous cannot reach the anterior chamber (**Figure 6.83**). The exact mechanism for ciliary block glaucoma is not fully understood.

Signs and symptoms

The clinical appearance of both conditions is similar. The cornea is usually hazy. The anterior chamber is very shallow or flat, and the intraocular pressure is very high. However the most common cause for a shallow anterior chamber is a leaking wound, in which the intraocular pressure is low (see table on page 188).

Treatment

The patient should be given treatment to lower the intraocular pressure (Acetazolamide tablets or preferably by injection and beta-sympathetic blocking drops) and strong mydriatics to dilate the pupil (Cyclopentolate 1% and Phenylephrine 10% hourly). Mydriatics also cause the ciliary muscle to relax and so may relieve the malignant glaucoma. If the anterior chamber deepens and the intraocular pressure falls, no further treatment is necessary, but if possible the mydriatrics should be continued for some months.

If there is no improvement urgent surgery is needed. The aim of surgery is to restore the normal aqueous circulation. Pupil block should be treated by an iridectomy to make a hole in the iris to by-pass the block. Ideally this is done with a Yag laser but if this is not available a surgical iridectomy should be done. If the anterior chamber still does not deepen, this confirms the cause as malignant (ciliary block) glaucoma.

The recommended treatment for malignant glaucoma is to insert a vitrectomy probe or a wide bore needle through the pars plana (**Figure 6.83**). (After intracapsular extraction this can be done through the incision and the iridectomy). The needle is passed deep into the eye and a small amount of vitreous is aspirated. This should allow the aqueous to circulate again and

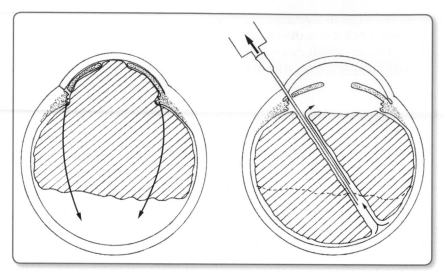

Figure 6.83 Malignant glaucoma. To show how the aqueous passes backwards pushing the vitreous forwards and a diagram of the treatment

cure the malignant glaucoma. Vitrectomy instruments are ideal for this procedure if they are available. Unfortunately these eyes are difficult to treat surgically. It is always very risky to operate on an eye with raised intraocular pressure, and yet it is often impossible to bring the pressure down without an operation. The main complication is a disastrous haemorrhage as the pressure in the eye suddenly falls.

Delayed complications

Retinal detachment

This is particularly common after vitreous loss or in a myopic patient. It is rare after an uncomplicated extracapsular extraction.

Signs and symptoms

There is loss of vision, often spreading like a curtain across the patient's field of vision. On examining the retina with an ophthalmoscope the characteristic changes are seen. Notably the red reflex is grey and the retina appears folded.

Treatment

Urgent surgical treatment is required. If treated quickly and correctly the results are good.

With delay in diagnosis or treatment the results of surgery become progressively worse. The surgical treatment of retinal detachment is outside the scope of this book and will not be described.

Cystoid macular oedema

In this condition oedema fluid collects around the macula probably as a result of a protein leak from the surrounding retinal blood vessels. The macula develops cystic changes and the visual acuity falls to around 6/60. It usually develops 1-6 months post operatively and is probably quite common in a mild form which usually recovers. Only a few patients progress to develop permanent central visual loss. The cause of cystoid macular oedema is not known, but it is more common after intracapsular than extracapsular extraction. Vitreous loss and post operative iridocyclitis both increase the risk of cystoid macular oedema. No treatment is known, but if it can be detected in the early stages a course of systemic steroids for a few weeks may be beneficial, and some surgeons advise a course of acetazolamide.

Permanent corneal oedema

This is the end-stage of severe striate keratopathy. The endothelial cells of the cornea are very active metabolically and transfer fluid from the cornea to the aqueous. If too many of these are destroyed excess fluid collects in the cornea, which becomes hazy so the patient cannot see properly (see plate 7). Small blisters containing fluid constantly form on the anterior epithelial surface of the cornea. These are known as bullae and when they rupture there is pain and inflammation of the eye.The condition is sometimes called **bullous keratopathy**.

Bullous keratopathy is a particularly distressing complication of cataract surgery because it is almost always due to poor surgical technique. It has unfortunately become more common with the introduction of intraocular lenses, particularly anterior chamber lenses. An eye with a cataract is blind but painless, but an eye with bullous keratopathy is blind and continually painful as well.

Treatment

The only treatment that can restore the vision is a full thickness corneal graft, and often the corneal graft fails or rejects after some years. If a graft is not possible the pain will be relieved by bringing down a conjunctival flap to cover the cornea (see page 274). The conjunctiva contains lymphatics which will drain the fluid away and prevent the recurrent blisters and ulcers on the cornea that cause so much discomfort. However this will not restore the vision. Treatment with an excimer laser, a very expensive laser used to correct myopia, can also relieve the pain by limiting the recurrent ulcers that form on the cornea. Multiple needle punctures to the surface of the cornea may also help.

Thickening of the posterior lens capsule (see plates 12–15)

This only occurs after an extracapsular cataract extraction. With extracapsular extraction becoming more popular, especially with lens implants, this is becoming a more common complication. The thickening of the lens capsule usually develops after one or two years but may happen at any time. It is more common in younger patients than older, but can occur at any age. Some slight thickening occurs after most extracapsular extractions, but only causes significant loss of vision inup to 25% of cases. The posterior capsule itself is transparent but there are two ways in which it can thicken and become opaque.

- Fibroblasts may grow on its front surface to make a thin opaque membrane.
- New lens cells may grow and spread on the front surface of the lens capsule so that its surface becomes irregular and scatters the light entering the eye. Very careful removal of all the lens cells at the time of surgery, sometimes called polishing the posterior capsule, will lessen the risk of this happening.
- Often both fibroblasts and new lens cells grow together on the posterior capsule.

Signs and symptoms

As the capsule opacifies the visual acuity falls. The thickened capsule is best seen by examining the red reflex of the eye through a dilated pupil with an ophthalmoscope using a lens of about + 5 and viewed from approximately 20 cms (see plates 14 and 15).

Treatment

Slight thickening of the posterior capsule requires no treatment, but if the capsular thickening causes significant blurring of vision a capsulotomy should be performed. If available an Nd:YAG laser is the best way to perform a capsulotomy, it is a painless, safe and simple procedure. Where lasers are not available a surgical capsulotomy should be performed.

Method for eyes without an intraocular lens

1. Anaesthetic. Usually just topical local anaesthetic drops provide adequate anaesthesia, but for an anxious patient or an inexperienced surgeon a retrobulbar and facial block may be required. A small sponge is soaked in topical anaesthetic and left on the surface of the eye provides better anaesthetic than just a drop.
2. The pupil should be dilated and a speculum used to retract the eye-lids.
3. Steady the eye with fine toothed forceps at the medial limbus. Then make a puncture wound at the lateral limbus with the capsulotomy knife, so as to enter the anterior chamber obliquely to form a self-sealing opening.
4. Pierce the capsule and make a short linear cut in it at the centre of the pupil. This is done by moving the handle of the capsulotomy knife and using the entry point at the limbus as the fulcrum of a lever (**Figure 6.84**). Only a relatively small hole in the capsule is necessary and with skill the aqueous should not drain out of the eye. If the capsule is very thick it may be necessary to make a cross shaped incision with one horizontal and one vertical cut. If during the capsulotomy the anterior chamber does drain away it will reform very quickly and usually no stitches are necessary to close the tiny puncture wound.
5. If a capsulotomy knife is not available the capsulotomy can be performed with an irrigating cystitome. First make a small incision at the limbus using a scalpel or razor blade fragment, but not the full depth of the cornea. Then introduce into the anterior chamber an irrigating cystitome mounted on a syringe full of balanced salt

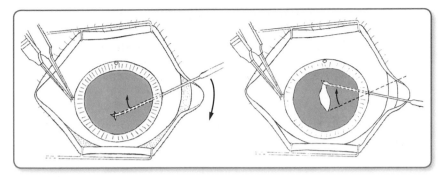

Figure 6.84 Posterior capsulotomy

solution or normal saline. If this is pushed through the groove of the incision it will make a self-sealing wound. Use the tip of the cystitome to pierce the capsule whilst the anterior chamber is maintained by irrigation. If the wound does leak, a single suture may be required to close it.

6. Very rarely the capsule is a very thick fibrous membrane. This may occur following a penetrating injury to the eye or a badly performed extracapsular extraction. In these cases the pupil is often constricted and adherent to the capsule. Very thick capsule remnants may require more extensive surgery. After a full local anaesthetic block a small incision is made in the limbus. Intraocular scissors are passed into the eye and used to cut a hole in the capsule, and sometimes to free synechiae. Visco-elastic fluids are very helpful in these cases. A full iridectomy may also be necessary.

Method for eyes with an intraocular lens

If the eye contains an intraocular lens, changes in the technique may be needed. If the pupil is well dilated, it may be possible to perform the capsulotomy through the limbus by passing the cystitome or the capsulotomy knife behind the optic of the lens and in front of the capsule. Because it is curved and not straight, a cystitome is easier than a capsulotomy knife to manoeuvre between the IOL and the capsule. When the tip has reached the centre of the capsule, it can be rotated so that the tip points backwards and makes a small cut in the centre of the capsule.

Very often a limbal approach and cutting the capsule from in front will not be possible because of adhesions between the lens and the capsule, or the pupil will not dilate enough. In such cases it is better to perform the capsulotomy through the pars plana, and cut the capsule from its posterior surface rather than its anterior surface. For a pars plana incision, a small injection of local anaesthetic subconjunctivally is helpful. The entry point is 4 mm behind the limbus. It is best to insert the capsulotomy knife in the infero temporal or superotemporal quadrant. (at 1.30 , 4.30 , 7.30 or 10.30 o'clock positions). This avoids the anterior ciliary vessels which enter the eye near the lateral rectus muscles.

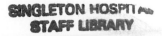

Preventing posterior capsular thickening

The risk of capsular thickening postoperatively is lessened by a careful re-moval of all the cortical lens fibres at the time of cataract extraction. Another possible way is to make a primary posterior capsulotomy at the time of the cataract extraction. Most people do not recommend this, but if a patient has cataract extractions in both eyes and lives far from medical care, it may be a useful technique.

At the end of the cataract extraction, when the IOL is in place and the wound sutured, the irrigating cystitome can be inserted between two of the sutures and then gently advanced behind the IOL and in front of the posterior capsule. It is then rotated so the tip points backwards into the posterior capsule, and a small tear made in the centre of the posterior capsule. If this is done in one eye, it means that the patient will not get posterior capsular thickening in both eyes.

A primary posterior capsulotomy may also be helpful if during the extrac-tion there is a posterior capsular opacity which will not "rub off" during irriga-tion and aspiration, and YAG lasers are not available.

Glaucoma

A few patients develop chronic glaucoma after cataract surgery. The usual reason for this is the delayed effect of a leaking wound. The mechanism is as follows:

The leaking wound post operatively causes a delayed reformation of the anterior chamber. This causes much of the periphery or base of the iris to ad-here to the periphery of the cornea, thus closing off the trabecular meshwork. These adhesions are called peripheral anterior synechiae. The leaking wound eventually seals itself and the anterior chamber reforms, but the aqueous is prevented from reaching the trabecular meshwork because of these adhe-sions, and chronic glaucoma develops.

If the eye is blind no treatment is possible. If there is still useful sight the treatment is the same as that for chronic glaucoma, a trabeculectomy opera-

Management of a flat anterior chamber			
		Treatment	
Cause	Symptoms and signs	Medical	Surgical
Excess aqueous leakage (common)	Painless. Intraocular pressure low or normal. Seidel's test positive	Mydriatics and a pressure pad	Find and close the leak and reform the anterior chamber
Pupil block glaucoma (rare)	Painful. Intraocular pressure raised. Hazy cornea	Intensive mydriatics and acetazolamide	Iridectomy
Malignant glaucoma (very rare)			Vitrectomy or vitreous needling

tion. Unfortunately the results of trabeculectomy are rather uncertain in a patient who has had a previous cataract extraction, particularly an intracapsular extraction.

Chronic postoperative uveitis

There is the possibility that the eye might become infected with an organism of low virulence during cataract surgery. This is a very rare occurrence, but if it does happen it is almost always following an extracapsular extraction with an IOL. The organism is usually a bacteria called Propionobacter which lives quite harmlessly on the skin (known as a commensal bacteria), but in the eye it can cause chronic slight inflammation. The bacteria get in the folds of the posterior capsule or between the capsule and the IOL, where the defence systems of the body cannot reach them. The eye shows all the signs of chronic uveitis, but on careful examination, there may be little patches of inflammation on the posterior capsule or behind the IOL. If the eye does not respond to conventional treatment for uveitis, the IOL and the posterior capsule may have to be removed in order to get the inflammation to subside.

A check list for post-operative eye examination

Symptom or sign	Probable causes
Pain	Endophthalmitis Pupil block glaucoma Iridocyclitis Irritation from the sutures Epithelial corneal ulcer
Eyelid swelling	Endophthalmitis Retrobulbar haemorrhage from the L.A. block Eyelid haemorrhage from the facial block Allergy to topical medication
Conjunctival vasodilation and oedema (chemosis)	Endophthalmitis Allergy to topical medication Non-specific reaction to surgery or to retrobulbar local anaesthetic block
Sub-conjunctival haemorrhage	Surgical trauma Retrobulbar haemorrhage from L.A. block
Corneal haze	Striate keratopathy Endophthalmitis Raised intraocular pressure
Anterior chamber shallow or absent	Leaking wound Pupil block glaucoma
Anterior chamber turbid or cloudy	Hyphaema Iridocyclitis Lens fragments following extra capsular extraction Endophthalmitis
Pupil irregular	Iridocyclitis Iris prolapse or iris incarcerated in the wound

Secondary intraocular lens implantation

As IOLs are becoming increasingly more popular and the standard method of cataract treatment in less developed countries, patients are often coming having had a previous cataract extraction without an implant and asking for a lens to be implanted in that eye. Another common experience is a patient who has had cataract extraction without an implant in one eye and has developed a cataract in the second eye. The best treatment is usually to remove the cataract and insert an IOL, and also insert an IOL in the other aphakic eye.

There are three possible places for a secondary IOLs:
- In the posterior chamber
- In the anterior chamber
- Fixed to the sclera

Secondary intraocular lens implant in the posterior chamber

If the posterior capsule is intact, a posterior chamber IOL can be placed in the ciliary sulcus (see **Figure 6.7**). This is the best place for a secondary lens implant. The technique for secondary implant of posterior chamber lenses is as follows:
1. Dilate the pupil fully.
2. Choose an IOL which has a large haptic and a large optic (6.5 or 7 mm). This is because the lens will be resting in the ciliary sulcus and not in the capsular bag.
3. Make an incision just large enough to insert the lens. Add viscoelastic fluid or air to the anterior chamber and insert the IOL in the standard way (see pages 131–4). Close the wound and wash out the viscoelastic fluid or air, or any other debris released by the operation, before final wound closure.
4. The post-operative care is the same as for a cataract extraction with a posterior chamber lens implant.

There are certain possible problems which may need special attention.
- A hole in the posterior capsule
- Adhesions between the iris and the posterior capsule
- A thickened posterior capsule with growth of new lens fibres (Elschnigg's pearls)
- A thickened posterior capsule with fibrosis of the capsule

There may be a hole in the centre of the posterior capsule following a previous capsulotomy but as long as the peripheral part of the capsule is present and the suspensory ligament of the lens is intact, a posterior chamber IOL can be inserted. However, if the vitreous has come through the hole in the posterior chamber and a slit lamp examination shows some vitreous in the anterior chamber, all the vitreous should first be removed from the anterior chamber with a vitrectomy machine. If this is not available, it is possible to perform a "sponge and scissors" vitrectomy (see pages 130–1) but this is very much a second best option and may not clear all the vitreous from the anterior chamber. A viscoelastic injection into the anterior chamber as soon as the incision enters the anterior chamber may help to keep any vitreous away from the wound edges.

There may be adhesions between the iris and the capsule. These are best divided by injecting viscoelastic fluid between the iris and the capsule and using the pressure of the injected fluid to separate the two layers. It may be necessary to use capsular scissors to separate very firm adhesions between the iris and the capsule but this may make a hole in the posterior capsule. If the adhesions cannot easily be separated, it may be possible to insert the IOL and place the haptics so as to avoid the adhesions. If there are many adhesions, it may not be possible to insert a posterior chamber IOL at all.

New lens fibres, known as Elschnigg's pearls, may have grown on the posterior capsule and in that case, inserting the secondary IOL is a very good opportunity to remove these new fibres using the Simcoe two-way cannula, or using a small cannula with a specially roughened tip known as a capsule polisher.

The posterior capsule may be thickened with fibrous tissue which cannot easily be irrigated away or polished. In that case, a small central capsulotomy should be made, either with capsular scissors, a capsulotomy knife or the tip of a cystitome. It is easiest to make this before inserting the IOL but the anterior chamber should be full of visco-elastic fluid to prevent any vitreous coming forward into the anterior chamber when the hole in the posterior capsule is made. If the surgeon has access to a YAG laser, then it is best to do a YAG laser capsulotomy during the post operative period rather than a capsulotomy during the operation.

Secondary intraocular lens implant in the anterior chamber

In most cases, the previous operation will have been an intracapsular extraction and therefore a posterior chamber lens cannot be inserted. In these cases, an anterior chamber IOL is the easiest choice but there are certain precautions to observe.

- All anterior chamber IOLs may gradually damage the vital corneal endothelial cells so that over the course of years they become reduced in number. This risks causing bullous keratopathy, a very serious complication. Therefore anterior chamber IOLs should never be used on patients under 50 and only with great caution in patients under 60.
- If there are adhesions between the iris and the peripheral cornea (peripheral anterior synechiae), or if a full iridectomy has been performed, then it is very difficult to insert a secondary anterior chamber IOL.
- There may very often be vitreous present in the anterior chamber which needs careful and appropriate management.

The method for secondary IOL insertion in the anterior chamber is as follows:
1. Always constrict the pupil with pilocarpine.

2. Make a limbal incision just large enough to insert the anterior chamber IOL and as soon as the anterior chamber is entered, insert viscoelastic fluid or air to keep the vitreous face behind the pupil.
3. If vitreous was present in the anterior chamber pre-operatively, then ideally an anterior vitrectomy should be performed, or failing that a "sponge and scissors" vitrectomy.
4. Choose an anterior chamber IOL of the correct power and correct size (horizontal corneal diameter white-to-white plus 1 mm).
5. With a constricted pupil and a deep anterior chamber, a lens glide is not usually needed to insert an anterior chamber IOL but it may be helpful in difficult cases.
6. The lens is inserted as described on page 165–7. Make sure the pupil is round and not distorted. A distorted pupil means that one of the haptics has caught on the peripheral iris and is not properly placed in the angle. It may be possible to adjust it with a fine cannula.
7. Make sure that there is a **patent peripheral iridectomy** because the posterior surface of the lens can cause pupil block against the pupil.
8. The wound is closed and air and viscoelastic fluid carefully washed out of the anterior chamber. Take care not to engage the vitreous when doing this and maintain a deep anterior chamber at all times.
9. The post operative care is routine and the pupil can safely be dilated after the intraocular lens is in place.

Sclerally fixated IOLs

If the eye is aphakic and an anterior chamber lens contraindicated, either because the patient is young or because it cannot be inserted, then a sclerally fixated lens is the only option (see **Figure 6.9**). The operation is more difficult, takes longer and needs some special equipment but the long term results are better than with anterior chamber IOLs. In particular, the lenses will not cause any long term damage to the endothelial cells of the cornea.

There are several different ways of inserting and securing the lens but the most common method is as follows:
1. After opening up a small conjunctival flap, make two small half-thickness triangular flaps in the sclera. These should be over the pars plana, 3–4 mm from the limbus and usually in the upper nasal and lower temporal quadrants of the eye (**Figure 6.85**).The pupil should be dilated.
2. Make a 7mm limbal incision to insert the IOL later.
3. Using a vitrectomy machine, through the limbal incision remove all vitreous from the anterior chamber and also from just behind the pupil. A vitrectomy machine is essential to do this. "Sponge and scissors" vitrectomy is not really good enough.
4. A 10-0 polypropylene or polyester suture is now passed from one scleral pocket to the other across the centre of the eye. *This suture must not be nylon as nylon will degrade inside the eye and after a few months, the suture will break.* There are various ways of passing this stitch across the eye but the following method is probably the easiest.

5. The suture is mounted on a long, thin, straight needle. The needle is inserted through the upper scleral pocket and when the tip is seen at the pupil margin, it is grasped with forceps placed through the wound and pulled out of the eye (**Figure 6.86**).

6. A small hypodermic needle is now inserted through the lower scleral pocket so the tip of the hypodermic needle is just visible in the pupil margin. The straight needle is then reinserted through the wound and its tip inserted into the tip of the hypodermic needle (**Figure 6.87**). The hypodermic needle is then carefully removed from the eye so that the tip of the straight needle comes out through the lower scleral pocket.

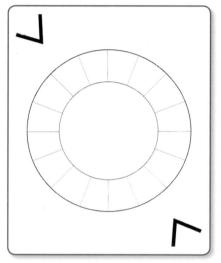

Figure 6.85 To show the position of the two small half-thickness scleral pockets

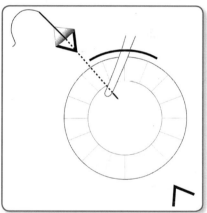

Figure 6.86 Inserting the polyester or polypropylene suture on a straight needle

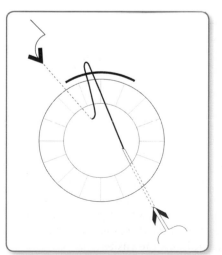

Figure 6.87 Completing the insertion of the suture across the eye

In this way, the 10-0 suture has been passed right across the eye and is also looped out through the incision.

It is possible to combine steps 5 and 6 and pass the needle straight across the eye from one scleral pocket to the other. Alternatively, after step 5, the thread can be cut and the needle inserted through the lower scleral pocket from outside the eye to inside just as in **Figure 6.86**.

7. The next step is to cut the loop of the suture and tie each end to the haptic of a posterior chamber lens, which is placed on the surface of the cornea. Ideally a special lens with loops on the haptic is used but if this is not available, the tip of the haptic can be heated with a cautery point to make it into a small lump so that the suture will not slip off the end of the haptic (**Figure 6.88**).

8. Once the suture has been tied to the end of each haptic, the two suture ends are pulled tight whilst the lens is gently manoeuvred through the wound, through the pupil, to lie behind the iris with the two haptics tied to the two suture ends.

9. The last stage is to secure these two suture ends to the sclera and also to make sure that the knot is buried in the sclera and not on the surface of the sclera where it will irritate and become infected, and cause infection to enter the eye. The way to do this is as follows (see **Figure 6.89**):

    • First tie a 10-0 polyester or polypropylene suture to close the superficial scleral flap, making sure that the stitch begins and ends inside the wound so that the knot is buried.

    • Then tie this knot to the 10-0 polyester or polypropylene suture which is attached to the sclerally fixated IOL (indicated by the black

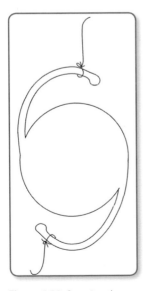

Figure 6.88 Securing the two suture ends to the intraocular lens lying on the surface of the eye

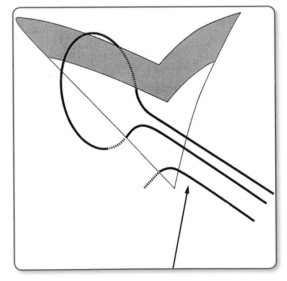

Figure 6.89 A method of burying the knot. Tie all three suture ends together to leave a knot buried inside the sclera

arrow in **Figure 6.89**). In this way, the entire knot is buried inside the sclera.

- Finally, close the limbal incision and apply routine post-operative care.

For further information

It is possible to obtain teaching videos of cataract surgery which are in many ways a better way of learning than from a book. The following can be recommended:-

"Extracapsular cataract extraction and intraocular lens implant for developing countries" by John Sandford-Smith from The Resource Centre International Centre for Eye Health, The London School of Tropical Medicine and Hygiene, 11 Keppel St., London,WC1E 7HT, U.K.

Small incision cataract surgery videos

A video from Aravind Hospital (1 Anna Nagar, Madurai, 625020 India) shows the technique using a loop described here.

The Hennig technique video is available from CBM (Nibelungstrasse 124, D6140 Bensheim, Germany). or the International Centre for Eye Health.

A 45 minute 'Sutureless ECCE' training DVD of a modified Hennig technique, together with slides and information on complcations; as well as an accompanying booklet is also available from CBM, the ICO and the ICEH. The International Council for Ophthalmology have also uploaded this entire training DVD onto their website. It is in sections, so is much easier to download or view portions of the video and slides where internet speed is not so fast. The website is:

http://icopedia.ophthalmologyblogs.org/2012/02/29/sutureless-extra-capsular-cataract-extraction-secce/

The Blumenthal method video is called "small incision cataract surgery – mini nuc" – and is available from "Visitec" (7575 Commerce Court, Saratoga, Florida U.S.A.34243–3212).

References

1.   Pascolini D, Mariotti SP. Global estimates of visual impairment: 2010. Br J Ophthalmol 2012;96:614-8.
2.   Global Initiative for the Elimination of Avoidable Blindness: action plan 2006-2011. Geneva: World Health Organization; 2007.
3.   Ruit S, Tabin G, Chang D, et al. A prospective randomized clinical trial of phacoemulsification vs manual sutureless small-incision extracapsular cataract surgery in Nepal. Am J Ophthalmol 2007;143:32-8.
4.   Gogate P, Deshpande M, Nirmalan PK. Why do phacoemulsification? Manual small-incision cataract surgery is almost as effective, but less expensive. Ophthalmology 2007;114:965-8.
5.   Schroeder B. Sutureless cataract extraction: complications, management and learning curves. Community Eye Health 2003;16:58-60.
6.   Hennig A. Sutureless non-phaco cataract surgery: a solution to reduce worldwide cataract blindness? J Comm Eye Health 2003;16:49-51.

7.   Ruit S, Paudyal G, Gurung R, Tabin G, Moran D, Brian G. An innovation in developing world cataract surgery: sutureless extracapsular cataract extraction with intraocular lens implantation. Clin Experiment Ophthalmol 2000;28:274-9.
8.   Waddell KM, Reeves BC, Johnson GJ. A comparison of anterior and posterior chamber lenses after cataract extraction in rural Africa: a within patient randomised trial. Br J Ophthalmol 2004;88:734-9.
9.   Yorston D. Using intracameral cefuroxime as a prophylaxis for endophthalmitis. Community Eye Health 2008;21:11.

Glaucoma

> **Objectives**
> - Signs and diagnosis of glaucoma
> - Medical treatment
> - Surgical treatment:
>   - Iridectomy
>   - Trabeculectomy: technique, post-operative care, complications

Glaucoma is a common disease and an important cause of blindness. This chapter will briefly describe the clinical picture of the different sorts of glaucoma and then concentrate on the surgical treatment of glaucoma. It is particularly important to understand the indications for surgery and the choice of operation. Medical treatment is important to prepare the eye for surgery but long-term medical treatment is not usually appropriate.

Glaucoma is globally the second most common cause of blindness.[1] Although the disease itself is not preventable, the blindness that glaucoma can cause is preventable if appropriate treatment is given in time, before vision is lost. There are about 4 million people blind from glaucoma in the world. Primary open angle glaucoma is the most common, and can sometimes come on quite quickly and at a young age especially in African eyes. Primary chronic angle closure glaucoma and acute angle closure glaucoma are more common in Asia.[2]

Glaucoma is a disease in which the optic nerve is damaged. This is nearly always caused by *raised intraocular pressure*, and the basic treatment is to lower the intraocular pressure. There are two common types of glaucoma, primary open angle glaucoma (sometimes called chronic simple glaucoma) and angle closure glaucoma. There are numerous other causes which are very much less common.

The normal intraocular pressure is 10–20 mm Hg (millimetres of mercury). The pressure is regulated by the production of aqueous in the eye and its drainage from the eye (see **Figure 7.1**). The aqueous is produced by the ciliary processes and passes between the lens and the pupil margin into the anterior chamber.

Once in the anterior chamber the aqueous is absorbed through the trabecular meshwork which is situated in the angle of the anterior chamber. From there it passes into the canal of Schlemm and so out of the eye. The trabecular meshwork acts as a kind of sponge allowing aqueous to pass slowly through it into the canal of Schlemm. If the trabecular meshwork is not functioning well the intraocular pressure will gradually rise. This is called ***primary open angle glaucoma*** (**Figure 7.2**) and it nearly always develops very gradually and slowly. It is the most common type of glaucoma.

If the anterior chamber is very shallow the iris may touch the back of the cornea, preventing aqueous from reaching the trabecular meshwork so the

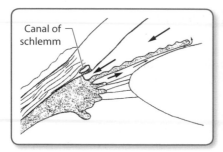

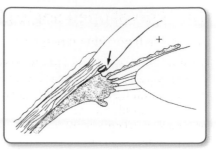

Figure 7.1 To show the production, circulation and drainage of aqueous fluid in the eye

Figure 7.2 The mechanism of open angle glaucoma. The aqueous drainage through the trabecular meshwork and into the canal of Schlemm (arrowed) is impaired, and so the intraocular pressure rises

pressure rises. If this persists, it will cause ***angle closure glaucoma*** (**Figure 7.3**). It can come on rapidly as in an angle closure attack (especially in people with 'small eyes' or people who are 'long-sighted'), with severe and acute symptoms. The trabecular meshwork may become blocked in other ways and result in some of the other less common types of glaucoma. It may be blocked by:

- White blood cells and protein exudate – secondary glaucoma from intraocular inflammation or uveitis.
- Red blood cells – secondary glaucoma from an intraocular haemorrhage (hyphaema).
- Growth of new blood vessels – neovascular or thrombotic glaucoma.
- Lens protein and macrophages – phacolytic glaucoma.
- A fine membrane of mesodermal tissue – congenital glaucoma.
- Post operative adhesions between the periphery of the iris and the cornea called peripheral anterior synechiae.

If the pupil is completely adherent to the lens, aqueous cannot even enter the anterior chamber. The iris bows forward and the intraocular pressures rises. This condition is called pupil block glaucoma (**Figure 7.4**), but it is much less common.

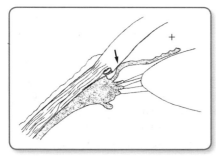

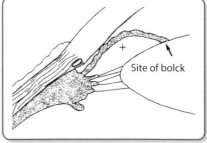

Figure 7.3 Angle closure glaucoma.The arrow shows where the iris is obstructing the flow of aqueous

Figure 7.4 The mechanism of pupil block glaucoma

The signs of open angle glaucoma

Raised intraocular pressure

Most patients with glaucoma have raised intraocular pressure. A pressure of between 20 to 30 mm Hg is increasingly suspicious of glaucoma. Pressure above 30 mm Hg is definite evidence of glaucoma. The intraocular pressure is measured with a tonometer. A "Schiotz" tonometer is reasonably accurate as long as it is kept scrupulously clean and used correctly. The Applanation or "Goldmann" tonometer is more accurate. Non-contact (or air-puff) tonometry machines are useful for screening; and portable Tono-pen or AccuPen can be helpful in a busy clinic, but these machines are expensive and need calibrating and maintenance.

This rise in intraocular pressure causes two other changes in the eye: atrophy of the optic nerve and defects in the visual field. These will be present in all patients with glaucoma. A few patients develop optic atrophy and visual field defects even though their intraocular pressure is normal. This is usually called normal tension (or low tension) glaucoma.

Optic atrophy

The optic nerve is the first structure in the eye to be damaged by raised intraocular pressure. The nerve atrophies and so the optic disc appears white. The atrophy follows a particular pattern and the optic disc also appears cupped or hollowed out. Many normal eyes have a small central portion of the optic disc which is pale and cupped. Because the optic disc varies in size from person to person, there is considerable natural variation in the size of this central cupped area in healthy normal eyes. In glaucoma this cupped and pale central portion enlarges because the nerve fibres atrophy and these make up the solid outer part of the optic disc atrophy. Finally the pale cupped area fills up the whole disc. It is usual to measure the cup/disc ratio. That is the proportion of the optic disc which is hollowed out by this pale area. The following disc changes are all very suspicious of glaucoma:

- A cup/disc ratio of greater than 0.6.
- A cup/disc ratio which is different in the two eyes by 0.2 or more.
- Notches or thin areas in the outer rim of the optic disc.

Visual field loss

As the optic nerve atrophies the vision is affected. The vision deteriorates in a characteristic way, with defects in the visual field spreading out from the blind spot but preserving the central vision and the visual acuity. Finally all the vision is destroyed, and the eye becomes completely blind. **Any sight loss is permanent and will never recover**, so glaucoma must be diagnosed in its early stages when the patient still has useful vision. Once the eye is blind no treatment will restore vision.

Unfortunately glaucoma is difficult to diagnose in the early stages for 2 reasons:

- *The patient* will not complain of any pain and may not be aware of the gradually increasing defects in the visual field.

- *The person examining the eye* may not notice the changes of glaucoma. The intraocular pressure needs to be carefully checked and the optic nerve examined. It needs time and patience to plot the visual field and detect small defects in it.

Open angle glaucoma is a *bilateral disease*, it nearly always affects both eyes. However it often affects one eye worse than the other, so that the patient may be almost blind in one eye and still have useful sight in the other.

Any patient with optic atrophy will have an *afferent pupil defect*. If one eye is worse affected than the other there will be a relative afferent pupil defect, as demonstrated by the swinging torchlight test (see footnote at the end of this chapter). Because glaucoma is the most common cause of optic atrophy and is often worse in one eye than the other, *the swinging torchlight test is a very simple and quick screening test that will detect many cases of glaucoma.*

The signs of angle closure glaucoma

In acute angle-closure glaucoma the intraocular pressure rises very rapidly to a high level so the clinical signs are very different. The symptoms usually come on very suddenly and acutely. There is rapid and severe loss of vision, and the patient may be in considerable distress. The eye is inflamed and very painful, the pupil is fixed and dilated and the cornea is oedematous and appears hazy. The anterior chamber is very shallow, and if a slit lamp is available an examination with a special mirrored contact lens called a gonioscope will be able to confirm that the iris is touching the back of the cornea.

Sometimes angle closure glaucoma will develop slowly and gradually rather than suddenly. This is called chronic angle closure glaucoma, and the symptoms and changes in the optic nerve are just like open angle glaucoma, and the treatment is the same as well.

Acute angle closure glaucoma is usually a *unilateral disease*, and only one eye is affected. However the other eye will also have a shallow anterior chamber, and so it is very likely that sometime in the next few years the other eye will also have an attack of angle closure glaucoma.

Acute angle closure glaucoma should always be treated surgically.

Diagnosis

It is important to diagnose glaucoma at an early stage, and also to identify the exact type of glaucoma from a careful history and clinical examination. This is not always easy without a slit lamp, but it is important as it affects the treatment. Consider for example a patient with one eye blind from glaucoma and the other eye apparently normal:

If the affected eye has gone blind from angle closure glaucoma, then the other eye must have an iridectomy.

If the affected eye has gone blind from open angle glaucoma, the other eye is likely to have early open angle glaucoma or could develop it in future years. It may need treatment now or at some stage in the future. The patient needs to be followed up carefully and regularly.

If the affected eye has gone blind from secondary glaucoma, the other eye probably needs no treatment or supervision at all.

It is helpful to remember that open angle glaucoma is more common and more severe in African eyes, and that angle closure glaucoma is common in Asians.[1, 3, 4] Both angle closure and open angle glaucoma become increasingly common with increasing age.

Patients with glaucoma are often not seen until they have already lost the sight in one eye. They often have great difficulty in understanding the surgeon's interest in the other eye which can still see. The patient is anxious about the *blind eye*, and hoping that something can be done to restore the sight. The surgeon is anxious about the seeing eye, and trying to decide the best plan to save what vision is left. This obviously requires a lot of patience and sympathy from the surgeon in explaining the situation to the patient.

Screening

It is difficult to screen for glaucoma on a large scale, as no single screening test with an appropriately high sensitivity and specificity exists.[5] However screening is important, and every patient, especially those over the age of 40 years seen in clinic should have their IOP checked routinely if the equipment is available.

Treatment

There are five treatment options possible for a patient with glaucoma:
1. Medical treatment
2. Surgical treatment
3. Laser treatment
4. Palliative treatment for pain
5. No treatment

Medical treatment

There are several drugs which will lower the intraocular pressure.
- Beta sympathetic blocking drugs lower the production of aqueous from the ciliary body. Timolol drops 0.25% or 0.5% twice daily is the most popular but there are others available. Betaxolol, Levobunolol and Carteolol are also beta blockers that may be available.
- Carbonic acid anhydrase inhibitors also lower the production of aqueous. Acetazolamide (also called Diamox) 250 mg by mouth up to 4 times daily, or intravenously 500mg once for acute closure-angle glaucoma. Dorzolamide 2% or Brinzolamide 1% drops three times daily can also be given. These should be given twice daily if given together with Timolol drops.
- Parasympathetic stimulating drugs constrict the pupil and also improve the flow of aqueous from the eye. Pilocarpine 1% to 4% four times daily is the drug of choice.
- Adrenaline (epinephrine) 1% twice daily drops lower the intraocular pressure by improving the outflow of aqueous. Brimonidine is a similar drug which has recently been introduced.
- Prostaglandin analogs: Latanoprost, Bimatoprost, and Travoprost are new drops, which improve the outflow of aqueous from the eye, and are

given once daily (usually at night time). They are very effective but like all newer medications are expensive.

- In severe cases osmotic diuretics will produce a short and dramatic fall in the intraocular pressure. Glycerol by mouth or Mannitol by i.v. injection are both osmotic diuretics. They may have unpleasant side effects and should be avoided if possible.

There are three indications for medical treatment.

1. In *glaucoma secondary* to uveitis. Both the uveitis and the glaucoma should be treated until the uveitis resolves. The intraocular pressure will then return to normal. (Pilocarpine should not be used for this type of glaucoma).

2. *To prepare the eye for surgery by bringing down the intraocular pressure to normal.* Operating on an eye with raised intraocular pressure has a risk of causing a sudden intraocular haemorrhage, and so for all glaucoma surgery the intraocular pressure should first be controlled with medical treatment if possible.

   In acute angle closure glaucoma, urgent and intensive treatment to lower the intraocular pressure is needed. Intensive Pilocarpine drops (every hour for a few hours and then four times a day) should be applied to the affected eye, as well as Timolol drops twice daily and Acetazolamide tablets four times daily. If the intraocular pressure has still not fallen, massaging the eye by indenting the central cornea or osmotic diuretics (see above) may lower the intraocular pressure, and so may giving a general anaesthetic. Steroid drops to the affected eye will help by suppressing the inflammation.

   Pilocarpine drops four times a day must be applied to the other eye whilst waiting for surgery, as this eye is at risk of developing angle closure glaucoma.

   When operating on an eye with primary open angle glaucoma it is best to lower the intraocular pressure preoperatively. This does not usually take more than a few days. Timolol and Pilocarpine should be used first and Acetazolamide also given if necessary.

3. *To give long-term control of the intraocular pressure in primary open angle glaucoma.* Medical treatment is usually recommended in developed countries as the treatment of choice. However medical treatment has several disadvantages.

- For medical treatment to succeed the patient must take the drops regularly for the rest of his or her life, and be checked regularly to ensure that the treatment is working, and that there are no side effects from the treatment.
- A life time of medical treatment and supervision is very costly.
- Medical treatment may work at first, but the glaucoma may get worse as the patient gets older.
- It seems that long term medical treatment causes inflammation in the conjunctiva so that if surgery is attempted later, the chance of success is less.

Obviously a life time of medical treatment is not appropriate for most patients in developing countries. Even where it is possible to give and supervise medical treatment, it seems the long-term results from surgery are as good as or better than those from medical treatment, except in mild cases or very elderly patients.

Surgical treatment

There are two operations which are commonly performed in glaucoma, a drainage operation and an iridectomy.

Drainage operations

The purpose of drainage operations is to make a pathway for the aqueous to leave the eye, so that it can be absorbed into the subconjunctival tissues, the blood vessels and the lymphatics (**Figure 7.5**). It forms a raised fluid "bleb" where the aqueous collects in the subconjunctival tissues. Some of the aqueous may drain into the cut end of the canal of Schlemm, and some may pass into the suprachoroidal space. However patients with a good bleb usually have a good result, and those with a poor bleb a poor result, so it would seem that most of the aqueous drains out subconjunctivally.

Many different types of drainage operation have been described for glaucoma such as a trephine, sclerectomy, Scheie's operation and trabeculectomy. They seem to be equally effective at achieving drainage, but the trabeculectomy allows the aqueous to drain from the eye in a more controlled manner. A trabeculectomy therefore has less post operative complications, and will be described here as the operation of choice. A Scheie's operation will also be described because it is easy to do, and may have a place when working in difficult circumstances (i.e. without an operating microscope), although it is generally considered as rather out dated and obsolete.

The indications for a drainage operation

The main indication is for primary open angle glaucoma where useful sight is still present. For useful sight the patient should at least be able to count fingers looking straight ahead. A simple functional test of the patient's vision is to see if they can navigate around obstacles in a room without bumping into them. If the vision in the eye is not good enough for this then surgery is pointless.

Another very difficult decision is whether to operate on an eye with borderline early glaucoma. Drainage operations are not free of complications, and it may be the patient's only eye. If the diagnosis is certain and especially if the other eye is badly affected, it is best to operate as without treatment the sight will almost certainly deteriorate in the next few years. If the diagnosis is uncertain, it is best to wait and review the patient in six months or a year's time. Sometimes this in itself may be difficult to arrange.

There are other situations in which a trabeculectomy operation is recommended:

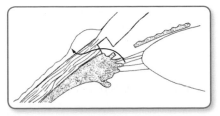

Figure 7.5 Open angle glaucoma cured by a "drainage" operation

- In acute angle closure glaucoma, if there is still useful sight in the eye, but the pressure has not come down to normal with medical treatment; or if an iridectomy has been performed but the pressure is still raised.
- In other types of glaucoma for example aphakic or pigmentary glaucoma, if the raised intraocular pressure is long-standing and there is still sight in the eye.
- In congenital glaucoma, a very rare condition, the recommended treatment is a goniotomy operation. This is difficult to perform and needs special equipment. Most surgeons have very little experience of goniotomy, and so rather than attempt this operation a trabeculectomy is recommended and usually works satisfactorily.

It is most important to **counsel patients very carefully before surgery for open angle glaucoma**. Most patients think that they are going to see better after an operation, and it must be very carefully and sometimes repeatedly emphasised to them that the purpose of the operation is not to help them to see better, but to stop them going blind in the future.

Often patients do not seek medical advice until one eye is blind and the other also affected, so surgeons must take particular care with glaucoma operations. *Any mistakes or complications mean that the last little bit of sight may be lost for ever rather than preserved.*

Iridectomy

The purpose of an iridectomy is to allow the aqueous to circulate inside the eye, from behind the iris to the anterior chamber (**Figure 7.6**). If done properly it is a very simple and successful operation with few complications.

- To treat an eye with acute angle closure glaucoma, if the pressure has come down and is well controlled on medical treatment with drops alone.
- To prevent angle closure glaucoma occurring in the second eye of a patient whose first eye has developed acute angle closure glaucoma. **An iridectomy must be performed in all these eyes**.
- For any sort of pupil block glaucoma, if the pupil block has not been cured with mydriatic drops.

Other operations

There are other possible operations to try to reduce the intraocular pressure in very severe cases, but usually they are not as successful as drainage operations.

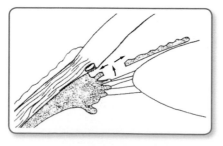

Figure 7.6 Angle closure and pupil block glaucoma cured by an iridectomy

- The ciliary body can be treated with diathermy, cryotherapy or laser in order to reduce the production of aqueous.
- A fine silicone tube sometimes attached to a valve can be inserted into the anterior chamber through a trabeculectomy incision to drain the aqueous out of the eye.
- A cyclodialysis cleft can be made from the angle of the anterior chamber into the supra choroidal space.
- Deep sclerectomy. In this recently described operation, some of the tissue around the trabecular meshwork and the canal of Schlemm is excised but the anterior chamber is not entered. It appears to be very successful but is difficult to perform.

Laser treatment

There are a few specialist hospitals and clinics where lasers are available. A YAG laser will make a small hole in the iris and so avoid having to do an iridectomy operation for angle closure glaucoma. An argon laser can be used to treat the trabecular meshwork in open angle glaucoma, and this will often help to lower the pressure in the eye. Trans-scleral cyclophotocoagulation may also be of benefit for difficult cases of glaucoma, but only if this expensive equipment is available.

Palliative treatment

If the eye is blind and painful there is no point in performing a drainage operation. The sight will not be restored, and severely inflamed eyes with very high pressures often develop complications from surgery. A blind painful eye often occurs in prolonged angle closure glaucoma or thrombotic glaucoma. For these patients steroid and atropine drops may relieve the pain. If not a retrobulbar injection of phenol or alcohol may help (see page 306). Finally if all else fails it may be necessary to remove the eye to cure the pain.

No treatment

If the eye is blind or virtually blind and free of pain there is no purpose in giving any treatment at all. It gives false hopes, it wastes the patient's and the doctor's time, and may discourage any of the patient's friends or relatives from seeking treatment if they have a treatable eye disease.

Surgical technique

Iridectomy

Principle

To remove a piece of iris to allow aqueous to circulate freely inside the eye. Usually a small piece is removed near the root of the iris. This is called a peripheral iridectomy.

Indications: These have been discussed in more detail on pages 203–4.

- To treat angle closure glaucoma.
- To prevent angle closure glaucoma.
- To treat pupil block glaucoma.

Preparation

1. Medical treatment will have been given to the eye as previously described on pages 201–2 to control the intraocular pressure and constrict the pupil.
2. The eye is prepared as for any intraocular operation.
3. A full local anaesthetic block should be given.
4. The eyelids are retracted with a speculum, and the surgeon may wish to insert a superior rectus suture to help turn the eye down. This may not be necessary.

Method

1. A small conjunctival flap is raised. This may be limbus based or fornix based (see page 37). Alternatively the incision can be in the peripheral cornea without raising a conjunctival flap at all. The operation is usually performed at the 12 o'clock position on the eye. If the eye has had an attack of acute angle closure glaucoma, some surgeons prefer to operate slightly to one side, at 10 o'clock or 2 o'clock. Then if the intraocular pressure remains high and a trabeculectomy is later needed, there is still space for it under the upper eyelid.
2. Very gentle cautery may be applied to the surface of the sclera at the incision site. This is only necessary if there are obvious blood vessels.
3. Using a scalpel blade or a razor blade fragment, an incision is made into the anterior chamber at the limbus (**Figure 7.7**). The site of the incision should be where the clear cornea meets the white opaque sclera. It needs to be only 3–4 mm in length. Make sure that the incision is almost perpendicular to the cornea (at right angles to the corneal surface) so that it enters the anterior chamber near the angle of the anterior chamber and at the root of the iris (see **Figure 7.8**). As soon as the blade enters the anterior chamber a small amount of aqueous will leak from the incision lowering the intraocular pressure. The iris will probably plug the wound. Because of this it is very easy for the opening in the deep part of the wound not to extend the whole length of the incision, and so be too small to allow the iris to prolapse from the eye. The best way to make sure that the incision is full thickness in its entire length is to reverse the scalpel or razor blade once the anterior chamber has been entered, and cut in the opposite direction just using the tip of the blade (**Figure 7.9**). Try to avoid pushing the tip of the blade right into the eye where it may injure the iris (a complication) or puncture the lens capsule (a disaster).
4. Now a small knuckle of peripheral iris root should be prolapsed through the wound. The iris may prolapse spontaneously. If it does not, then apply gentle pressure on the posterior (scleral) lip of the incision and it should prolapse (**Figure 7.10**). If the iris still does not prolapse, then make sure the incision has entered the eye along its entire length. If it still does not prolapse insert non-toothed iris forceps into the wound to grasp the

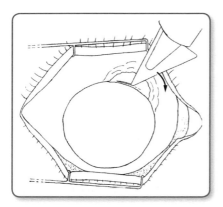

Figure 7.7 Making the incision at the limbus

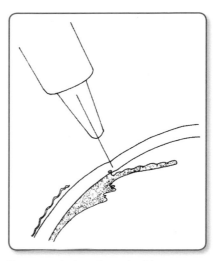

Figure 7.8 To show the angle of the incision

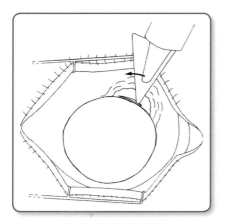

Figure 7.9 Reversing the blade of the knife to complete the incision

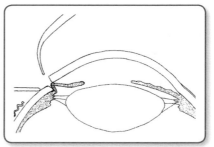

Figure 7.10 Pressure on the posterior lip of the wound to prolapse the iris

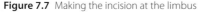

iris near its root and lift it out through the wound.Take great care not to even touch the surface of the lens with the forceps (see page 40–41).

5. Grasp the knuckle of prolapsed iris with a non-toothed iris forceps, and using a de Wecker's scissors excise this small iris knuckle (**Figure 7.11**). Make sure that a complete hole has been made in the iris including the black pigment on its deep surface. The iridectomy need only be very small, except in pupil block glaucoma when a larger iridectomy is advisable. Do not worry too much if by mistake the iris sphincter has been excised creating a full iridectomy, as the patient's vision will not be badly affected.There is usually no bleeding. If there is any bleeding, then by waiting patiently it will always stop in a few minutes.

6. The cut edges of the iris must now be replaced inside the eye. Gently massage the surface of the cornea just in front of the anterior lip of the wound with an iris repositor (see **Figure 7.12**). This usually succeeds in replacing the iris easily. When the iris is free from the incision, the pupil should be round and central. If this gentle massage does not succeed, and if a guaranteed source of sterile intraocular fluid is available, then gentle irrigation of the wound should free the iris from the wound edge. If sterile fluid is not available, the iris must be replaced by gently sweeping the wound edge with an iris repositor. Avoid pushing the repositor right into the anterior chamber.

7. Wound closure. Many people think that sutures are not necessary after an iridectomy as the wound is small and the edges soon seal with fibrin. If the operation has been done neatly through a small incision and the anterior chamber is still partly formed, this is indeed true. If there is any doubt about the wound closure, one corneo-scleral suture will close it adequately.

Post-operative care

At the end of the operation mydriatic drops are applied to dilate the pupil and prevent adhesions between the iris and the lens. Topical antibiotics and steroids are also given to prevent post-operative infection and iritis. A pad is usually applied for one day. Post operative complications are rare following iridectomy, but it is usual practice to keep the pupil dilated and apply topical antibiotics and steroids for a few days. Check the intraocular pressure before discharge. If the eye had suffered an acute angle closure glaucoma attack, there may be permanent adhesions in the anterior chamber angle preventing a satisfactory flow of aqueous from the eye. In such cases if the intraocular pressure remains high a trabeculectomy operation will be required.

Trabeculectomy

Principle

To improve the drainage of aqueous fluid from the eye. A piece of trabecular tissue is excised under a flap of superficial sclera. A peripheral iridectomy is also carried out. The aqueous drains into the sub-conjunctival space at a controlled rate, and is then probably absorbed into the conjunctival blood

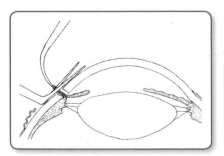

Figure 7.11 Performing the iridectomy

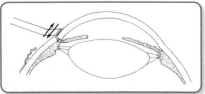

Figure 7.12 Gentle pressure and massage on the anterior lip of the wound to replace the iris

vessels and lymphatics (see **Figure 7.6**). Some of the aqueous may possibly pass directly into the cut ends of the canal of Schlemm.

Indications (these are discussed in more detail on pages 203–4):

- In primary open angle glaucoma to prevent further sight loss.
- In any other type of chronic glaucoma where the optic nerve is damaged by raised intraocular pressure.

Preparation

This is the same as for a peripheral iridectomy. Try to control the intraocular pressure preoperatively with medical treatment.

Method[6]

1. It is usual to rotate the eye downwards with a superior rectus suture (see pages 33–4). If the L.A. block has been very good, it may be possible to operate without a superior rectus suture. In particularly difficult cases of glaucoma some surgeons would advise rotating the eye downwards with a suture in the upper part of the cornea (see **Figure 7.13**). To do this a flat curved needle (with 7-0 or 8-0 silk or vicryl) is inserted into half the thickness of the cornea about 2 mm from the upper limbus. The reason for avoiding the use of a superior rectus suture is that it may damage the subconjunctival tissues where the aqueous is planned to drain from the eye. In particular it may cause a sub conjunctival haemorrhage and that would cause subconjunctival fibrosis and limit the benefits of the operation. However most surgeons still use a superior rectus suture and do not have any problems.
2. Then raise a flap of conjunctiva about 6 mm in length. This may be a fornix based or limbus based flap. For the reasons given on page 37 the fornix based flap is preferred. Lift up the conjunctiva with non-toothed forceps as near the limbus as possible at one end of the planned incision and make a small nick in the conjunctiva with scissors. Insert one blade of the scissors in this small hole, and cut round the conjunctiva and tenons insertion as near to its corneal attachment as possible (**Figure 7.14a**). Then use the scissors to undermine the conjunctival flap and separate it from the sclera

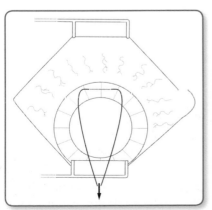

Figure 7.13 A traction suture inserted into the upper cornea to pull the eye downwards

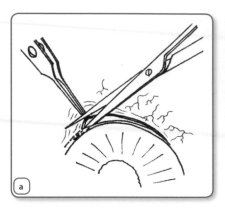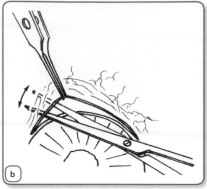

Figure 7.14a and b Dissecting a fornix based conjunctival flap

(**Figure 7.14b**). Allow the conjunctiva to retract back to leave a bare area of sclera. If the eye is pointing downwards because of traction on the superior rectus the conjunctiva will retract more.

3. There is a layer of loose connective tissue between the conjunctiva and sclera called Tenon's capsule. In young people this tissue forms a definite thin layer of connective tissue, but it atrophies in older patients. Tenon's capsule is inserted into the surface of the sclera about 2 to 3 mm back from the limbus, and it needs to be separated from the surface of the sclera where the trabeculectomy is to be done. The easiest way to do this is just to cut its insertion into the sclera with a pair of scissors and it will retract backwards out of the way. Once this is done, the side of a crescent blade can be used gently to scrape away any remaining small fibrous remnants still attached to the sclera.

4. Mark out a flap of superficial sclera to be hinged at the limbus (**Figure 7.15**). The exact size, shape and position of this flap does not matter as long as it is 4 mm wide at the limbus. It is usual to make it rectangular in shape but some people prefer a trapezoid or a triangular flap (**Figure 7.16**). Plan the position of the flap so as to avoid any obvious large blood vessels lying on the surface of the sclera, taking special note to avoid any 'penetrating' scleral vessels.

   Having chosen the place for this flap, apply only very minimal cautery or diathermy to the surface of the sclera over the area of the flap. Applying too much cautery will promote fibrosis and lead to bleb failure. This should be just sufficient to blanch the vessels without burning the sclera.

5. Use a scalpel blade or razor blade knife to cut lightly into the sclera along the edges of the flap. Dissect this flap back using a crescent blade or scalpel, to the limbus. Start at one corner lifting up that corner with fine toothed forceps and aim to dissect the flap both across to the other corner and down to the limbus (**Figure 7.17**).

   The flap should be about half the scleral thickness. If it is too thin the flap will appear transparent and may curl up and fray at the edges.

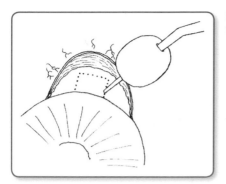

Figure 7.15 Using light cautery to coagulate the blood vessels in the area of the scleral flap

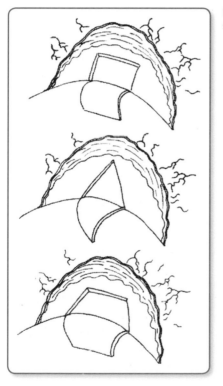

Figure 7.16 Possible shapes of the superficial scleral flap

If it is too thick the black of the choroid and ciliary body will be seen through the bed of the flap. The dissection is continued forwards until it just passes across from opaque sclera into clear cornea. Try to make this dissection in one smooth layer as this improves aqueous drainage.

6. Making a limbal puncture(paracentesis). At this stage it is helpful to make a small self sealing puncture wound into the anterior chamber at the limbus. This is done with a sharp tipped knife such as razor blade fragment or a 15 degree blade, or alternatively a fine hypodermic needle. The purpose of this is to be able to test the tightness of the wound later on by injecting saline or Ringer's solution into the anterior chamber (**Figure 7.18**). If a hypodermic needle is used its tip

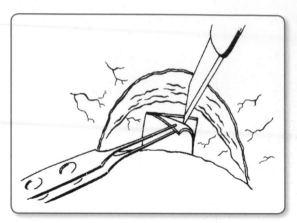

Figure 7.17 Dissecting the superficial scleral flap

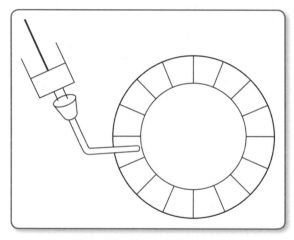

Figure 7.18 A small suture (arrowed) to bring down the conjunctiva incision

is directed downwards towards the six o'clock position and away from the lens so it will avoid damaging the lens or iris and help to make this puncture wound self sealing.

7. The deep block of (trabecular) tissue is now excised. The operation is called a "trabeculectomy" because this tissue is from near the trabecular meshwork, but it is best to take it from the peripheral part of the cornea. This should be a rectangle 3mm x 2mm (see **Figure 7.19**). The anterior cut should be at the anterior end of the dissection just in clear cornea and the posterior cut where the grey-blue limbal tissue meets the white sclera. This corresponds to the position of Schwalbe's line. (See page 35–37 for a description of the anatomy of the limbal area). If the surgeon has some doubt as to the landmarks and the exact place from where to remove this tissue, it is better to be more forward (anterior) in the cornea than back (posterior) in the sclera. An incision which is too far back is likely to damage the ciliary body or the base of the iris where the circular artery lies. This will cause bleeding into the eye at this stage or later on when the iridectomy is

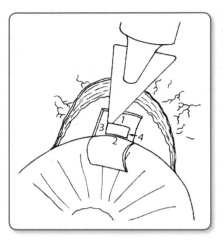

Figure 7.19 The position of the deep block of corneo-scleral tissue to be excised, and cutting through into the anterior chamber using a knife. For an explanation of the numbers see the text on page 213

performed. Removing this block of tissue nicely and neatly is probably the hardest part of the operation. The assistant should retract forwards the superficial scleral flap. Now mark out the edges of this deep block with gentle cuts which do not perforate into the eye. There are three different ways of excising this block of trabecular tissue:

A. Using a knife only

- Complete the posterior horizontal incision into the eye (**Figure 7.19-1**). There will be a small leak of aqueous and the base of the iris will plug the incision.
- Complete the anterior horizontal incision into the eye (**Figure 7.19-2**). Then grasp this bridge of tissue between the two incisions with toothed forceps and lift it upwards away from the eye (**Figure 7.20**).
- Complete one radial incision, (**Figure 7.19-3**) then by lifting the block of tissue excised on three sides any remaining attachments where the anterior and posterior cuts are not complete can be divided. Finally the block is removed by cutting along its fourth side (**Figure 7.19-4**).
- The advantages of this method is that no instrument enters the eye to risk damaging the iris or lens, and it only requires a razor blade

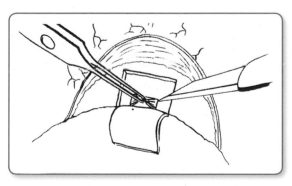

Figure 7.20 Excising the deep corneo-scleral tissue with a knife. This is the recommended method for most situations

fragment or a similar sharp knife blade and a pair of fine toothed forceps. There is no need to use fine Vannas scissors or a fine punch both of which easily become blunt.

B. Using a knife and Vannas scissors.

- Complete the two radial cuts down into the anterior chamber so there is a small leak of aqueous (**Figure 7.21a**).
- Insert one blade of Vannas scissors into the eye and cut across to join the anterior ends of the two radial cuts (**Figure 7.21b**). Lift this piece of tissue dissected on 3 sides backwards and complete the posterior cut with scissors (**Figure 7.21c**).
- The advantage of this method is that the position of the posterior cut can be seen and is not made "blind".

C. Using a Corneo-scleral punch, usually a "Kelly" punch.

This is probably the easiest method if a fine sharp punch is available. Only the anterior incision into the eye is made, (the incision labelled "2" in **Figure 7.19**). The tip of the punch is then inserted into the incision and a small piece of sclera punched out. Make sure that the punch is at right angles to the surface of the eye, so it cuts through all layers of the sclera.

8. *The peripheral iridectomy* A portion of peripheral iris is now excised directly under the trabeculectomy hole. The iris may already have prolapsed through this hole or it may be necessary to lift it out of the eye. Grasp the iris with fine iris forceps, and excise a segment with de Wecker's scissors (**Figure 7.22**). Take care not to cut into the extreme root of the iris or the ciliary body both of which will bleed. Also take care not to touch the surface of the lens with the forceps. Ideally the iridectomy should be the same size as the area of deep scleral tissue excised.

Particular care must be taken with the iridectomy if the operation is for congenital glaucoma. The fibres of the suspensory ligament of the lens are stretched and very weak in these patients, and can easily rupture when the iridectomy is done. The result is that vitreous will come into the wound and the operation fails. In these patients it is best to do the iridectomy well away from the base or root of the iris and more towards the pupil margin.

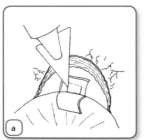
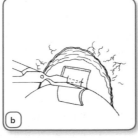
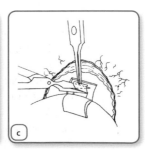

Figure 7.21 Excising the deep corneo-scleral tissue with a knife and Vannas scissors

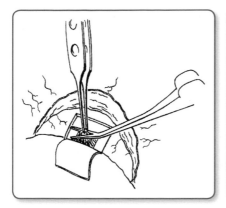

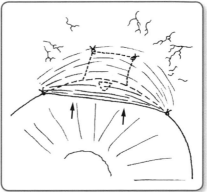

Figure 7.22 The iridectomy

Figure 7.23 Closure of the sclera and conjunctiva. It is very important that the conjunctiva presses tightly down against the corneal margin where shown with arrows so that aqueous does not leak out from the wound

9. *Suturing the sclera* Close the superficial scleral flap with two fine sutures at the corners (**Figure 7.23**). 8-0 virgin silk, or polyglactin (vicryl), or 9 or 10-0 monofilament nylon may be used. Nylon is probably the better suture as it will not provoke a tissue reaction. Make sure the knots and stitch ends are not sticking up, and are on the side of the incision furthest from the cornea. The knot of 10-0 nylon suture can be buried in the wound. These sutures should not be too tight because the aqueous fluid will need to drain out of the anterior chamber, through the incision in the superficial sclera and under the conjunctival flap. It is helpful to test that the aqueous can drain through the wound by inserting a fine cannula on a 2 ml syringe with Ringer's solution through the limbal puncture wound made at step 6. Gentle pressure on the syringe should allow fluid to come out through the scleral incision.

10. *Suturing the conjunctiva* Suturing the conjunctiva correctly and tightly is also a critically important part of the operation. By contrast to the scleral incision which needs to leak a little, the conjunctival incision needs to be watertight so that the aqueous does not leak out of the subconjunctival space at all. The conjunctiva is closed by pulling it down and suturing it at the two corners (see **Figure 7.23**). First the superior rectus suture should be loosened or removed at this stage to enable the conjunctiva to be brought down more easily. **It is extremely important that the conjunctiva is anchored very tightly at the corners and under slight tension, so that it presses closely on the corneaat the limbus. In this way the aqueous will not leak out under the edge of the conjunctival flap, or from the sides.**

    If virgin silk or vicryl is used to close the conjunctiva, the knot is probably best placed on the surface of the eye. A bite of limbal tissue is taken so the point of the needle enters the limbus at point A in **Figure 7. 24**, and emerges at the edge of the incision. A bite of the conjunctiva is then

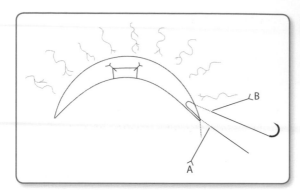

Figure 7.24 Closing the conjunctiva with a virgin silk or Vicryl suture

taken with the needle emerging at point B. When this suture is tied it will pull the flap of conjunctiva down over the cornea.

If nylon is used to close the conjunctiva, it is best to have the knot buried, otherwise the hard knot will cause quite a lot of irritation. To do this the tip of the needle is passed into the edge of the incision to emerge from the limbus at point A in **Figure 7.25**. The needle then enters the conjunctiva at point B to emerge under the conjunctiva. When this suture is tied the knot will automatically be buried in the wound.

When the two sutures at each end of the wound have been tied, the edge of the conjunctiva should be tight against the upper corneal margin as shown in **Figure 7.23**. If it is not, one or both sutures should be replaced and reinserted so as to take a bigger bite of the conjunctiva. Finally the wound should be tested to confirm that it is watertight. The fine cannula and syringe should again be inserted through the puncture wound in the anterior chamber and fluid injected into the anterior chamber. This time fluid should emerge through the scleral incision, but should balloon up under the conjunctiva if the conjunctival wound is watertight. If the conjunctival wound leaks, then

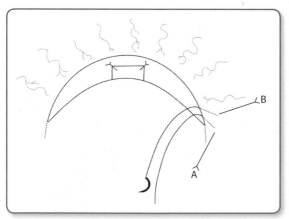

Figure 7.25 Closing the conjunctiva with a nylon suture

either extra sutures must be applied or the sutures readjusted until the wound is watertight.

Limbus based conjunctival flap

The operation described above creates a fornix based conjunctival flap with the incision in the conjunctiva at the limbus. In some circumstances a limbus based conjunctival flap may be made with the incision in the conjunctiva towards the fornix. there may be various reasons for this.

- Surgeon's preference. Some surgeons prefer this technique, because the conjunctival wound is further from the trabeculectomy site.
- Excessive conjunctival scarring at the limbus. If the conjunctiva is very scarred, the dissection will be very difficult either way but a limbus based flap may be easier.
- The use of anti-metabolite solutions (see pages 222–24). If these are being used a limbus based flap may have less complications.

To make a limbus based flap the eye is rotated downwards with a superior rectus or corneal fixation suture as described in step 1 above. A conjunctival incision is then made about 7 mm from the limbus (**Figure 7.26**). The edge of the conjunctiva is then lifted up with non-toothed forceps, and the spring scissors used to dissect just under the surface of the conjunctiva towards the limbus (**Figure 7.27**). This dissection is made easier if the conjunctiva is kept taut and stretched by lifting it up and pulling it back with the forceps. Take very great care not to make a hole in the conjunctiva. It is essential that the flap is intact and doesn't have hole in it. Once the dissection has reached the limbus then Tenon's capsule is separated from its insertion into the sclera about 2–3 mm from the limbus.

Step 4 to 9 are then performed as already described. The conjunctival incision is then sutured with interrupted or a continuous stitch, and the wound tested to make sure that it is watertight.

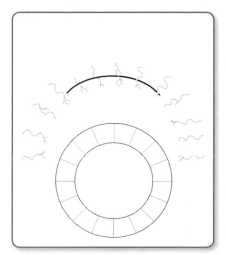

Figure 7.26 The position of the conjunctival incision for a limbus-based conjunctival flap

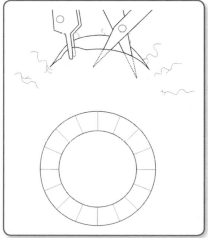

Figure 7.27 Dissecting the limbus based conjunctival flap

Post operative care for trabeculectomy

- *Mydriatics.* These should be applied at the end of the operation and continued for at least a week (Atropine 1% daily or Cyclopentolate 1% twice daily are used). Mydriatics help to prevent post operative uveitis and adhesions forming between the iris and the lens. They also help the anterior chamber to deepen by relaxing the ciliary muscle. If there are post operative complications, they should be used for longer.
- *Topical steroids and antibiotics.* These should also be applied at the end of the operation and must be continued regularly, four times (or more often) a day, for at least a month. The purpose of the steroids is to prevent post operative uveitis and also to suppress fibrosis and scarring which occurs around the drainage bleb. Because some degree of postoperative fibrosis is such a common problem, many surgeons would advise using topical steroids for up to 3 months. The antibiotics are to prevent infection.
- *Padding.* The eye should be firmly padded for one day. Provided the anterior chamber is fully or even partly formed no further padding is needed (see below).
- The eye should be carefully examined after a month to make sure that the drainage bleb is well formed and the intraocular pressure controlled.
- *Suture removal.* If the conjunctival sutures have not fallen out after a month, it is best to remove them, especially if they are causing any irritation. After drainage operations there is always the slight risk that bacteria will enter the eye by the same route that the aqueous drains out of it, and this risk is increased if a foreign body like a piece of suture is present.

Post operative complications

These can be divided into early complications – within the first two weeks of surgery, and delayed complications – appearing a month or even some years post operatively.

Early complications

Delayed reformation of the anterior chamber (see plates 18–21)

This is the commonest post operative complication. It occurs to some degree in many patients because the aqueous at first drains too rapidly out of the eye. It is acceptable for the anterior chamber to be shallow on the first post-operative day, and gradually reform over the next 3 to 4 days.

If the aqueous is draining too fast, the anterior chamber will not reform at all and the eye becomes soft. A soft eye causes protein exudate to leak from the choroidal vessels, and accumulate in the supra choroidal space. This fills up the space in the rigid sclera, which further delays the anterior chamber from reforming. Such accumulations are called choroidal detachments and can be seen with an ophthalmoscope. If the anterior chamber remains flat for a long time (a week or more), further problems may develop. Firstly a cataract may form quite rapidly. Secondly, when the fluid circulation in the eye eventually recovers, the normal drainage pathway into the trabecular meshwork will be completely closed and the drainage pathway created by the operation may also seal off, so that the operation fails. *Making sure that the conjunctival wound is watertight at the end of the operation is the best way of avoiding all these complications.*

Management

Instill fluorescein drops into the conjunctival sac to see if there is any aqueous leak seeping from the wound (see plates 3 and 4).Try to decide if the anterior chamber is just shallow, or completely absent with the anterior surface of the lens touching the back of the cornea. This is easy to decide with a slit lamp but otherwise quite difficult.

Apply topical treatment, mydriatics and steroids and antibiotics, and then tightly cover the eye with a firm pad and bandage and leave it for one day. Examine the eye daily, and as long as the anterior chamber remains shallow or is gradually reforming, continue to treat with daily medication and a pad and bandage. If available a bandage soft contact lens works better than padding the eye. These lenses are soft and very thin and have a large diameter of 14 mm. They will press on the conjunctiva and help to seal a small leak. They can be left in the eye for a week but should then be removed.

If the anterior chamber appears to be completely flat for 2 days or more, surgical treatment is advised as follows:

1. If a leak of aqueous from the conjunctiva can be identified, try to close it by suturing the conjunctiva more tightly. Reapply a pad and bandage and wait for a day or two to see if the anterior chamber reforms.

2. If no obvious aqueous leak can be demonstrated, then reform the anterior chamber with air. (If they are available, visco-elastic fluids like sodium hyaluronate are better than air). Make a small puncture wound at the limbus into the anterior chamber with a razor blade fragment, a 15 degree blade or sharp hypodermic needle, and inject air into the anterior chamber. This is quite a difficult manoeuvre because the anterior chamber is flat, and therefore it is easy to puncture the iris or the lens with the tip of the needle. If possible inject through the same limbal puncture wound (paracentesis) as was made during the operation If the air immediately leaks out of the anterior chamber this may demonstrate a hole in the conjunctiva which needs closing.

3. Some people also advise draining the choroidal effusion through a small radial incision in the sclera about 5 mm from the limbus, usually in the inferotemporal quadrant. The protein rich choroidal effusion which is coloured yellow will drain out, and more air can then be inserted into the anterior chamber. This may be difficult to do and is often not necessary.

   (Steps 1 and 2 can be performed using just topical anaesthetic drops and a small sub conjunctival injection of local anaesthetic in a relaxed patient. Step 3 requires a full retrobulbar block, as does Step 1 and 2 in a nervous patient. A facial block is advisable for all patients.)

Failure of the aqueous to drain

This is the second most common post-operative problem. There will be no bleb of aqueous under the conjunctiva, the anterior chamber will be fully formed and the intra ocular pressure remain high. There are various reasons for the drainage of aqueous to fail. The trabeculectomy hole may be blocked with the iris or with fibrin and blood. The scleral sutures may be so tight that the aqueous cannot drain through the wound.

Management

There is no harm in waiting for one day to see if the aqueous will start draining spontaneously. If there is still no drainage ocular massage should be done. The best way of doing this is to apply topical anaesthetic drops to the conjunctiva and press on the sclera just above the incision in the sclera with a glass rod or a blunt instrument. This will raise the pressure in the eye and also help to open up the scleral incision. In this way the aqueous is forced out of the eye and usually a drainage bleb will form. Often the aqueous will then continue to drain by itself or the massage may be repeated. Sometimes it may be helpful to get the patient to massage their own eye once or twice a day. This is done by looking down, shutting the eyelid, placing two fingers on the eyeball and pressing with first one finger and then the other.

If massage fails, the sutures in the scleral flap should be cut. For those with the luxury of an argon laser, this can be done by focussing the laser beam with a glass rod on to the nylon suture. Alternatively the sutures can be cut by passing a hypodermic needle through the conjunctival wound, under the conjunctiva and using the sharp edge of the tip of the needle to cut the suture.

The use of releasable sutures

This technique has developed in the last few years as a way of having better postoperative control of the intraocular pressure. One or more of the sutures on the scleral flap are tied very tightly so as to lessen the risk of excessive drainage, but by a method so that they can be released very easily if there is inadequate drainage. Different suturing techniques have been described, they are all slightly complex and some good fine instruments and the patient's co-operation is needed if they have to be removed. One method is shown in **Figure 7.28**. Monofilament 10-0 nylon must be used. The needle enters the sclera at "A" to emerge in the peripheral cornea at "B". It re-enters through the cornea at "C" to come out of the superficial scleral flap at "D". It then passes across and through the wound edge from "E" to "F". The knot is tied by winding the suture beyond "F" at least three times round a suture tying forcep and then grasping the loop between "D" and "E" with the tip of the suture forcep. This is pulled very tight to close the wound between "E" and "F" and also tighten the small loop of the suture lying on the cornea between "B" and "C". The needle is cut off and the ends at "A" and "F" are left under the conjunctiva. If postoperatively the aqueous is leaking through the scleral wound then the suture is left in position. If there is no drainage and the pressure is high then topical anaesthetic drops can be applied, and the loop of suture on the cornea between "B" and "C" is grasped and pulled. This will undo the slip knot and the whole stitch will come out.

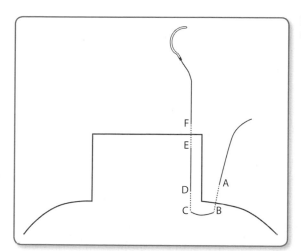

Figure 7.28 To show how a releasable suture is inserted

Hyphaema

A small hyphaema is quite common. It usually occurs because the iridectomy has been done too near the circular artery at the root of the iris. It will absorb in time without any serious effect.

Malignant glaucoma

Malignant glaucoma and its treatment is discussed on page 183. It is fortunately extremely rare. The vitrectomy probe or needle should be inserted through the pars plana and a small amount of vitreous aspirated. The anterior chamber should then be filled through a limbal puncture wound.

Delayed complications

Inflammation and fibrosis around the drainage bleb

Inflammation may appear around the drainage bleb about 2 weeks post operatively, and this inflammation may persist for some weeks. During this stage the intraocular pressure is often raised. This inflammation may resolve and the intraocular pressure fall, with the formation of a good drainage bleb subconjunctivally. Sometimes the inflammation may progress to form a fibrous scar which prevents the aqueous leaving the eye, so there is no drainage bleb or a thick wall of scar tissue around it. The intraocular pressure remains permanently raised and the operation will fail. This excessive inflammatory reaction causing the operation to fail is more common in certain circumstances:

- If patients have received drops for glaucoma, especially those who have been treated for a long time or those given adrenaline or similar drugs.
- Patients who have had previous surgery especially involving the conjunctiva.
- Young patients.
- Patients who are Afro-Caribbean seem to have a more marked postoperative inflammatory response.

During the stage of inflammation it is important to continue with regular and intensive topical steroid treatment until the inflammation subsides.

If there are signs of inflammation around the drainage bleb it is best to give topical steroids every two hours for up to two months. Occasionally the trabeculectomy appears to be a complete success, with a good drainage bleb, but the intraocular pressure remains high. This may be a complication of the steroid drops, because topical steroids can occasionally cause raised intraocular pressure.

Medical treatment to lower the intraocular pressure (Timolol, Acetazolamide etc.) may also be required during this period.

Preventing postoperative fibrosis and failure of the drainage bleb

Good surgical technique will greatly reduce the risk post-operative fibrosis. The following details are particularly important:
- Haemostasis so there is no subconjunctival bleeding
- Only minimal cautery or diathermy. Too much cautery causes fibrosis
- No loose sutures or stitch ends to cause inflammation
- A watertight conjunctival wound to prevent hypotony

Intensive postoperative topical steroids as described above also help to prevent postoperative fibrosis. A more effective method is the use of antimetabolite or cytotoxic drugs which inhibit the multiplication of the fibroblasts. These are the cells which make the fibrous tissue which causes the bleb to fail. Two different drugs are recommended, 5-fluorouracil, and mitomycin C. There is still some uncertainty as to what exactly is the best way to deliver the drugs and what is the correct dose. **Be very careful during the operation with anti-metabolies: The aim is to treat a posterior area of sclera. Do not spill any on the cornea, or edges of the conjunctiva (or you will risk causing a chronic corneal abrasion or wound leak).**

5-Fluorouracil (usually supplied in ampoules of 250 mgs in 10 ml of water).This can be applied during the operation. A small eye swab is soaked in this solution and tucked under the conjunctival flap (see **Figure 7.29**).This is done after the conjunctiva has been dissected off the sclera but before any incision has been made in the sclera (between step 3 and step 4 on pages 210). In this way the drug inhibits the fibroblasts under the conjunctiva and on the surface of the sclera. The swab is left in place for five minutes, although some surgeons recommend replacing it with a fresh swab every minute. Finally the wound should be thoroughly irrigated with saline solution (at least 20mls, if not more) to wash away any residual chemical.

There seem to be very few complications from giving 5-fluorouracil in this way. Some surgeons are advising that it should be given routinely in all trabeculectomies.

Alternatively, 5-fluorouracil may be given as a sub-conjunctival injection of 5 mgs shortly before the operation or postoperatively daily for one week and then on alternate days for one week. Giving multiple injections like this may obviously be difficult to arrange, and a full course may not be possible. These injections should not be given too close to the bleb site.

Mitomycin C. 1mg of mitomycin is diluted in 5 ml of water (making a solution of 0.2 mg per ml). Mitomycin C is a more potent drug than 5-fluorouracil

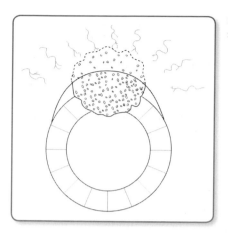

Figure 7.29 To show the position of a small sponge soaked in 5-fluorouracil

and has a stronger effect on inhibiting cells which are dividing and multiplying. Therefore very great care must be taken so that the solution does not touch the edge of the conjunctival wound. If it does it can prevent the wound healing so that there is a permanent leakage of aqueous through the conjunctival wound. Therefore the best way of applying it is as follows:

- First place a very small piece of dry sponge under the conjunctiva, but place this high up so it is not near the edge of the wound.
- Draw up a very small amount of mitomycin solution in a 1 or 2 ml syringe attached to a very fine cannula.
- Lift up the edge of the conjunctival wound and inject the mitomycin directly on to the sponge. (**Figure 7.30**)
- Make sure that the solution does not spill over on to the edge of the wound but try to treat as large an area as possible.
- After 5 minutes remove the sponge and irrigate the wound thoroughly with saline.
- Because mitomycin is such a strong drug, some surgeons advise that it should always be used with a limbal based conjunctival flap and not a fornix based flap. In this way even if there is some delayed wound healing, this will not occur right over the site of the trabeculectomy.

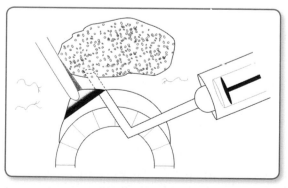

Figure 7.30 To show the position of a small sponge soaked in mitomycin and how to avoid the mitomycin coming into contact with the edge of the conjunctival wound

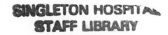

Even then the surgeon should place the sponge and the mitomycin so that it does not touch the cut edges of the conjunctiva.

Recommendations for preventing fibrosis and failure of the drainage bleb

- *Low risk cases* – Carry out a routine trabeculectomy and give routine postoperative topical steroids.
- *Moderate risk cases*, for example African patients, young patients or patients who have had several years of medical treatment. –Apply 5 fluorouracil by preoperative Injection or on a sponge at the time of the operation. It may also be given as postoperative sub conjunctival injections, if there is evidence of marked postoperative inflammation.
- *High risk cases*, for example patients who have had an unsuccessful previous operation or who have chronic uveitis – Apply mitomycin C on a sponge at the time of the operation, and if necessary postoperative sub-conjunctival injections of 5-fluorouracil as well

Future prospects. Quite a lot of active research is being done at present to try to modify the postoperative reaction in the conjunctiva. This would enable a trabeculectomy to be a more reliable operation and lessen the risk of failure or excessive drainage.

A single dose of **beta radiation** (750 centigray) from a strontium 90 applicator placed on the conjunctiva over the trabeculectomy site immediately postoperatively will suppress post-operative fibrosis. This is probably safe and effective, but strontium 90 applicators are not widely available at present.

There is also research into antibodies which can prevent fibroblast activity.

Encysted bleb

Sometimes there is a good drainage bleb but a fibrous capsule develops around it so that the aqueous cannot get absorbed from the subconjunctival tissues and the intraocular pressure remains high. This situation may be helped by a needling of the bleb.

- Apply plenty of topical anaesthetic drops, and povidone iodine to sterilise the conjunctiva.
- Insert a fine hypodermic needle under the conjunctiva about 4mm away from the bleb, inject some lignocaine with adrenaline to cause the conjunctiva to balloon a little, and slowly advance the tip of the needle through the fibrous wall of the bleb and out the other side, but without puncturing the conjunctiva itself. Take great care to avoid any blood vessels and not to cause a sub conjunctival haemorrhage.
- Inject 5mg of sub-conjunctival 5-fluorouracil well clear of the bleb.

Cataract

There is an increased risk of developing cataract after a drainage operation. A cataract may develop some years later, even if the surgery is completely uncomplicated. If there are complications at the time of operation or post operatively, then cataract formation is more likely and may develop quite quickly. The cataract should be treated surgically just as any other cataract, but a corneal incision avoiding the drainage bleb or a temporal incision is recommended. After trabeculectomy sutured extracapsular, and not suture-less cataract surgery should be performed as the scleral tunnel will cause scarring and interfere with the drainage bleb of the trabeculectomy operation, unless performed from a temporal approach.

Intracapsular, cataract extraction should be not performed as the vitreous would become trapped in the drainage site.

Endophthalmitis

After a drainage operation, aqueous passes from the eye into the sub-conjunctival space. There is always a risk that infection will pass in the opposite direction, from the conjunctiva into the eye. The infection may just reach the drainage bleb, sometimes called "bleb-itis" with pus and inflammation around the drainage bleb (see plate 17). It may spread further into the eye causing endophthalmitis. (See plates 9 and 10 for a description). Any episode of unexplained inflammation or iritis in an eye after a drainage operation might signify an intraocular infection needing urgent treatment.

If the infection is just in the bleb then intensive topical, sub conjunctival and systemic antibiotics should be given (see page 180). If there is an endophthalmitis, then intravitreous antibiotics should be given (see page 177–9 and Table on page 181).

Excessive drainage of aqueous and hypotony

Excessive drainage of aqueous causing a very low intraocular pressure (hypotony) is quite common in the first few days after the operation. It nearly always recovers by itself. If a very large drainage bleb and a very soft eye persist for more than a few weeks, a long mattress suture of 10-0 nylon may make the drainage bleb smaller and restore the intraocular pressure to normal levels (**Figure 7.31**). These may be placed on one side or both sides of the bleb.

Note: If the reader is uncertain of the significance of the relative afferent pupil defect or how to test for it, please see "Eye Diseases in Hot Climates" 5th edition published by JP Medical Ltd (for address see page iv).

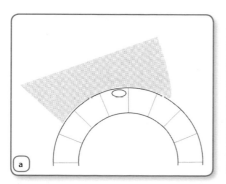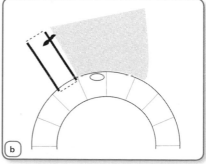

Figure 7.31 A mattress nylon suture placed to reduce the size of the drainage bleb if it too large

References

1. Cook C. Glaucoma in Africa: size of the problem and possible solutions. J Glaucoma 2009; 18:124-8.
2. Foster PJ. Advances in the understanding of primary angle-closure as a cause of glaucomatous optic neuropathy. Community Eye Health 2001;14:37-9.
3. Quigley HA, Broman AT. The number of people with glaucoma worldwide in 2010 and 2020. Br J Ophthalmol 2006;90:262-7.
4. Nolan WP. Prevention of primary angle-closure glaucoma in Asia. Br J Ophthalmol 2007;91:847-8.
5. Cook C, Cockburn N, van der Merwe J, Ehrlich R. Cataract and glaucoma case detection for Vision 2020 programs in Africa: an evaluation of 6 possible screening tests. J Glaucoma 2009;18:557-62.
6. Murdoch I. How I approach trabeculectomy surgery. Community Eye Health 2006;19:42-3.

Surgery of the eyelids

Objectives
- Surgical anatomy of the eyelids
- Surgical pathology of the eyelids
- Basic principles of eyelid surgery
- Entropion and trichiasis operations
- Lower lid entropion
- Ectropion
- Treatment of eyelid tumours

Eyelid disorders are common and their treatment is often surgical. Most eyelid diseases will produce three possible effects:

1. *Cosmetic deformity*. This may vary from being mild to quite severe causing serious disfigurement.
2. *Conjunctivitis*. Eyelid diseases often cause conjunctivitis if the conjunctiva is exposed or irritated by the eyelid deformity. The patient will complain of irritation and discharge from the eye.
3. *Corneal ulcers and scarring*. The eyelid protects the cornea and severe eyelid disease can damage the cornea. The cornea may become progressively more scarred and opaque from keratitis and corneal ulcers eventually causing loss of sight. Obviously loss of sight is the most important consequence of any eyelid disease.

There are many different operations that can be performed on the eyelids. This book cannot begin to describe them all, and there are already many excellent textbooks available describing eyelid surgery. Only common conditions will be described, especially those which cause loss of sight by damaging the cornea. Upper lid entropion and trichiasis as a result of trachoma is the most important cause of corneal scarring. It is more common than all other eyelid disorders in tropical countries. Facial palsy is also important particularly in leprosy. Surgical treatment of other eyelid conditions will be discussed here in much less detail.

As with any other surgery, the surgeon must first understand the structure of the tissues (surgical anatomy) and the nature of the disease (surgical pathology) before considering the details of the individual operations.

Surgical anatomy of the eyelids

The eyelid tissues can be divided into four layers from front to back (**Figures 8.1** and **8.2**).

1. The skin
2. The orbicularis oculi muscle
3. The tarsal plate
4. The conjunctiva

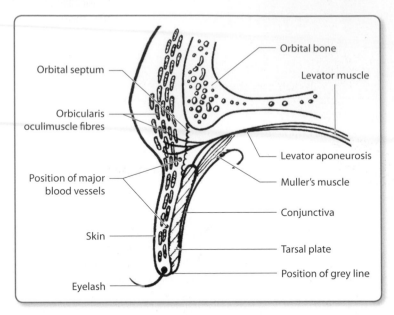

Figure 8.1 A cross section of the upper eyelid to show its four layers. Note also the position of the orbital septum, the levator muscle and its aponeurosis, and the position of the main blood vessels

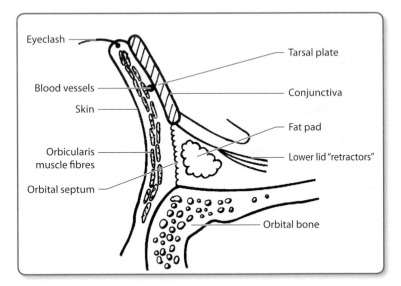

Figure 8.2 A cross section of the lower eyelid to show its four layers. Note the position of the orbital septum and lower lid retractors

The skin

There are several important features about eyelid skin:
- Eyelid skin, especially in the upper lid, is thinner, more elastic and more mobile than skin anywhere else in the body. It is also very loosely attached

to the underlying connective tissue, so that oedema fluid or blood can easily collect under the eyelid skin. Eyelid swelling is very common after surgery or trauma and may develop following infection or inflammation near the eyelid. Eyelid oedema may also occur in systemic diseases, which cause fluid retention particularly when the patient lies flat.

- There is little or no subcutaneous fat under the eyelid skin especially in the upper lid. This means the upper eyelid is a good source of skin for a free skin graft. Because the upper lid skin is so mobile and loose there is often enough to spare to fill a defect in another eyelid. There is usually no spare skin in the lower lid. In old age or after some chronic diseases like leprosy the eyelid skin, especially upper lid skin, may hypertrophy and stretch. Excess skin can easily be excised if it is causing problems.

- The eyelid has an extremely good blood supply. This means that wounds following surgery or trauma heal well and quickly without infection. Because of the good blood supply it is rarely necessary to excise traumatised or damaged eyelid tissue. It also means that free skin grafts applied to the eyelids will usually "take" satisfactorily.

In general, incisions into the eyelids should be made horizontally along the line of the skin creases. In this way they will heal well with minimal scarring. There is often spare skin in the upper lids, but by contrast there is usually none to spare in the lower lids. Therefore if any skin needs to be excised from the lower lid (for example to remove a skin tumour) it is best to make vertical not horizontal incisions to prevent contraction and ectropion.

The orbicularis oculi muscle (Figures 8.1–8.3)

This muscle is responsible for closing the eyelids. It forms a circular sheet of fibres that pass around the eyelids, and is inserted into the medial canthal tendon and surrounding bone of the lacrimal crest and the medial wall of the orbit. It is divided into 3 parts:

1. *Orbital.* The muscle fibres sweep around the orbital rim and are responsible for forced closure of the eye.
2. *Palpebral.* These muscle fibres pass over the orbital septum (the pre-septal fibres) and also over the tarsal plates (the pre-tarsal fibres). Together they are responsible for the movement of blinking. Sometimes in old age the fibrous tissue septa between these muscle fibres atrophy, so that when the muscle contracts the pre-septal portion rolls up over the pretarsal portion contributing to senile or spastic entropion in the lower lid (See **Figure 8.7**).
3. *Lacrimal.* These are a few fibres surrounding the lacrimal sac. They have a pump action sucking tears into the lacrimal sac and down to the nose.

The orbicularis muscle is supplied by the Facial nerve (the 7th cranial). The nerve fibres enter the muscle from its deep surface. Local anaesthetic injections should be placed deep to the muscle in order to paralyse it.

Incision through the muscle layer should be made horizontally in the line of the fibres. Vertical incisions will damage the muscle fibres and the wound edges will tend to gape from contraction of the muscle.

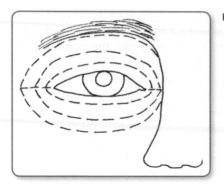

Figure 8.3 The orbicularis oculi muscle

The tarsal plates

The tarsal plates are composed of dense fibrous tissue and keep the eyelids rigid and firm. They are attached at each end to the medial and lateral canthal ligaments which join the eyelids to the bone of the orbit. The upper tarsal plate is larger than the lower. The upper lid is lifted by the Levator Palpebrae muscle which is supplied by the third cranial nerve. The muscle ends in a thin fibrous sheet or aponeurosis. This inserts into the upper border and anterior surface of the tarsal plate. It also breaks up to be inserted into the upper lid skin. Muller's muscle which is supplied from the cervical sympathetic nervous system also helps to lift the upper lid. It lies between the Levator aponeurosis and the conjunctiva and is inserted into the upper border of the tarsal plate. The lower lid has a few weak muscle fibres, called the "lower lid retractors", which also help to retract it. The Meibomian glands are embedded in the tarsal plate and produce an oily secretion which forms part of the tear film. Each gland opens on to the lid margin with a row of tiny ducts.

The conjunctiva

The conjunctiva forms a mucous membrane lining the inside of the eyelids. It stretches from the limbus, round the conjunctival fornix and to the eyelid margin. It is very firmly attached to the tarsal plate, and chronic inflammation particularly from trachoma will cause fibrosis and contracture here, so that the tarsal plate buckles and thickens. This makes the eyelid turn inwards.

The eyelid margin where the conjunctiva joins the skin is an important area. In the middle of the eyelid margin is a line of thin skin called the "grey line" because of its colour (**Figure 8.1** and **Figure 8.4**). It runs on the eyelid margin from the outer canthus to the inner canthus. Just in front of the grey line the eye lashes emerge through the skin of the eyelid margin. Just behind the grey line on the conjunctival side of the lid margin there are the openings of the Meibomian glands. If the eyelid is massaged, small beads of Meibomian secretion will appear. The tears flow along the eyelid margin from lateral end where they are produced by the lacrimal gland, to medial end where they drain into the lacrimal puncta. The oily Meibomian secretions prevent overflow of tears and help form the tear film on the surface of the cornea.

An incision into the eyelid margin along the grey line splits the eyelid into 2 parts (**Figure 8.5**). The anterior part is the skin and orbicularis muscle with the eye lashes. It is sometimes called the *anterior lamella*. The posterior part is the tarsal plate and conjunctiva, and is sometimes called the *posterior lamella*. This is a useful plane for making incisions into the eyelid margin. It does not damage the eye lash roots or the Meibomian glands and there is relatively little bleeding. As the incision is continued in this plane it will separate the orbicularis oculi muscle fibres from the front of the tarsal plate. This artificial division of the eyelid into an anterior and *posterior lamella* helps in understanding the principles of entropion surgery. If this splitting is continued still further upwards it splits the levator aponeurosis into 2 parts, the front part is attached to the eyelid skin and the back part with Muller's muscle to the tarsal plate (**Figure 8.5**).

The eyelids have a very rich blood supply which comes from both the ophthalmic artery which is a branch of the internal carotid artery, and the facial arteries which are branches of the external carotid. The arteries run between the orbicularis muscle and the tarsal plate. There is a main artery at the lateral and medial edge of the lid, and in the upper lid these two arteries are joined together by two arterial arcades which run transversely across between the muscles and the tarsal plate. One is about 3mm above the eyelid margin and the other just above the upper edge of the tarsal plate. In the lower lid there is one arterial arcade about 3mm from the eyelid margin. The veins from the eyelid pass both into the facial veins which drain into the external jugular vein and the ophthalmic veins which drain into the cavernous sinus.

It is easy to anaesthetise the eyelids with local anaesthetic. Adrenaline 1:100,000 should always be added to the local anaesthetic because the lids are so vascular. For superficial surgery to the eyelids the local anaesthetic can be injected just under the skin. For surgery to the deeper parts of the eyelids topical anaesthetic drops to the conjunctiva should also be given. If there is

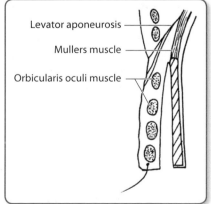

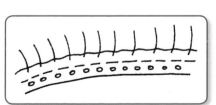

Figure 8.4 The margin of the eyelid. The position of the grey line is shown by the dotted line

Figure 8.5 The artificial division of the eyelid into an anterior and posterior lamella by an incision at the grey line

still some pain the anaesthesia can be increased with an injection through the conjunctiva into the conjunctival fornix. This is easily done in the lower lid. However the upper lid should be everted in order to give this injection.

Post operatively the good blood supply to the eyelids ensures good healing. There is usually some post operative haemorrhage into the tissues because the lids are so vascular and the connective tissues in the lids are so loose. Therefore good haemostasis is important particularly if the arterial arcades have been cut. To minimise post operative haemorrhage and tissue swelling some surgeons like to apply a firm pad and bandage for 24 hours after eyelid surgery. It should not be necessary to keep the eye padded any longer except in special cases (e.g. a skin graft). Always make sure that the pad is not rubbing against the cornea.

Surgical pathology of the eyelids

It is important to have a clear understanding of the different words used to describe abnormalities of the eyelids.

Entropion

This means that the eyelid turns inwards so that the eyelid margin and eyelashes rub against the cornea. There are two common causes:

1. Contracture of the tarsal conjunctiva and distortion of the tarsal plate causing the eyelid to turn inwards (**Figure 8.6**). This is often called "cicatricial" entropion (a cicatrix is an old fashioned word for a scar). It is much more common in the upper lid than the lower. By far the most common cause in tropical countries is long-standing trachoma. Trachoma is an infection of the conjunctiva caused by the organism *Chlamydia trachomatis*. There is a chronic inflammatory reaction in the tarsal conjunctiva and sub-conjunctival tissues. This inflammation leads on to scarring, particularly in the upper tarsal plate and conjunctiva. As the scar tissue contracts it distorts the tarsal plate and causes it to buckle inwards. The tarsal plate often becomes thickened as well and the Meibomian glands may be destroyed or blocked.
2. Laxity of the connective tissue and the tarsal plate of the lower lid in old age (**Figure 8.7**). Because the tissues are lax and the tarsal plate has lost its rigidity, when the orbicularis oculi muscle contracts to close the eyelids, the muscle fibres roll upwards and so the eyelid turns in. This is usually called "spastic" or "senile" entropion and only occurs in the lower lid.

Trichiasis

The normal eyelashes point forwards. Trichiasis means that some of the eyelashes are pointing backwards and so rub against the cornea. Obviously every patient with entropion will also have trichiasis. However there may be some misdirected lashes turning inwards without the whole eyelid turning in (i.e. trichiasis without entropion).

Trichiasis like entropion is usually a result of previous trachoma. Scar tissue from the chronic infection causes contracture around the eyelash roots and distorts them so the lashes point inwards.

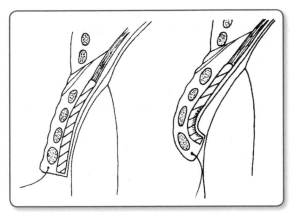

Figure 8.6 A small suture (arrowed) to bring down the conjunctiva incision

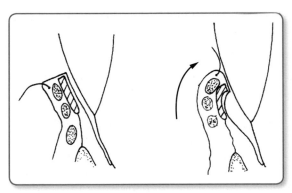

Figure 8.7 Senile or "spastic" entropion. The normal eyelid is shown on the left. As the orbicularis muscle contracts during eyelid closure the tarsal plate buckles inwards

Ectropion

This means that the eyelid is turned outwards (everted) so that the eyelid margin does not rest against the eyeball (**Figure 8.8**). In severe cases the eyelid will be so everted that the conjunctiva lining the inside of the lids will be exposed and face outwards. There are four causes of ectropion:

1. *Cicatricial ectropion.* A cicatrix is an old fashioned name for a scar. A contracture or loss of eyelid skin will cause the lid to turn outwards and is often called a "cicatricial" ectropion. It is fairly common in the lower lid because the lower lid has little or no excess skin. The lower lid does not cover the cornea, and therefore lower lid ectropion will only cause discomfort, irritation and discharge but rarely causes any damage to the cornea or loss of sight.

- Cicatricial ectropion is rare in the upper lid because the upper lid has so much spare skin. If however it does occur, the cornea is unprotected and exposed, and there is a great risk of corneal ulceration and permanent damage to the sight.
- There are several possible causes of eyelid skin contracture leading on to an ectropion. The commonest are:
- Burns–thermal or chemical causing destruction of the skin and subsequent scarring.

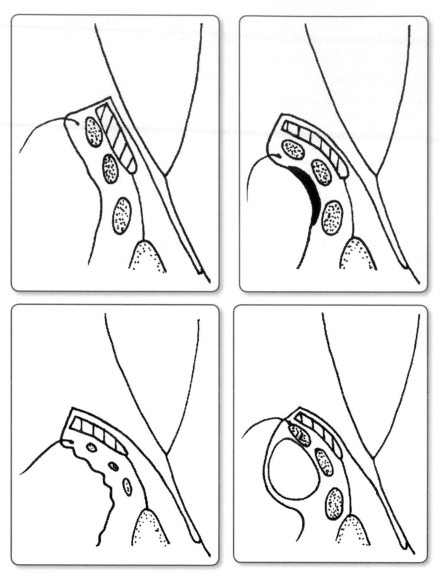

Figure 8.8 The causes of ectropion

- Trauma from injury or surgery.
- Chronic skin infection or fistulas from infected nasal sinuses.
2. *Paralytic ectropion.* Paralysis of the Orbicularis Oculi muscle which closes the eye will make the lower lid sag and fall away from the eyeball. This is called a "paralytic" ectropion and is caused by a paralysis of the Facial nerve.
3. *Senile ectropion.* This results from stretching of the lower eyelid tissues in
   old age.
4. *Mechanical ectropion.* This is caused by a tumour or thickening of the lower eyelid which by its weight pulls the eyelid away from the eyeball.

Once ectropion from any of these causes has occurred, the exposed conjunctiva becomes chronically inflamed, thickened and hypertrophic, and in this way makes the ectropion worse.

Lagophthalmos

This is the traditional word used when the eyelids will not close due to paralysis of the Orbicularis Oculi muscle. The word literally means "eye of a hare" because the ancients thought that hares went to sleep with their eyes open. The Orbicularis Oculi muscle is supplied by the Facial nerve and so a better name for lagophthalmos is *Facial Palsy*. In a mild case the eye will look normal, but when the patient tries to blink or close the eyes the weakness will become apparent. In severe cases the whole side of the face will be affected and droop from loss of function of the facial muscles. The lower lid will sag so it does not rest against the eye (paralytic ectropion). In this way facial palsy and ectropion often occur together. If the eyelids will not close properly there is a risk that the cornea will become ulcerated. This usually occurs when the patient is asleep and the eyelids are not closed. Corneal damage is particularly common in facial palsy from leprosy because the sensation of the cornea is also affected. In this way both the motor and sensory parts of the protective reflex for the cornea are absent. Most other causes of facial palsy do not also affect corneal sensation.

Ptosis

Ptosis means a drooping of the upper eyelid and it can have many causes. The most common are:
- A congenital abnormality of the levator muscle which elevates the upper lid.
- A paralysis of the third cranial nerve supplying the levator muscle, this usually causes a severe ptosis.
- A paralysis of the cervical sympathetic nerve supplying Muller's muscle, which will cause a slight ptosis.
- Senile stretching of the insertion of the levator muscle into the upper lid.
- Myopathy or myaesthenia affecting the levator muscle.
- Trauma to the upper lid.

Eyelid retraction

This is when the eyelids are abnormally open or retracted so that they do not close easily. It can occur when the eyelids have been scarred following disease or injury, or may be a complication of thyroid eye disease, which causes the levator muscle to become thickened and contracted.

Eyelid tumours

A great variety of "lumps and bumps" may be found in the eyelids. They may be congenital abnormalities, cysts, inflammatory masses, benign or malignant tumours. They may arise from any of the many different tissues present in the eyelids. The most common lesion is a retention cyst of a Meibomian gland (often called a chalazion). Malignant tumours are fortunately rare, except for a basal cell carcinoma or "rodent" ulcer. This occurs almost entirely in fair skinned people and is usually a consequence of excessive exposure to sunlight.

Basic principles of eyelid surgery

The reader should first revise the basic principles of extraocular surgery described in chapter 3. There are several other points worth mentioning or emphasising.

1. Always use adrenaline 1/100,000 in the local anaesthetic as the eyelid blood supply is so good.
2. Eyelid surgery is much easier if the lid is taut and fixed. This can be done for most eyelid operations with a lid guard (**Figure 8.20a**) or with a lid clamp (**Figure 8.20b**) (see page 255). As well as holding the lid steady and secure, these also help to protect the eye and especially the cornea from accidental damage during the operation. They also lessen the bleeding. The clamp should be applied just tight enough to occlude the marginal arteries, but not so tight that it damages the tissues permanently. The lid guard can be used as a lever to stretch the lid and push it forward. This will help lessen the bleeding by shutting off the marginal arteries.
3. Try to close the skin and conjunctiva so as to avoid any "bare areas" not covered by skin or conjunctiva.(In some operations this is not possible). If there is a bare area it will fill up with granulation tissue, which will later turn to fibrous tissue. This may contract causing the deformity to recur some months later. This is a particular problem with tarsal rotation operations for upper lid entropion.
4. Try to avoid sutures and especially knots on the inside surface of the conjunctiva where they will irritate the cornea.
5. Sutures which are closing skin wounds can be removed early (4 to 5 days) because the skin heals very quickly. However some sutures, especially mattress sutures, may be used to rotate or to alter the position of some tissue. These should be left in for about two weeks to ensure a permanent correction. If the patient cannot return in two weeks then absorbable mattress sutures can be used. Buried sutures ideally should be absorbable but can be non-absorbable.
6. Make sure there is good haemostasis from the marginal arteries at the medial and lateral margins of the tarsal plates, and try to avoid excess padding of the eye postoperatively.

Entropion and trichiasis of the upper eyelid

Upper lid entropion and trichiasis is nearly always a complication of trachoma. Repeated infection from trachoma can cause subsequent scarring and several different pathological changes in the lid.

- *Entropion.* The upper tarsal plate and the tarsal conjunctiva become scarred and contracted causing the eyelashes to rub against the cornea (see **Figure 8.6**) This is the most important complication of trachoma to affect the eyelids and one of the most common.

- *Trichiasis.* Scarring around the eyelash roots causes them to lose their alignment and some or all of them point inwards.
- *Scarring in the tarsal plate.* The tarsal plate may become thicker and the Meibomian glands may enlarge because of obstruction to their ducts and retained secretions. Sometimes the tarsal plate and the Meibomian glands may atrophy.
- *Changes to the cornea.* This is why patients lose their vision. The eyelashes rub against the cornea causing inflammation and ulceration, and this is made worse by damage to the conjunctiva and the tear film. The cornea becomes scarred and vascularised, this gradually progresses until the patient goes blind from corneal scarring.
- Shortening and retraction of the upper lid. This is not common but may occur especially after previous failed surgery. It will leave the cornea exposed and therefore at risk of being damaged. The treatment is discussed on page 250.
- *Stretching of the lateral canthal tendon.* This is also not common and is discussed on page 256–7.

The surgical correction of upper lid entropion and trichiasis is a most important subject for three reasons:

1. *Blindness from trachoma is very common.*
2. *Most of this blindness can be prevented by early surgery.*
3. *Entropion and trichiasis cause a lot of discomfort as well as sight loss.*

Trachoma is the third commonest cause of world blindness after cataract and glaucoma, and nearly all those who are blind from trachoma have had upper lid entropion for some years. If the entropion is corrected when the patient can still see, there should be no further irritation to the cornea and so no risk of the vision getting worse.

Even if the cornea is already scarred, the inflammation and scarring may gradually become less once the constant irritation from the eyelashes ceases. Therefore there may even be some gradual improvement in the vision after entropion surgery.

As well as blindness, the ingrowing eyelashes constantly rub against the very sensitive cornea, causing a great deal of irritation and discomfort. Patients who have had successful surgery for entropion are some of the most grateful, and it is still worth operating even if the eye is blind.

Trachoma surgery also has three practical problems that confront the surgeon.

1. *Trachoma is a disease of the rural areas and of poor hygiene.* Therefore trachoma surgery is often performed in poorly equipped clinics with large numbers of patients. The prevalence of blindness from trachoma appears to be falling gradually worldwide as public health is slowly improving. However there is still a huge number of patients needing entropion and trichiasis surgery, an estimated 8 million people worldwide.[1]
2. *The tissues are usually scarred and inflamed.* The surgery may be quite difficult because the anatomy is distorted and the tissues bleed easily. What seems an easy operation in a textbook may not be easy to carry out in practice.

3. *There is no general agreement about the best operation for entropion.*
    There have been very few reliable follow up studies or comparisons of
    trachoma surgery and it is difficult to choose the best operation.[2]

There are basically two possible ways of treating trichiasis and entropion:
1. To remove the lashes.
2. To operate to alter the direction of the lashes, and correct the deformity
    in the tarsal plate.

Removal of the lashes

This is only recommended if there is trichiasis without entropion and if only
a few lashes are affected.
    There are various ways of trying to remove the lashes:
*   Epilation
*   Cutting the lashes
*   Electrolysis
*   Cryotherapy
*   Excision of lash follicles or small clumps of lashes

Epilation

If the offending lashes are plucked out with tweezers, the patient obtains
temporary relief. Nearly always the lash grows again and the symptoms recur. It is possible for patients with only slight trichiasis to keep their eyes
comfortable by repeated epilation. In some cases it is best just to give the
patient or their relatives a pair of tweezers, especially patients who decline
surgery, or if surgery is unavailable.[3]

Cutting the lashes

Some patients cut off the offending lashes with scissors. This is worse than
useless as it makes the eyelash end sharper and more irritant.

Electrolysis

The principle of electrolysis is to pass a fine needle along the eyelash up to
the root of the lash. A low voltage current is then passed through this needle
causing a localised burn and the lash root will be destroyed.

Method
1. Infiltrate the eyelid with local anaesthetic.
2. Insert the electrolysis needle into the eyelash follicle along the direction
    of the eyelash to a depth of 3 mm. Switch on the current and tiny
    bubbles should appear on the surface of the eyelid where the needle
    enters the skin. Allow the current to flow for at least 5 seconds. Often
    patients feel some discomfort from the passage of current even when
    the local anaesthetic block is adequate.
3. If the lash root has been destroyed the lash can be lifted out of the
    tissues with an epilation forceps without any resistance at all. If there is
    some resistance the electrolysis should be repeated.

4. Continue until each ingrowing eyelash has been treated.

Repeated treatment with electrolysis may be necessary but it is a satisfactory way of removing a few ingrowing eyelashes.

Cryotherapy

Principle

The eyelash follicles are permanently destroyed if the eyelid margin is frozen to a temperature of about -20 degrees Centigrade with a cryoprobe. What matters is the temperature of the tissues not the temperature of the probe. The best way to measure the tissue temperature is with a fine needle thermocouple inserted into the roots of the lashes. However most units do not have such a thermocouple. It is thought that freezing twice is more effective than freezing once.

Method

1. Infiltrate the lid margin with local anaesthetic.
2. Apply the cryoprobe to the lid margin making sure the cornea is not frozen.
3. If a thermocouple is available freeze till the tissue temperature falls to –20 degrees Centigrade. Allow the tissues to thaw and then freeze again to –20 degrees Centigrade.
4. If no thermocouple is available a standard cryo unit using nitrous oxide or carbon dioxide gas should achieve a tissue temperature of –20 degrees Centigrade in 30 seconds. Therefore freeze for 30 seconds, thaw and refreeze for 30 seconds.
5. Repeat the process wherever the eyelashes need to be removed.

The advantage of electrolysis and cryotherapy is that no surgery is performed. However there are several *disadvantages*:

- Expensive equipment is required.
- The lashes may grow again following either electrolysis or cryotherapy.
- Electrolysis often needs repeating and may be quite painful. It may remove the offending lashes but can cause scarring in the surrounding tissues so that other eyelashes start turning in.
- Cryotherapy causes quite a lot of inflammation and swelling in the eyelids. It will often produce depigmentation of the frozen skin. Rarely it can cause some atrophy of the eyelid margin.

Cryotherapy can be combined with an anterior lamellar resection to help destroy the lash roots (see page 245).

Excision of misdirected lashes

This is a possible alternative to electrolysis or cryotherapy in mild cases of trichiasis. Occasionally there are just one or two small tufts of abnormal eyelashes and it is possible to excise these lashes and their roots without affecting the rest of the eyelid (**Figure 8.9**).

Method

1. Infiltrate the eyelid margin with local anaesthetic and adrenaline.
2. Incise along the grey line for just the length of the tuft of abnormal eyelashes to a depth of 3 mm.

3. Make 2 vertical cuts in the eyelid skin at either side of a tuft of lashes
    and remove the small strip of eyelid skin and lashes. Allow this small
    wound to heal by granulation.

Operations for entropion and trichiasis which realign the eyelashes

Very many operations and modifications have been described and it might
be helpful to give a summary of the different types of operation and what
each is trying to achieve. After that some recommended operations will
be described in more detail. The reader should first revise the pathological
changes caused by trachoma (page 236–7) and shown in **Figure 8.6** and also
the anatomy of the eyelid described at the beginning of this chapter. Note
especially the division of the eyelid into an anterior lamella (the skin and orbicularis muscle) and a posterior lamella (the tarsal plate and conjunctiva)
as already described.

There are basically six different methods for trying to realign the lashes.
Some operations are a combination of more than one of these methods.

Anterior lamellar shortening (Figure 8.10)

The aim is to remove some skin and orbicularis muscle so as to shorten the
anterior lamella and so help the eyelashes to evert. Mattress sutures placed
as shown in **Figure 8.17d** help to maintain the everted position of the eyelid.
This is an easy operation to do, but it does not correct any contracture of the
conjunctiva and tarsal plate. It is therefore only recommended in mild cases
of trichiasis without any entropion or serious scarring of the tarsal plate.

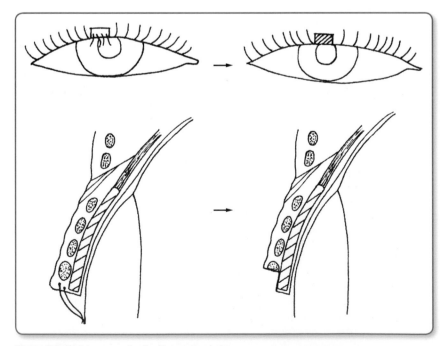

Figure 8.9 Excising a small tuft of ingrowing lashes

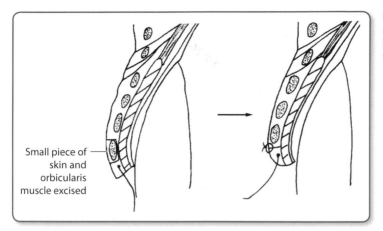

Figure 8.10 Anterior lamellar shortening

Small piece of skin and orbicularis muscle excised

Posterior lamellar lengthening (Figure 8.11)

The conjunctiva and tarsus is lengthened with a graft. This can be of mucous membrane from the mouth or cartilage plus mucous membrane from the nose. This specifically corrects the deformity and so in theory is a good operation. Unfortunately in practice it is difficult to perform. The grafted tissue may be difficult to take, to handle and to insert and secure with sutures on the inside of the eyelid. The sutures on the inside of the eyelid may lead to irritation of the cornea. For these reasons it cannot be generally recommended. However it may be worth considering for a patient with recurrence after other operations.

Splitting the grey line so that lashes can rotate forward (Figure 8.12)

This will redirect the lashes successfully, and so can correct trichiasis but will not alter any entropion. The problem is how to maintain the lashes in their new position. This can be done quite easily with some kind of eversion suture. **Figure 8.12a** shows an eversion suture tied over a small bolster made of gauze or cotton wool. This allows the split to fill with granulation tissue, but

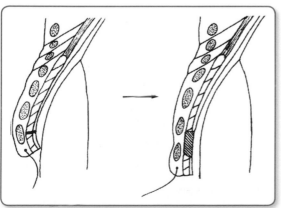

Figure 8.11 Posterior lamellar lengthening

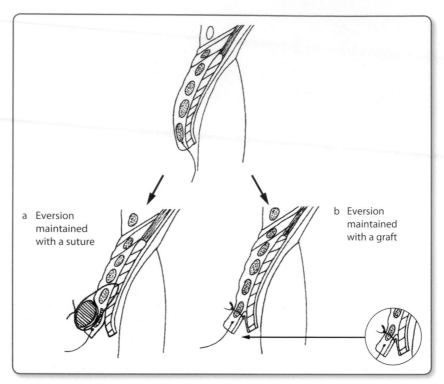

a Eversion maintained with a suture

b Eversion maintained with a graft

Figure 8.12 Splitting the grey line

unfortunately the granulation tissue tends to contract so the eyelid often returns to its original shape, thus causing a recurrence. Splitting the grey line can be combined with an anterior lamellar resection for patients who have trichiasis and no entropion.

Alternatively the split can be filled with a graft of mucous membrane (**Figure 8.12b**). This will effectively maintain the lashes in their new position but involves all the practical problems of taking and fixing a graft. Certainly it is easier to put a graft in the eyelid margin than it is to put a graft in the tarsal plate (a posterior lamellar lengthening operation).

Tarsal grooving (Figure 8.13)

A wedge is cut out of the anterior surface of the tarsus. Sutures are placed to close the wedge. This also will correct the basic defect but again the correction is sometimes hard to maintain post-operatively. One disadvantage of this operation is that tissue from the tarsal plate is excised, and the Meibomian glands are divided. It is possible to excise too much tissue leaving the eyelid shortened.

Tarsal grooving combined with anterior lamellar shortening and a grey line split is an operation known as Snellen's operation. It is a popular operation and effective for trichiasis and mild entropion or entropion when only part of the eyelid is involved. It is described in detail on page 246.

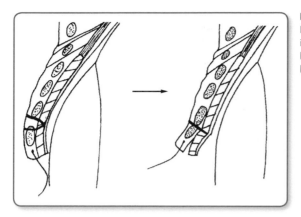

Figure 8.13 Tarsal grooving. In this diagram tarsal grooving is combined with an anterior lamellar shortening and a grey line split

Tarsal rotation (Figures 8.14 and 8.15)

The purpose of a tarsal rotation operation is to divide the tarsal plate just above the eyelid margin. This frees the lower end of the tarsal plate bearing the eyelashes to rotate outwards, so it can be fixed with sutures in its new position. This will correct the deformity very well and no tissue is excised or grafted which makes the operation more straightforward. There are however 3 disadvantages of tarsal rotation.

- There is a large bare area left on the conjunctival surface. This will fill with granulation tissue and eventually become covered with conjunctival epithelium. However the granulation tissue may later contract causing a recurrence of the entropion. According to basic surgical rules it is not good to leave an area uncovered by skin or conjunctiva at the end of an operation.
- This granulation tissue may hypertrophy causing granulomas, and these occasionally prevent wound healing and need to be excised.
- The ducts of the Meibomian glands are cut through. In practice this does not seem to cause any complications, possibly because the glands are usually damaged by the inflammatory process. However in theory it must lessen the production of Meibomian secretion.

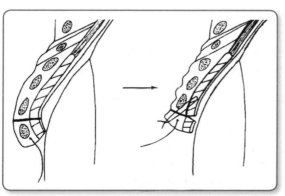

Figure 8.14 Tarsal rotation, anterior approach

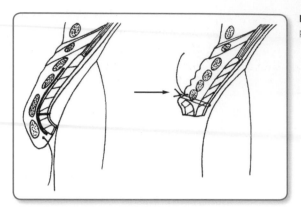

Figure 8.15 Tarsal rotation, posterior approach

In spite of these possible disadvantages tarsal rotation is a popular operation and in a prospective randomized controlled trial the results were better than for any other procedure.[4] Two methods of tarsal rotation will therefore be described in detail.

Firstly, from the anterior or skin surface (**Figure 8.14**).This operation is called the bilamellar rotation or Ballen operation. (Ballen was the first surgeon in the modern literature to describe it, and because both the anterior and posterior lamellas of the eyelid are divided it is called the bilamellar rotation). It is a fairly simple and straightforward operation and appears to produce fairly reliable and good results.

Secondly, from the posterior or conjunctival surface (**Figure 8.15**).This is called the Trabut operation, after the surgeon who described it in the nineteenth century. It is a slightly harder operation to perform but produces an extremely good reliable correction even in severe cases of entropion. It also preserves the skin and muscle layer.One advantage of theTrabut operation is that it can correct eyelid shortening (see below page 250).

Tarsal slide (Figure 7.16)

The lid is split from the grey line right up to the top edge of the tarsal plate into an anterior and posterior lamella. The two layers are then brought together with mattress sutures so that the posterior lamella comes further down than the anterior lamella. This automatically everts the lashes, although it does not correct the primary deformity in the tarsal plate and conjunctiva. It also leaves a bare area where there is no skin or mucous membrane on the surface of the eyelid which is a bad surgical principle. This is not an operation that has become very popular, but it is relatively easy to perform and appears in theory to be a sensible approach.

Conclusions and recommendations

1. A ***tarsal rotation*** procedure is recommended if there is entropion and a significant deformity of the tarsal plate.Tarsal rotation procedures seem to give the most reliable correction. The World Health Organisation (W.H.O.) has recommended the ***bilamellar rotation***

(Ballen operation) for "field conditions" where a simple, easy-to-teach and easy-to-do operation is needed. It is difficult to disagree with an international organisation like the W.H.O. but the *Trabut operation* seems in some ways better than the bilamellar rotation. It does not cut right through all layers of the eyelid, and it can correct vertical eyelid shortening.

2. *Grafting operations*, either a posterior lamellar graft or grafting into a grey line split have excellent results in expert hands but are hard to perform so they will not be described in detail.

3. If there is trichiasis only and the tarsal plate is normal, a tarsal rotation operation is not recommended because it is too destructive. Instead an *anterior lamellar resection* with a grey line split is recommended.

4. *Snellen's operation* is recommended if there is trichiasis and very slight entropion, or if only a small segment of the eyelid is affected. It is also useful if the tarsal plate is very thickened. The outward rotation of the lashes from a Snellen's operation is less than from a tarsal rotation. The advantages of Snellen's operation are that it leaves no raw granulating wounds and it is useful if the tarsal plate is badly thickened. The main disadvantages are that it does not usually correct severe entropion, and removing too big a wedge from the tarsal plate may cause lid shortening.

Details of surgical technique

These will be given for the four operations recommended, the anterior lamellar resection, the Snellen's operation, the bilamellar rotation and the Trabut's operation.

The anterior lamellar resection with a grey line split

Indications

This is a good operation to correct trichiasis if there is a fairly healthy and unscarred tarsal plate.

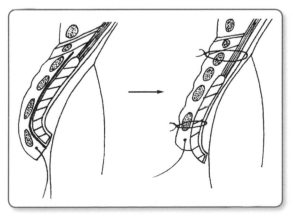

Figure 8.16 Tarsal slide

Principle

An ellipse of skin and muscle is excised from the front of the eyelid, and a grey line split also performed.With carefully placed mattress sutures, this helps to evert the inturning lashes.

Method

1. After injection of the local anaesthetic, a lid guard is inserted as a gentle lever to push the lid forward away from the eye by gentle pressure on the lower end of thelidguard (**Figure 8.17a**).This tightens the tissues and helps haemostasis.If the assistant also pulls gently on the eyelid margin with forceps this will help the exposure. An incision is made in the skin crease about 5.mm from the lid margin.
2. Cut down to the tarsal plate and separate the orbicularis muscle from the surface of the tarsal plate with blunt dissection until the black roots of the eyelashes can be seen (**Figure 8.17b**).
3. Now insert but do not tie a row of mattress sutures to evert the lashes. The sutures should enter the skin just above the lash line, then take a horizontal bite of the tarsal plate about 2 or 3 mm higher up ,and emerge again through the skin (**Figure 8.17c**). About 4 mattress sutures are needed.
4. Now make an incision about 1 to 2 mm deep in the grey line with a scalpel, and tie the mattress sutures. This will both lift up the lashes and evert them (**Figure 8.17d**).
5. Finally an ellipse of skin 2 mmwide is excised from the lower edge of the original incision.The skin incision is then sutured (**Figure 8.17e**).

There is a useful modification of this operation if patients do not mind losing their eyelashes. After step 2. when the black eyelash roots can be seen, cryotherapy can be applied directly to the lash roots as described on page 239. This will destroy the lashes and lessen the risk of recurrence.

The Snellen operation

Indications

Trichiasis with slight entropion or only involving part of the eyelid. Entropion with a very thickened tarsal plate.

Principle

A wedge is excised from the front of the tarsal plate so that the margin of the tarsal plate can rotate outwards. An ellipse of skin and muscle from the front of the eyelid is usually excised also, and a grey-line split performed as well. This helps the eyelashes to evert further.

Method

1. Step 1 is the same as for the anterior lamellar resection (page 245).
2. Step 2 is the same as for the anterior lamellar resection (page 245).
3. Keeping the lid guard in place and taut, use a scalpel blade to cut a wedge out of the tarsal plate just above the line of the eyelash roots right across the entire tarsal plate (**Figure 8.18a**). It is difficult to cut this wedge neatly and cleanly. It should not perforate the conjunctiva, but if it does perforate in places, it does not matter too much.

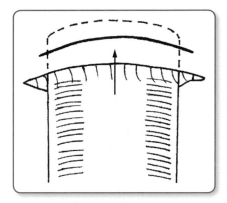

Figure 8.17a Inserting the lid guard and incising the skin

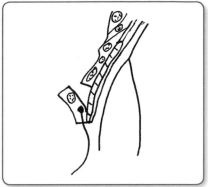

Figure 8.17b The dissection to expose the eyelash roots

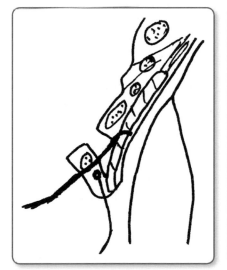

Figure 8.17c The position of the mattress sutures

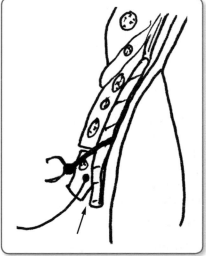

Figure 8.17d The grey line split is made (shown by the arrow) and the mattress sutures tied

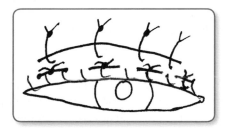

Figure 8.17e The mattress sutures and the skin sutures tied

4. Insert the mattress sutures (as shown in **Figure 8.18b** and **8.18c**). It is very important to put these sutures in correctly. They both close up the wedge in the tarsal plate and also lift the eyelashes upwards and outwards. First pass the needle through the skin just above the line of the eyelashes. Then take a short vertical bite in the main (upper) part of the tarsal plate passing the needle towards the eyelid margin. Then take a horizontal bite in the lower part of the tarsal plate just above the lashes. Where the needle comes out another short vertical bite in the upper part of the tarsal plate should be taken this time passing the needle away from the lid margin. Finally bring out the needle through the skin just above the eyelashes to complete the mattress suture. Make a row of 3 or 4 mattress sutures in all.
5. A small ellipse of skin should now be excised from the edge of the skin incision.
6. Now make an incision 1 to 2 mm deep in the grey line and tighten and tie the mattress sutures. This should close up the wedge in the tarsal plate, lift up the lashes and also evert them. Finally close the skin incision with interrupted sutures (**Figures 8.18d** and **8.18e**).
7. The sutures in the skin incision can be removed after 5 days. The mattress sutures should be left for at least 2 weeks. If it is not possible for the patient to return, then use an absorbable material so that the sutures can fall out in due course.

Division and rotation of the lower end of the tarsal plate from the conjunctival surface

Indications

Upper lid entropion of any severity, especially if there is eyelid shortening.

Principle

The tarsal plate is divided from the inside, the conjunctival side. The lower end of the tarsal plate is dissected free and then rotated right round through up to 180 degrees and fixed in the new position with sutures. This will correct entropion of any severity.

Method

1. After infiltrating with local anaesthetic and adrenaline, evert the eyelid so as to expose the conjunctival surface. The best and easiest way is to use a Cruickshank or Erhardt clamp (**Figure 8.19a**). This grasps the skin of the lid margin and holds the lid nicely everted (**Figures 8.19b** and **c**). If the clamp is not available the lid can be stretched over a Desmarres retractor held by an assistant, but this is not quite so satisfactory.
2. From the conjunctival surface incise the tarsal plate 2–3 mm from its margin along its entire width (**Figures 8.19c** and **d**). Cut right through the tarsal plate, but no deeper. At the medial end make a vertical cut down to the eyelid margin just avoiding the lacrimal punctum. At the lateral end extend the incision to the lid margin at the lateral canthus.
3. Grasp the proximal cut edge of the tarsal plate (the edge furthest from the lid margin) with toothed forceps, and using a scalpel or scissors dissect the front of the tarsal plate from the orbicularis

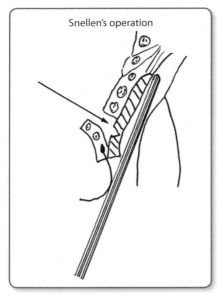

Snellen's operation

Figure 8.18a The lid guard is in place and the wedge excised from the tarsal plate is shown by the arrow

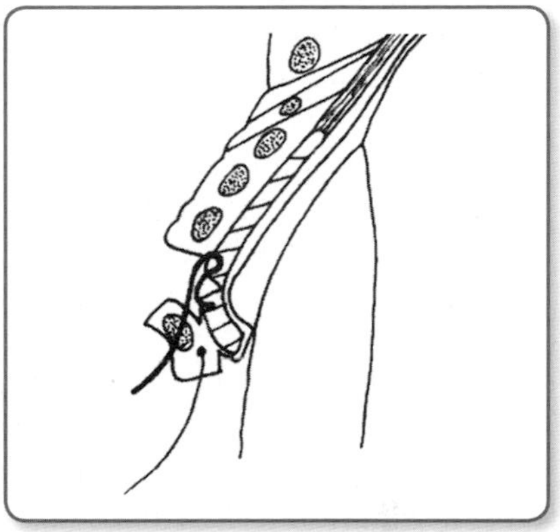

Figure 8.18b Inserting the mattress sutures

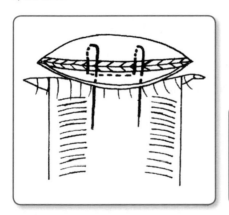

Figure 8.18c Inserting the mattress sutures

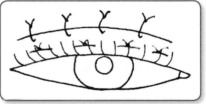

Figure 8.18d The mattress sutures and skin sutures tied

muscle (**Figure 8.19e**). Continue separating the tarsal plate from the orbicularis muscle almost up to the upper end of the tarsal plate. There is often arterial bleeding at the medial or lateral end which may need clamping and ligating, or diathermy.

4. Now grasp the distal cut edge of the tarsal plate (the edge nearest the lid margin) with toothed forceps, and with a scalpel dissect the front of the tarsal plate from the orbicularis muscle until the roots of the eyelashes are reached (**Figure 8.19f**). Be very careful with the dissection at this stage. There is often bleeding at the two ends of the wound. Try especially not to damage the eyelash roots.

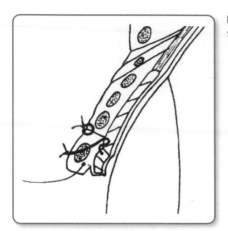

Figure 8.18e The mattress sutures and skin sutures tied

5. The eyelid margin should now be completely free from the rest of the tarsal plate. It should be possible to remove the eyelid clamp, and the lid should stay everted on its own with all the eyelashes pointing forwards (**Figure 8.19g**). If the eyelid margin still tends to turn in, a further dissection must be carried out to separate the front of the tarsal plate from the orbicularis muscle. Both the upper and lower part of the tarsal plate must be freed.
6. The eyelid margin is now rotated through 180 degrees and anchored in that position with a row of 4 mattress sutures. The needle should enter the skin through the lash line, and then take a horizontal bite of the main part of the tarsal plate and back out through the lash line again (**Figures 8.19h** and **8.19i**). Because the skin has not been incised no other sutures are needed.
7. Post operatively the mattress sutures in the lid margin should be left for about 2 weeks or if they are absorbable they can be left to fall out spontaneously.

The problem of eyelid shortening

A tarsal rotation operation will shorten the vertical length of the eyelid by about 1 to 2 mm. However a Trabut operation will usually naturally compensate for this. At step 3 (see **Figure 8.19e**) the orbicularis muscle is separated from the front of the tarsal plate. Some of the fibres of the levator muscle which lifts up the upper lid are also inserted here into the front of the tarsal plate. These fibres will automatically be separated from the front of the tarsal plate by carrying out step 3 of the Trabut operation. Therefore the eyelid tends to come down a little bit and this compensates for the natural shortening produced by the operation.

A few cases of entropion may be complicated by eyelid shortening preoperatively. It may be caused by contracture of the tissues from fibrosis or by previous surgery which has failed. Eyelid shortening means that the upper eyelid does not cover the cornea properly when the eyes are closed gently as in sleep. If the eyelid closure is inadequate there is a great risk that the cornea will be damaged and it is important to lengthen the eyelid.

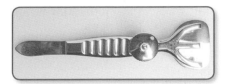

Figure 8.19a The Cruikshank or Erhardt clamp

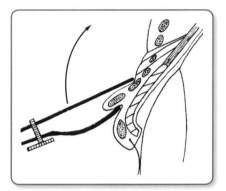

Figure 8.19b Applying the clamp

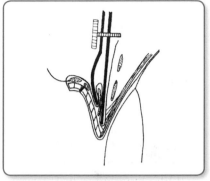

Figure 8.19c The lid is held everted by the clamp and the position of the incision through the conjunctiva and the tarsal plate is shown

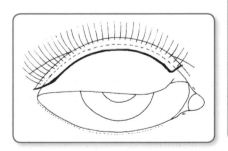

Figure 8.19d The line of the incision through the tarsal plate

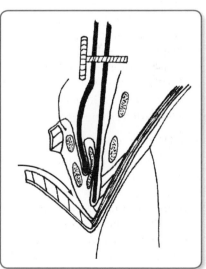

Figure 8.19e Separating the proximal tarsal plate from orbicularis muscle. The arrow shows the plane of dissection

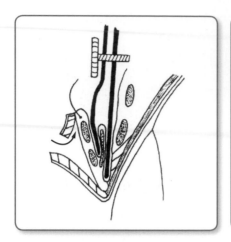

Figure 8.19f Separating the distal tarsal plate from orbicularis muscle

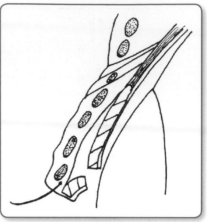

Figure 8.19g The dissected eyelid should rest with all the lashes pointing forwards

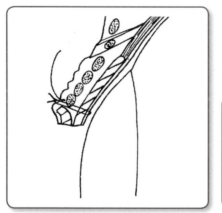

Figure 8.19h To show the position of the mattress sutures

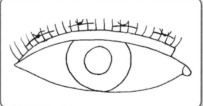

Figure 8.19i To show the position of the mattress sutures

If there is obvious eyelid shortening or retraction before the operation then the levator muscle can be more extensively divided to correct this. During step 3 (**Figure 8.19e**) the orbicularis muscle (and with it some of the insertion of the levator muscle) should be separated from the front surface of the tarsal plate right up to the upper edge of the tarsal plate. If the eyelid shortening still doesn't seem corrected, Muller's muscle should be divided (See **Figure 8.20a** and **Figure 8.5** on page 231). This will lengthen the lid by about an extra 2 mm. Muller's muscle is inserted into the upper edge of the tarsal plate, and great care is needed not to divide the conjunctiva to which it is closely attached. There may be some bleeding from the upper arterial arcade which runs at this level. The correction is maintained by inserting an extra row of 2–3 mattress sutures high up in the eyelid (**Figures 8.20b** and **c**)

The main advantage of the Trabut procedure is that it produces an extremely good correction however severe the entropion may be. If eyelid shortening

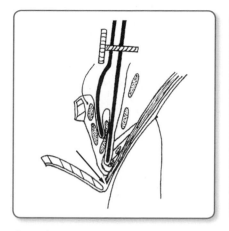

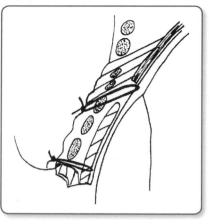

Figure 8.20a Dividing Muller's muscle, see also fig. 7.5 page 208

Figure 8.20b The position of the mattress sutures to maintain the eyelid lengthening

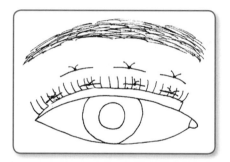

Figure 8.20c The position of mattress sutures to maintain the eyelid lengthening

is a problem it can be modified to lengthen the lid a little. The main disadvantage is the large granulating area which is left on the posterior surface of the eyelid which takes a long time to heal. Occasionally small granulomas develop, which may need to be excised. Another disadvantage is that quite extensive dissection is required from the conjunctival surface so the operation is not quite so easy to perform, especially if a Cruickshank or Erhardt clamp is not available.

Bilamellar or full thickness tarsal rotation (Ballen operation)

Indications

Entropion of any severity.

Principle

The eyelid is divided transversely through all layers. The lid margin can then be resutured in an everted position.

Method

1. After infiltration with local anaesthetic and adrenaline a lid guard or spatula is inserted between the eyelid and the eyeball (**Figure 8.21a**).

If the assistant presses gently on the lower end of this, it will act as a lever pushing the eyelid forward and tightening it. This helps to prevent bleeding.Alternatively a large lid clamp (**Figure 8.21b**) will both secure the lid and prevent bleeding. However using a lid clamp makes it difficult to reach the lateral and medial ends of the lid which are caught in the clamp.The incision may need to be extended when the clamp has been removed. The W.H.O. description of the operation uses artery forceps at the medial and lateral end of the eyelids both to fix the lid and prevent bleeding(**Figure 8.21c**).

2. Make a transverse skin incision 3–4 mm above the lid margin the whole length of the lid, and down to the tarsal plate.

3. Separate the orbicularis muscle fibres from the surface of the tarsal plate towards the margin of the lid until the lash roots are just visible (**Figure 8.21d**). This will be about 2–3 mm from the lid margin.

4. Cut right through the tarsal plate and conjunctiva at this level 2 mm from the lid margin (**Figure 8.21e**). This incision must be started with a scalpel. It can be completed with either a scalpel or scissors. Take great care that this incision runs exactly parallel with the lid margin just above the eyelash roots and that it runs the whole length of the lid. Check for bleeding and ensure haemostasis especially at the lateral and medial ends of the incision. Remember that the blood supply to the eyelid margin will now come from either end of the separated strip of eyelid tissue. Therefore take great care not to damage the tissue at each end of the lid margin (**Figure 8.21f**).

5. Place 4 mattress everting sutures from the skin just above the lashes, into the upper tarsal plate and back through the skin (**Figure 8.21g and h**). Tie the stitches snugly and the eyelid should freely evert. Aim for a slight overcorrection so that the lid margin appears slightly everted. If the entropion appears under-or overcorrected at this stage the stitches should be readjusted. If they are placed higher up in the tarsal plate the correction will be increased and if they are placed lower down in the tarsal plate the correction will be diminished.

6. Place interrupted skin stitches to close the incision (**Figure 8.21h**).

7. The use of a specially designed lid clamp:[5]

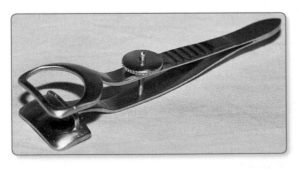

A special lid clamp for upper lid entropion has recently been designed – the Waddell Clamp. Obtainable from Collton Hailsham Ltd, UK; email: colltonhailsham@btinternet.com; telephone: +44 (0) 1323743629 www.colltonhailsham.com

The lid is placed in it with the lid margin up against the prominent ridge and the small markers on the clamp show the point at which to make the cut

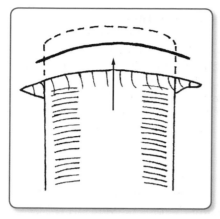

Figure 8.20a The skin incision using a lid guard

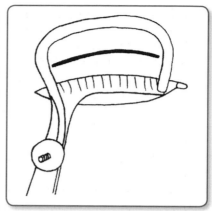

Figure 8.20b The skin incision using a lid clamp

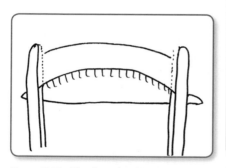

Figure 8.20c The show the skin incision using two artery forceps

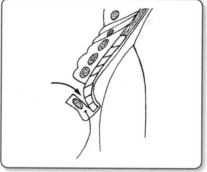

Figure 8.20d Dissection through the skin and muscle

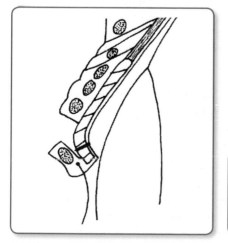

Figure 8.20e To show the incision through the tarsal and conjunctiva

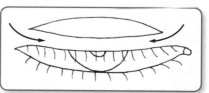

Figure 8.20f The blood supply to the separated eyelid margin

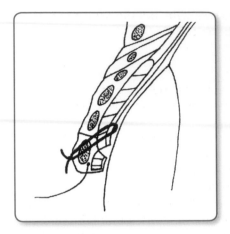

Figure 8.21g The position of the mattress sutures to evert the lid margin

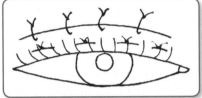

Figure 8.21h The mattress sutures and the sutures closing the skin incision

in the defective tarsal plate. The operation is shown in the DVD which accompanies the book.

The main advantage of this operation is its simplicity. It has produced good results under "field" conditions. Even in ideal circumstances operations are not as easy as the diagrams in a textbook and therefore the simplest operation is often the best. Entropion surgery is often carried out in far from ideal circumstances where simple operations have even more advantages.

The main disadvantage is that it leaves a granulating wound on the conjunctival surface of the lid like the Trabut operation.

Post operative care

Post operative care for all the operations described is identical. Antibiotic ointment is always applied to the eye. A pressure pad and bandage is usually applied for 24 hours to minimise bleeding. There is often considerable post operative swelling, and applying a firm pad and bandage will minimise this swelling and prevent early eyelid movement. Once the pad has been removed the eye should be kept open and antibiotic ointment applied. Skin stitches can be removed after five days but the mattress sutures which are used to hold the eyelid everted should be left for at least 2 weeks. If absorbable sutures are used they will cause a little more tissue reaction than either silk or polypropylene sutures, but eventually they will fall out so the patient will not have to return for removal of the mattress sutures.

Stretching of the lateral canthal tendon

Some patients may have suffered with upper lid entropion for many years, and the constant irritation and squeezing of the eyelids may cause stretching of the lateral canthal tendon so that the eyelid becomes very loose and floppy. The entropion should be corrected but it may be helpful at the end of the operation or later to tighten the lateral canthal tendon. **Figure 8.29** shows how to expose the tendon. A non-absorbable suture can then be placed from the lateral edge of the tarsal plate into the periosteum at the lateral orbital margin to tighten up the tendon.

Lower lid entropion

Entropion of the lower lid is usually caused by stretching and atrophy of the lower lid tissues as a result of degeneration from ageing. Several different changes occur together.

- There is atrophy of the tarsal plate so it buckles inwards when the orbicularis muscle contracts on eyelid closure.
- Atrophy of the septa between the muscle fibres in the orbicularis causes the muscle to bunch up and roll in on lid closure.
- Horizontal stretching or laxity of the lower lid makes it weak and floppy.

The best way to test for horizontal stretching of the lower lid is to pull it downwards away from the eyeball. If on releasing it does not snap back into place, there is horizontal lid laxity.

Many different procedures have been described to tighten up the lower lid. One fairly easy and successful operation is a transverse full-thickness lid incision closed with everting mattress sutures, known as the Wies procedure. If there is horizontal lid laxity, and in most cases there is, some tissue should be excised at the same time to tighten the lid.

The wies procedure

Principle

A transverse incision is made through all layers of the lower lid. Everting mattress sutures are then placed across the incision. The scar of the incision helps to stop the muscle fibres rolling up. The everting sutures help correct the entropion. At the same time the weak muscle fibres called the retractors of the lower lid are tightened. This holds down the lower border of the tarsal plate and stops the lid turning in.

Method

1. After injecting the tissues with local anaesthetic and adrenaline, either insert a lid guard between the lower lid and the eye (**Figure 8.22a**) or clamp the lid with a broad lid clamp (**Figure 8.23a**). These tighten and stretch the lid making the surgery easier. They also stop bleeding and protect the eye.
2. Incise horizontally through all layers of the lid 4–5 mm from the lid margin with a scalpel (**Figure 8.22a and b**). The line of incision should be at the lower end of the tarsal plate. It may be easier to complete the incision with scissors.
3. Apply 3 or 4 everting mattress sutures of 4-0 or 5-0 catgut. These go through the skin just below the lash line, then into the conjunctiva fairly far down towards the inferior fornix and then back through the skin again just below the lash line (**Figure 8.22c**).
4. Remove the lid guard or clamp, and then tighten and tie the mattress sutures (**Figure 8.22d**) starting from the lateral end so the lid is just everted giving a slight ectropion. This will correct itself within a few

days. Then suture the skin incision with interrupted sutures (**Figure 8.22e**). Usually there is no need to pad the eye. The skin sutures can be removed after a week but the mattress sutures should be left to fall out. (If they are non-absorbable they should be left in for at least two weeks to encourage some scar tissue to develop which strengthens the lax tissues).

5. If there is horizontal lid laxity, about 3mm of the lid margin should be excised after step 2 (**Figure 8.22f**). The cut edges of the eyelid are then sutured before prceeding to step 3.

Cicatricial lower lid entropion

Occasionally lower lid entropion can be caused by scarring and contracture of the conjunctiva and tarsal plate. In other words cicatricial entropion may occur in the lower lid just as in the upper. Cicatricial entropion of the lower lid can be corrected by a similar operations to the Wies operation for senile entropion. However at step 2 the eyelid should be incised horizontally through the scarred tarsal plate about 3 mm from the lid margin as shown in **Figure 8.22g**. (Compare this with the incision shown in **Figure 8.22b**) The everting mattress sutures should be placed in the lower part of the tarsal plate, as shown in **Figure 8.22g**, rather than in the conjunctiva below the tarsal plate.

Pentagonal wedge excision

If the lower lid is very lax or if the entropion has recurred after the above operation then a Pentagonal Wedge Excision will tighten the lid and in this way correct the entropion (**Figure 8.23**). One way of demonstrating lid laxity is to pull the lower lid downwards away from the globe. It should spring back to rest snugly against the globe. If it does not there is lid laxity.

Method

1. After local anaesthetic and adrenaline injection insert a lid guard or lid clamp (**Figure 8.23a**).
2. Excise a full thickness pentagon of tissue from the lateral part of the eyelid using scissors (**Figure 8. 23b**). Each edge of the pentagon should be about 4 mm long. The two edges of the wound should come together so the lid rests firmly against the eye but is not under excessive tension.
3. Suture the deep layer (the tarsal plate and conjunctiva) with interrupted absorbable sutures (**Figure 8.23c**). Make sure that the knots are not on the conjunctival surface or they will irritate the eye. The eyelid margin must be very carefully sutured so that the two edges come together without a notch. Then suture the skin using interrupted sutures (**Figure 8.23d**). The segment that is removed from the eyelid is deliberately shaped like a pentagon. In this way the lower part of the tarsal plate is tightened more than the margin of the tarsal plate. This helps prevent the tarsal plate from rolling over, which happens in entropion.

A similar operation will cure lower lid ectropion due to eyelid laxity. However for this a segment of the eyelid removed should not be a pentagon but a slightly different shape (**Figure 8.23e**).

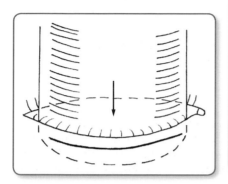

Figure 8.22a The skin incision using a lid spatula

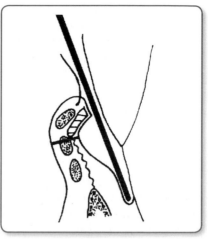

Figure 8.22b The position of the incision

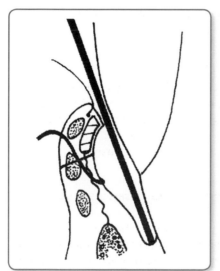

Figure 8.22c The position of the mattress sutures

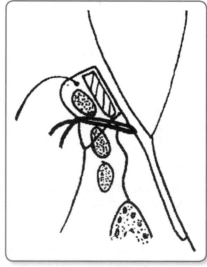

Figure 8.22d The lid margin everts as the mattress sutures are tightened

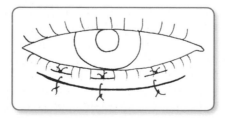

Figure 8.22e The mattress sutures and the sutures closing the incision

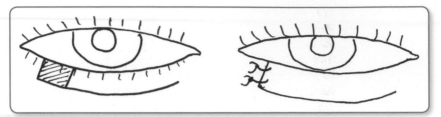

Figure 8.22f To show the piece of tissue from the eyelid margin which is excised to correct the horizontal lid laxity

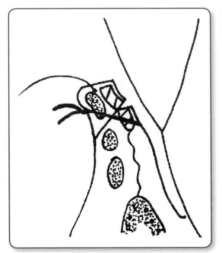

Figure 8.22g The position of the eyelid incision and mattress suture for cicatrical entropion of the lower lid

Ectropion

For a cicatricial ectropion resulting from scarring of the skin 2 procedures will be described, the Z plasty and the skin graft.

The Z plasty

If there is only a localised linear scar it may be possible to release the contracture caused by the scar with a Z plasty (**Figure 8.24**).

Method

Two triangular flaps of skin are cut either side of the scar and the triangles transposed after undermining the skin flaps. The effect of this is that the scar is lengthened and tissue brought in from the sides. In **Figure 8.24** the scar line EF is made longer and the distance CD is made shorter. It is possible to make several Z-plasties rather than just one along the line of a scar. If the scar is very thick, it may help to excise the scar itself with parallel incisions down each side of it, before carrying out the Z-plasty.

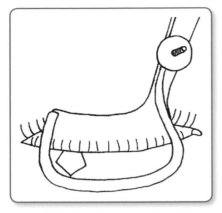

Figure 8.23a The skin incision using a lid clamp

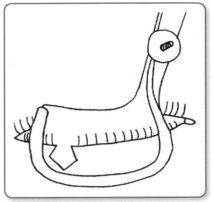

Figure 8.23b The full thickness wedge of eyelid removed

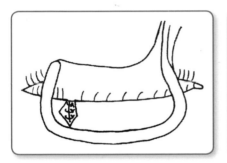

Figure 8.23c Suturing the tarsal plate

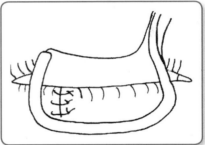

Figure 8.23d Suturing the skin

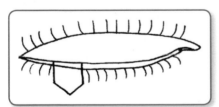

Figure 8.23e Eyelid excision for senile ectropion

Skin graft

If there is an extensive loss of skin, a skin graft is necessary. Because the blood supply to the lids is so good a full thickness graft will usually take but make sure the graft contains no fat.

Method

1. Prepare the bed for the graft. Incise along the edge of the scar so as to free the tissues completely (**Figure 8.25b**). Make absolutely sure there is no bleeding from the bed where the graft will be placed. Haemorrhage

will separate the graft from its bed and cause it to fail. The other common cause for graft failure is infection in the bed of the graft.

2. A piece of sterile silver paper or similar material is cut to match the shape of the area to be grafted. This is used to make sure that the donor skin is the right shape and size. The donor skin will shrink by 10% and so should be cut slightly larger than the defect.

3. Cut the graft. The best donor site is the upper lid if you are sure there is enough skin to spare. If the lower lid is being grafted with skin from the upper lid on the same side, a small pedicle can be made which ensures the blood supply of the graft remains intact. If there is any doubt about using skin from the upper lid the next best site is the area immediately behind the ear. This of course must be a free graft. Having cut the graft using a scalpel and scissors make sure there is no fat on its undersurface, and if there is trim it off. This is done by laying the graft skin side downwards on a board and using scissors to trim off any subcutaneous fat. Keep the graft moist in normal saline and close up the defect in the donor site.

    For a very large defect a split skin graft from the arm or the thigh may be needed if there is not enough skin behind the ear.

4. Apply the graft to the graft bed and suture it in place (**Figure 8.25c**). Keep some stitches long and use these to tie a bolster of moistened sterile cotton wool or Vaseline gauze over the graft (**Figure 8.25d**). This

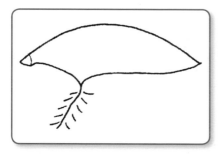

Figure 8.24a The shortened scar

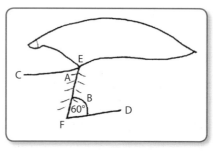

Figure 8.24b Marking out the Z with cuts at 60 degrees to the scar line

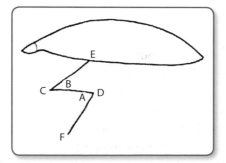

Figure 8.24c Transposing the flaps after they have been undermined

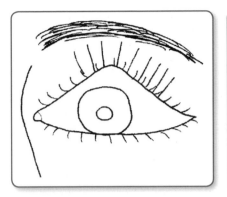

Figure 8.25a Cicatricial ectropion of the upper lid

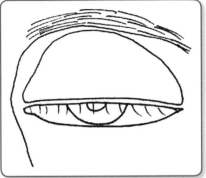

Figure 8.25b Incision along the edge of this scar to free the lid margin leaving a bare area to be grafted

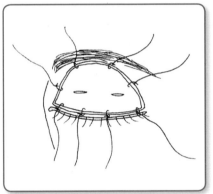

Figure 8.25c Suturing the graft in place and making two small holes in it

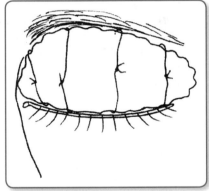

Figure 8.25d The sutures tied over a bolster

is to keep the graft in place resting tightly on the graft bed. Make 2 or 3 small holes in the graft to drain any possible haematoma.

5. Apply a bandage and leave for at least 5 days. Remove the bandage and the bolster with very great care. Some surgeons advise systemic antibiotics to prevent the graft becoming infected.

Senile ectropion

If the ectropion is due to laxity of the lower lid a wedge can be excised usually from its lateral end as already described.

Lateral tarsal strip

A popular technique for the correction of lower lid ectropion, especially when the ectropion is associated with laxity of the lateral canthal tendon, is a lateral tarsal strip procedure.

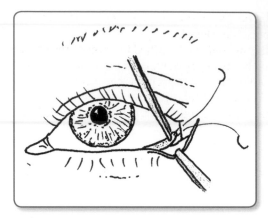

Figure 8.26 The lateral tarsal strip is sutured with double-armed non-absorbable suture to the peri-osteum.

The procedure aims to shorten the lid, and create a 'new' lateral canthal tendon from the lateral edge of the lower tarsal plate.

Firstly, make a horizontal incision through the skin at the lateral canthus. Then cut the lower part of the lateral canthal tendon, but leave the upper part of the lateral canthal tendon alone.

To create the 'new tendon', carefully excise skin, orbicularis muscle fibres, the lashes and the conjunctiva from the lateral part of the tarsal plate. The length of this new tendon will depend on the degree of laxity, but should be only a few millimetres.

Using blunt dissection, expose the peri-osteum over the lateral orbital rim.

Using a double armed 4-0 or 5-0 non-absorbable suture (Prolene is very good), pass the needles through the edge of the new lateral tarsal strip. Then pass each arm of the suture into the peri-osteum, starting behind the orbital rim. When the suture is tightened, the lateral tarsal strip is pulled towards and posterior to the orbital rim. Finally, tie the sutures firmly.

Close the wound by passing absorbable (Vicryl) 6/0 suture through the orbicularis. Then close the skin with interrupted sutures.

Tarsorrhaphy

A tarsorrhaphy closes the eyelids with sutures. It is usually performed to help protect the cornea from ulceration when the eyelids will not close following a facial palsy. Leprosy patients are particularly at risk because they often have no corneal sensation as well as a facial palsy. Sometimes a tarsorrhaphy is done to close the lids temporarily to help a long-standing corneal ulcer to heal.

The position and size of the tarsorrhaphy will vary according to the disease. Nearly all patients with a permanent facial palsy will benefit from a permanent lateral tarsorrhaphy of about one third of the total eyelid length. Many will also benefit from a medial canthoplasty to tighten the inner end of the eyelid as well. Sometimes the lower lid becomes very stretched with a permanent facial palsy causing ectropion and these patients may also need a wedge excision to tighten up the lower lid (see **Figure 8.23e**, page 261).

A temporary tarsorrhaphy to heal a chronic corneal ulcer is usually done near the centre of the lids to keep them closed.

There are other more complex operations described in order to restore the ability of the eyelids to shut. The two most popular are either to use the temporalis muscle and tendon to close the eye when the temporalis muscle contracts, or else to insert the hypoglossal nerve which supplies the tongue muscles into the facial nerve of the same side. These are both highly specialised procedures.

Lateral tarsorrhaphy

Suturing together the lateral ends of the eyelids is both an effective and easy treatment for facial palsy.

Method

1. Incise along the grey line for the lateral one-third of the length of the eyelids. For a permanent tarsorrhaphy excise a triangle of skin and eyelashes from the lower lid and a corresponding triangle of tarsal plate and conjunctiva from the upper lid (**Figure 8.27a**).
2. Overlap these two triangles, and sew them together with mattress sutures. To provide a wide area of pressure these sutures may be tied over a small rubber bolster (**Figure 8.27b**). Leave the sutures for 2 weeks.

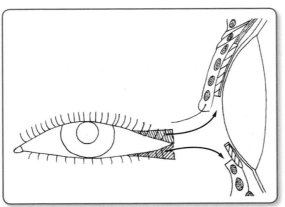

Figure 8.27a Lateral tarsorrhaphy to show the tissue excised

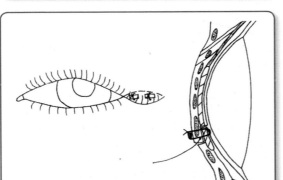

Figure 8.27b Lateral tarsorrhaphy. The lids are sutured together with mattress sutures over a small bolster

3. For a temporary tarsorrhaphy incise the grey line of each eyelid but do not excise any tissue. A temporary tarsorrhaphy may be at the lateral end of the lid for facial palsy or in the middle of the lid to heal a chronic corneal ulcer. Insert mattress sutures over bolsters to join the two raw surfaces (**Figure 8.27c**).

Many leprosy patients and some patients with other neurological diseases may have corneal anaesthesia as well as a facial palsy, thus putting the cornea at very great risk of damage. These patients may need a very large lateral tarsorrhaphy and also a further tarsorrhaphy medial to the pupil, just leaving a tiny hole in the lids to see through (**Figure 8.27d**). It is better to look as if the eye is almost shut than to go blind from exposure changes to the cornea. When doing a medial tarsorrhaphy near the lacrimal puncta or canaliculi great care must be taken not to damage the lacrimal passages.

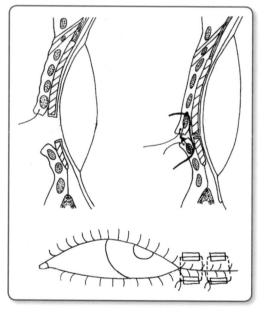

Figure 8.27c Temporary tarsorrhaphy

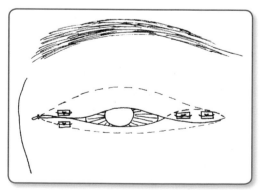

Figure 8.27d Extensive lateral and medial tarsorrhaphy for severe corneal exposure and corneal anaesthesia

Medial canthoplasty

Even after a successful lateral tarsorrhaphy many patients still have slight ectropion of the inner end of the eyelid. This causes excessive watering of the eye because the lacrimal punctum does not touch the globe. Also the lacrimal pump is not working because of the facial palsy. A medial canthoplasty is a simple way of helping tear drainage in a patient with permanent facial palsy. It tightens the medial end of the lid and also brings the lacrimal punctum up against the eye.

Method

1. Make a shallow cut along the medial edge of each eyelid medial to the puncta. Take very great care not to damage the lacrimal canaliculi which are close to the edge of the eyelid. Lacrimal probes must first be placed in the canaliculi to identify and protect them from damage (**Figure 8.28b**).
2. A small Z plasty is now marked out on the skin by incising as shown to make two small skin triangles (**Figure 8.28c**).These small triangles of skin are dissected free.
3. The two conjunctival surfaces are sewn together with very fine absorbable sutures (**Figure 8.28d**).
4. The two skin flaps are transposed and sutured as shown (**Figure 8.28e**). This pulls the lower punctum up and in towards the eye.

The drainage of tears may be helped by enlarging the lower lacrimal punctum with a punctoplasty (see page 302).

It is possible to do a tarsorrhaphy medial to the pupil but lateral to the puncta for very severe cases of corneal exposure and damage (**Figure 8.27d**).

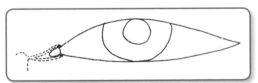

Figure 8.28a The lacrimal canaliculi are very close to the margin of the eyelid

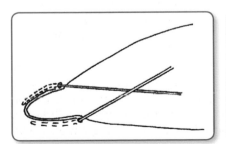

Figure 8.28b The incision with a probe in each canaliculus

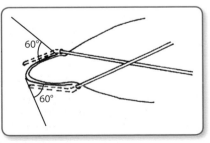

Figure 8.28c Cutting the flaps for the Z plasty

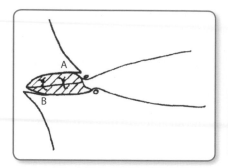

Figure 8.28d Suturing the conjunctival surfaces

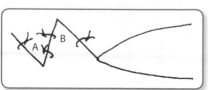

Figure 8.28e Transposing and suturing the flaps of skin

Meibomian cysts

These are very common and often get better spontaeneously with time. They can be incised and curetted quite easily.

1. After infiltration with local anaesthetic and adrenaline apply a Meibomian clamp and evert the lid (**Figure 8.29a**).
2. Incise vertically through the conjunctiva into the tarsal plate (**Figure 8.29b**) and use a curette to scoop out the cyst contents (**Figure 8.29c**).
3. Apply a pad until the bleeding stops and then give antibiotic ointment twice daily.

Treatment of eyelid tumours

The management of many eyelid tumours is quite complex and will depend basically on the nature of the tumour, its site and its size. Because it is a complex subject only the basic principles will be described here.

The type of tumour

The majority of eyelid tumours are benign and excision is the recommended treatment for them. If histopathology services are available it is very helpful to carry out a small biopsy first to know what the nature of the tumour is and plan appropriate treatment. The most common malignant tumour is a *basal cell carcinoma* or rodent ulcer which is found in fair skinned races when exposed to excessive sunlight.

When suspecting a malignant tumour, a rim of about 4 mm of healthy tissue should also be excised to make sure all the tumour cells have been removed. When excising a basal cell carcinoma it is better to excise too much tissue and leave the patient with a scar, then to excise too little and risk tumour recurrence. This is especially true for young patients with basal cell carcinoma. If the luxury of a local pathology service is available, these cases are best managed with frozen section histology at the time of the operation.

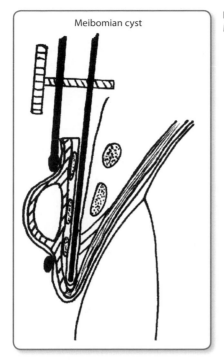

Meibomian cyst

Figure 8.29a Incision and curettage of a Meibomian cyst

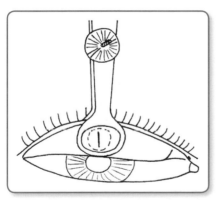

Figure 8.29b Applying the clamp and incising into the cyst. Make the incision vertical and avoid the lid margin

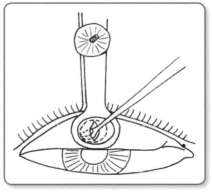

Figure 8.29c Curetting the cyst

The site

Tumours involving only the skin can usually be removed without excising the deeper tissues of the lid. Any lower lid skin excision should be repaired with a vertical suture line to prevent ectropion. An upper lid skin excision can usually be repaired with a horizontal suture line unless there is extensive skin loss. If there is extensive skin loss a graft is necessary (see page 261–3). Tumours near the lid margin, especially basal cell carcinomas will require full thickness lid excision.

The upper lid is essential for a healthy cornea but the lower lid can be sacrificed without loss of sight. Therefore the lower lid can be used to repair the upper lid, but usually not the other way round. Lesions of the medial end of the lids are difficult to excise because of the risk of damaging the lacrimal canaliculi.

The size

Up to one third of the total length of the lid can be excised and the wound closed with direct sutures in 2 layers. A lateral cantholysis will help to bring the wound edges together. This is done by making a horizontal skin incision in the region of the lateral canthus (**Figures 8.30a** and **b**) and then dividing with a vertical cut the lateral canthal tendon of the affected lid (see **Figure 8.30c**).

If more than a third of the upper lid has been removed a rotation flap from the lower lid can be used to help fill in the defect. When planning this flap be very careful to take it from the correct part of the lower lid so that it will rotate properly into the defect. Alternatively tissue can be transferred from the lower lid to the upper by an advancement flap. After 3 weeks the pedicle for either of these flaps can be divided.

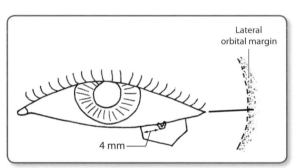

Figure 8.30a Incising over the lateral canthal tendon

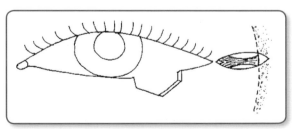

Figure 8.30b Identifying the tendon

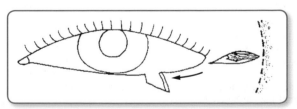

Figure 8.30c Cutting the tendon to the affected eyelid will mobilise that eyelid

If more than a third of the lower lid has been removed, a rotation or an advancement flap from the upper lid can be used to fill the defect. However the upper lid is more important to the health of the eye than the lower. Therefore this may not be appropriate, and must be done very carefully so as not to damage the healthy upper lid. A rotation flap from the cheek can also be used to replace the lower lid. It may be lined with mucous membrane from the mouth. There are many possible flaps recommended for different types of eyelid defects.

For further reading and resources

There are many text books on eyelid surgery, but "A Manual of Systematic Eyelid Surgery" by J.R.O. Collins, Churchill Livingstone. 4th Ed. London 2012, is strongly recommended.

The W.H.O. have produced a monograph entitled "Trichiasis Surgery for Trachoma – the Bilamellar Tarsal Rotation Procedure" Geneva, Switzerland: WHO; 1993 (1998;WHO/PBL/93.29) (Reacher M, Foster A, Huber J). It describes in detail this one operation to correct upper lid entropion which is such a major cause of blindness.

The International Centre for Eye Health have produced a free DVD which contains step-by-step teaching videos of both bilamellar tarsal rotation and posterior lamellar tarsal rotation procedures. In addition, there is extensive supporting material, such as the assessment and counselling of patients, setting up an operating theatre, sterilising instruments and post-operative care. It can be obtained free of charge from TALC (Email info@talcuk.org) and is available in English and French.

References

1. Mariotti SP, Pascolini D, Rose-Nussbaumer J. Trachoma: global magnitude of a preventable cause of blindness. Br J Ophthalmol 2009;93:563-8.
2. Rajak SN, Collin JR, Burton MJ. Trachomatous trichiasis and its management in endemic countries. Surv Ophthalmol 2012;57:105-35.
3. Rajak SN, Habtamu E, Weiss HA, et al. Epilation for trachomatous trichiasis and the risk of corneal opacification. Ophthalmology 2012;119:84-9.
4. Reacher MH, Munoz B, Alghassany A, Daar AS, Elbualy M, Taylor HR. A controlled trial of surgery for trachomatous trichiasis of the upper lid. Arch Ophthalmol 1992;110:667-74.
5. Waddell K. A new clamp for bilamellar torsal rotation for trachomatous trichiasis. Community Eye Health 2009. March; 22(69): 13

Surgery of the conjunctiva and cornea

> **Objectives**
> - Conjunctival flaps to cover the cornea
> - Pterygium excision
> - Conjunctival tumour excision
> - Removal of a sub-conjunctival loa-loa worm
> - Surgery for corneal scars

The conjunctiva lines the surface of the eye and the inside of the lids. It is a mucous membrane which protects the eye from infection and keeps its surface moist. It is vital for the health of the cornea. Under the mucosal surface of the conjunctiva there are numerous patches of lymphoid tissue, and a rich supply of blood vessels and lymphatics. The conjunctiva is closely related to the cornea both in structure and function. At the limbus the conjunctival epithelium becomes the corneal epithelium.

The cornea

Corneal diseases are very common in hot climates, and in many cases will cause loss of vision from corneal scarring. Indeed blindness from corneal scarring is very common in developing countries but rare in developed ones. There are many reasons for this, some from the climate of the tropics and some from poor hygiene and nutrition:

- Excess solar and ultra violet radiation causes pterygium and solar keratopathy.
- In desert areas the sand and dust constantly irritate the eye and can cause foreign bodies which scar and ulcerate the cornea.
- Where the climate is hot and humid, bacteria and fungi can easily multiply and cause corneal abscesses.
- In rural communities there is a higher risk of scratching the cornea with a twig or thorn.
- Poor hygiene and overcrowding encourages the spread of eye to eye infections. Trachoma is the most common of these but other organisms like adenovirus, herpes simplex and bacterial conjunctivitis are spread in the same way.
- Measles often affects the cornea, where measles vaccination is not available.

- Malnutrition causes vitamin A deficiency which can cause devastating corneal ulcers in young children.
- Traditional eye medication may be given by untrained healers and some of these medications can be toxic to the cornea.

The conjunctiva is on the surface of the eye, and so there is no difficulty in surgical access. Anaesthesia is usually easy, topical anaesthetic drops will anaesthetise the conjunctival surface and a sub conjunctival injection of local anaesthetic will provide additional anaesthesia. Dilute adrenaline should always be added because the conjunctiva is so vascular. The sub-conjunctival local anaesthetic injection also separates the conjunctiva from the underlying sclera and so makes surgery easier. Retrobulbar anaesthesia is rarely necessary.

There are several indications for conjunctival surgery. The most important are:

- A flap of conjunctiva can be used to cover diseased or damaged cornea.
- Excision of a pterygium or a conjunctival neoplasm.
- Reconstruction of damaged or scarred conjunctiva after disease or injury.

Conjunctival flaps to cover the cornea

The conjunctiva can provide a very useful protective covering for the cornea. Being vascular tissue, it brings cells such as fibroblasts and white cells into the cornea which help corneal ulcers and wounds to heal. It also provides a physical cover to the ulcer or wound. When the healing process is complete the conjunctiva will often spontaneously retract back to the limbus. If it does not, then the flap can easily be replaced. Naturally an opaque scar will be left in the damaged cornea but hopefully the eye will be saved from worse damage and will heal quicker.

The common indications for a conjunctival flap are:

- A long-standing and deep corneal ulcer which is not healing, particularly if the ulcer has perforated or is about to perforate. Sometimes a perforated ulcer can be sealed with tissue glue (see page 288).
- A penetrating corneal wound with iris prolapse which has presented too late for a primary repair (see page 319).
- Bullous keratopathy which is nearly always caused by damage to the corneal endothelium during cataract surgery (see page 185). The patient experiences recurrent and severe pain from the bullae or ulcers in the corneal epithelium. If the corneal epithelium is replaced with conjunctiva which has lymphatics and blood vessels, the ulceration ceases and the pain subsides. However the vision will not improve, for this a corneal graft is needed.

There are different ways of getting the conjunctiva to cover the cornea. The best is to advance a flap of conjunctiva from the limbus to cover the cornea. This is a versatile and simple operation by which the conjunctiva can be used to cover either a small peripheral lesion or the entire cornea. For peripheral lesions the conjunctiva can be advanced from the adjoining limbus (**Figure 9.1**). To cover the central cornea or the whole cornea, it is usual to advance the conjunctiva from the upper limbus because there is more conjunctiva to spare in the upper fornix (**Figure 9.2** and **9.3**). Also the conjunctiva here is protected by the upper lid.

Surgical technique for a conjunctival flap

1. Insert a speculum, apply topical anaesthetic drops and inject into the subconjunctival tissues with local anaesthetic and adrenaline.

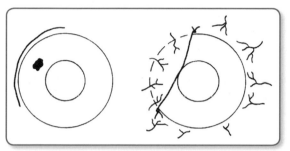

Figure 9.1 A conjunctival flap to cover a peripheral corneal lesion

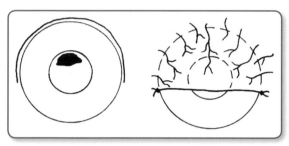

Figure 9.2 A conjunctival flap to cover a central corneal lesion

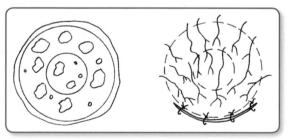

Figure 9.3 A conjunctival flap covering the entire cornea

The three secrets to performing a successful conjunctival flap:

1. The conjunctiva must be fully mobilised and dissected from Tenon's capsule.
2. The epithelium of the cornea should be removed to help the conjunctiva to stick to the cornea.
3. The flap must be secured tightly. It should be sutured so that it presses down tightly against the cornea and does not move around as the eye moves.

2. Plan the site and the size of the flap to cover the required part of the cornea.
3. Incise the conjunctiva at the limbus using non-toothed forceps and fine scissors (see **Figure 6. 11**, page 111). To cover a peripheral corneal lesion this incision should be about one-third of the circumference of the limbus. To cover a central corneal lesion it will need to be about two-thirds of the circumference of the limbus, and to cover the entire cornea the incision should be the entire circumference of the cornea (see **Figures 9.1–9.3**).
4. The conjunctiva should now be dissected free from Tenon's capsule and the sclera, dissecting backwards from the limbus towards the fornix. (Tenon's capsule is the layer of fibrous tissue which joins the under-surface of the conjunctiva to the sclera, it is more obvious in young people and gets thinner with old age). This is done by inserting both blades of the scissors under the conjunctiva at the limbus, pulling on the edge of the conjunctiva with non-toothed forceps to make it taut, and opening and closing the scissors just under the conjunctival surface to cut through the deep attachments of the conjunctiva (**Figure 9.4**). For a conjunctival flap which is to cover the whole cornea the conjunctiva should be dissected back almost to the upper conjunctival fornix, about 15 mm from the limbus.

    If a big flap is being made there are two common problems which occur. The first is not separating the conjunctiva properly from the Tenon's capsule, and this is the most common mistake. The conjunctiva should lie over the lesion without tension at the end of the dissection. If the flap is planned to cover the whole cornea, then the flap should cover the whole cornea without retracting upwards by itself. *It should rest over the lesion without being under tension and it should not retract spontaneously.* If this happens further dissection is necessary, by continuing to separate the many attachments of Tenon's capsule from the under surface of the conjunctiva.

    The second is accidentally making a small "button-hole" in the conjunctiva. If that happens it doesn't matter too much, but if the button-hole is rather large it may have to be closed with sutures.
5. The corneal epithelium should be scraped off from the area to be covered by the flap. This helps the conjunctiva to stick to the cornea. It is best done by using a flat scalpel blade as a scraper, and it may be helpful to gently scrape any mucus or plaque from a chronic corneal ulcer as well. For bullous keratopathy the entire corneal epithelium must be scraped away, but it usually peels off quite easily.
6. Fixation of the conjunctival flap. This is done by suturing the edge of the flap tightly and firmly to the limbus. For a flap covering part of the cornea this is achieved with 2 sutures placed where the edge of the flap crosses the limbus. The sutures should take a deep secure bite of limbal tissue to anchor the flap firmly, and so that it presses tightly against the corneal surface. The suture material should be as fine as possible (preferably 8-0 virgin silk or polyglactin) (**Figure 9.5**). If 10-0

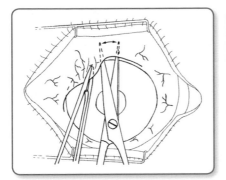

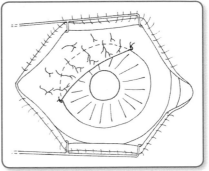

Figure 9.4 Dissecting the conjunctival flap to separate it from Tenon's capsule and the eyeball

Figure 9.5 The edges of the flap are sutured tightly to the limbus

monofilament suture is used, it is best to start and finish with suture inside the tissues so that the knot is buried.

For flaps that cover the whole cornea, the conjunctiva is pulled down from above and anchored to the lower limbus with several sutures. An incision at the lower limbus helps the edge of the flap to stick down to the lower limbus, and again deep bites should be taken to anchor the sutures (**Figure 9.3**).

Post-operative care

A subconjunctival antibiotic injection should be given at the end of the operation if it was performed for a chronic corneal ulcer or a corneal injury. Antibiotic drops or ointment should be applied and the eye padded for 24 hours. At first the conjunctival flap looks very vascular and opaque but with time it will become thinner and more transparent. The healing process is usually complete after about 2 months. If the flap has not retracted back to the limbus spontaneously it can easily be dissected free.

Pterygium

A pterygium (literally a wing) is an opaque wedge of conjunctival epithelium and blood vessels, which grows across the cornea from either the medial or lateral limbus, but more often the medial. A pterygium behaves like a piece of conjunctival scar tissue. It develops in response to excess exposure from ultra-violet light, and so it occurs mostly in the tropics.

It is extremely common to have a small pterygium at the limbus, and this may often grow into the peripheral cornea. Fortunately the pterygium only rarely grows beyond the pupil margin where it may begin to affect the sight. In young patients the pterygium looks quite thick and "fleshy" with numerous blood vessels, but in older patients the pterygium often becomes thinner and more transparent with less blood vessels. It is quite easy to remove a pterygium, but unfortunately it nearly always grows again. There seem to be two reasons for such a high incidence of recurrence following excision.

1. The pterygium is scar tissue which contains *fibroblasts*, so excising it only stimulates these fibroblasts, especially in young people whose fibroblasts are more active. Indeed the pterygium which regrows following excision is often bigger and more vascular than before. The fibroblasts are less active in elderly patients and so the risk of recurrence is less. The appearance of the pterygium also gives some indication as to the risk of recurrence. If the pterygium is thick, fleshy and opaque, it is much more likely to recur; if it is thin and transparent it is less likely to recur.
2. The *limbal stem cells* are special cells at the limbus which make the epithelium of the cornea develop normally. These stem cells are probably damaged after prolonged exposure to sunlight, so the conjunctiva grows across the limbus instead of corneal epithelial cells. Simply excising the pterygium doesn't alter either of these two basic pathological reasons which made the pterygium grow in the first place. Therefore surgical excision of a pterygium is not advised unless it has reached beyond the pupil margin. Even if surgery is necessary, patients should be warned of the serious risk of recurrence, especially if they are young, or have a thick fleshy pterygium.

Preventing recurrence of pterygium after excision

There are two ways of trying to lessen this high risk of recurrence, either by suppressing the activity of the fibroblasts, or by transplanting some limbal stem cells to suppress the growth of new blood vessels and the activity of the fibroblasts.

The activity of the fibroblasts can be suppressed in different ways.

*   *Topical steroid drops*. These will suppress fibroblast activity, and so should be given postoperatively fairly frequently (six times a day) for about 4 to 6 weeks until the wound is fully healed.
*   *Mitomycin C.* This is a much more powerful drug which will completely inhibit the activity of all the fibroblasts. It prevents natural wound healing as well as the recurrence of the pterygium, and must therefore be used with great caution. Mitomycin drops are available commercially but may be hard to locate, or they may be made up in a hospital pharmacy. The recommended strength is a 0.02% solution in normal saline (0.2 mg per ml). It is an extremely effective and powerful drug, but can cause side effects, especially failure of the wound to heal and atrophy of the sclera. Also the precise dose and the best way of giving the treatment have not yet been completely worked out. It is usually given during the operation by applying a small sponge soaked in mitomycin solution to the wound for 3 to 5 minutes. After applying the mitomycin the wound should be copiously irrigated with saline to wash away any excess and prevent complications. Mitomycin has also been given as postoperative drops 4 times daily for 5 days. It is probably safer to give it just once during the operation because of it being such a powerful drug and the risks of it not being used properly postoperatively by the patient.
*   *Thiotepa*. This is similar to mitomycin but a little weaker in its action. Thiotepa drops are recommended as a 0.05% solution in normal saline

(0.5 mg per ml). They should be applied postoperatively 4 times daily for 4 to 6 weeks. The drops will probably have to be made up in a hospital pharmacy.

- *Beta radiation.* These are electrons which have only very superficial penetration. As they are absorbed by the tissues they inactivate cells which tend to divide, whilst not damaging resting cells. The usual source of beta radiation is a strontium 90 applicator. This must be kept in a radiation proof container and applied to the limbus over the base of the pterygium. The recommended maximum dose is 2000 rad (20 Grey), but 1500 rad (15 Grey) is probably sufficient. It can be given in one application immediately post operatively. This dose should not be exceeded because of the risk of causing delayed radiation damage to the eye, and in particular lens opacities.

Delayed wound healing and necrosis of the sclera. Mitomycin C, thiotepa and beta radiation can all cause delayed wound healing and necrosis of the sclera. However if used in the correct manner and the correct dose this is not common. It is equally important to avoid excessive cautery or diathermy to bleeding points as this will also cause necrosis of the sclera.

Transplanting limbal stem cells

The technique for this is described below. The best method is to take a free graft of healthy conjunctiva and limbal tissue from the upper and outer quadrant of the same eye. There are other ways of covering with conjunctiva the bare area left after excising the pterygium. These are slightly easier to do but less effective.

These are useful techniques to help prevent recurrence but they have two disadvantages:

- They take quite a lot of time especially the free graft of conjunctiva.
- The sutures that must be used to secure the graft or cover the defect will act as foreign bodies, and provoke the fibrosis which the operation is trying to prevent.

Conclusions

- All cases must be given some treatment to try to prevent recurrence.
- Topical steroids are always available and have few side effects when used for only six weeks. They should be given to every patient as a full postoperative course.
- Young patients, patients who have had previous surgery for a pterygium, or patients with a thick fleshy pterygium have a very high risk of recurrence after surgery (about 70 to 80%). Topical steroids alone will not be enough to prevent recurrence. These should receive either a limbal stem cell graft or mitomycin, thiotepa or beta radiation according to availability.
- Try to cause as little surgical trauma as possible. The less traumatic the excision, the less likely it is to provoke postoperative inflammation and a recurrence. Excessive surgical trauma and excessive use of the cautery will also risk causing delayed wound healing and scleral necrosis especially if mitomycin or beta radiation is used.

Technique for excision of pterygium

1. Apply topical anaesthetic drops and inject local anaesthetic with adrenaline into the body of the pterygium.
2. Grasp the pterygium near its tip with fine toothed forceps and with a razor blade fragment or scalpel shave off the tip of the pterygium from the cornea (**Figure 9.6**).
3. Continue to cut the pterygium from the surface of the cornea, keeping the plane of dissection as superficial as possible, preferably just under the epithelium and not into the corneal stroma. Once the dissection has reached the limbus, the base of the pterygium can easily be separated from the sclera. With scissors divide the pterygium across its base to leave a small bare area of sclera about 3 mm from the limbus (**Figure 9.7**).

    Apply gentle cautery or diathermy to seal any conjunctival or sub conjunctival bleeding points at the base of the pterygium. Take great care that this is just enough to seal the vessels and does not damage the sclera, or cause necrosis of the tissues. Some of the reports of scleral

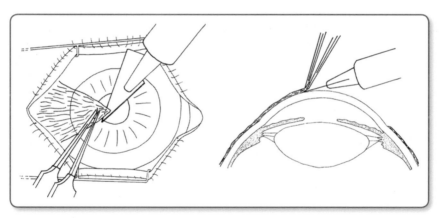

Figure 9.6 Starting to dissect a pterygium off the cornea

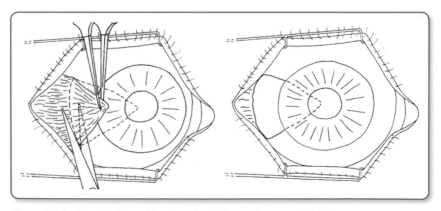

Figure 9.7 Excising the base of the pterygium to leave a bare area of sclera

necrosis after mitomycin and beta radiation may be partly due to excess cautery, diathermy or surgery and not to the actual treatment.
4. Some surgeons find it easier to dissect the pterygium off the eye from the opposite direction. In this method scissors are used to divide the base of the pterygium so that it is only adherent to the cornea. It can then be peeled off the cornea by grasping its base and dissecting it free with a scalpel blade. Whichever method is used it is important to preserve all the superficial layers of the sclera and cornea and only remove the pterygium.
5. If mitomycin is being used it should now be applied for 3 to 5 minutes and then the wound and the conjunctival sac copiously irrigated with saline.
6. Wound closure. With the bare sclera technique no further surgery is done, and the sclera is left bare. The sclera may be covered by a free autograft of the conjunctiva or by mobilising the surrounding conjunctiva.

Free autograft of the conjunctiva

(An autograft means grafting some tissue from the patient's own body.) There have recently been encouraging reports about the use of a free graft of conjunctiva to prevent pterygium recurrence as an alternative to cytotoxic drops or beta radiation. A piece of bulbar conjunctiva from the upper outer quadrant of the eye is excised and used to cover the bare area of sclera left by the removal of the pterygium (see **Figure 9.8**). The technique is a little time consuming but quite straightforward. Local anaesthetic with adrenaline is injected under the donor conjunctiva which is carefully dissected off the underlyingTenon's capsule right up to the limbus. It may help to use a knife to shave off a very small layer of the peripheral cornea as well as the conjunctiva. This gives the graft some stability so it doesn't wrinkle up and become very hard to handle. It also ensures that the vital limbal stem cells are included in the graft. The donor site is left bare and soon becomes spontaneously covered with conjunctiva. The conjunctival graft is carefully sutured into the bare area using fine interrupted sutures. If possible the sutures at the corneal side should be 10-0 nylon with buried knots so as not to cause any postoperative inflammation. Take great care to maintain the

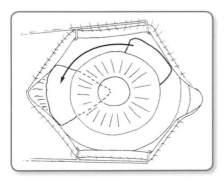

Figure 9.8 To show the site of the conjunctival transplant

correct orientation of the graft so that the limbal conjunctiva is attached to the limbus, and equally important that the graft is not turned upside down. It may help to get the right orientation by inserting one or two sutures in the graft before completely separating it from its bed.

Other methods of covering the bare area of sclera

Sometimes there may be some scarring over the donor site so that a conjunctival autograft cannot be done. There are also simpler ways of covering the bare area of sclera after excising the pterygium, if operating time is limited.

- The conjunctiva may be mobilised by incisions at the limbus so as to cover the defect. This is the easiest method. (**Figure 9.9**) Some surgeons routinely do this if mitomycin has been applied to lessen the risk of poor wound healing.
- A flap of conjunctiva from above the wound may be rotated down into the defect (**Figure 9.10**).
- Which ever method is used, the risk of recurrence is less if the suture knots are buried or the sutures are very carefully trimmed so as not to act as foreign bodies.

Post operative care

The postoperative care has already been discussed. It may be helpful to pad the eye for a day especially if a conjunctival graft has been performed.

Excision of conjunctival tumours

These are found mostly at the limbus but they may occur elsewhere. In most cases they can be cured by local excision, and removing a small margin of healthy conjunctiva as well. Limbal lesions should be removed with a small margin of superficial corneal tissue, dissecting in the same manner as for a pterygium. Usually it is fairly easy to shave these lesions off the marginal cornea using a scalpel blade or razor blade fragment. In some areas conjunctival tumours have become quite common in patients who are HIV positive.

With extensive lesions it may be necessary to excise eyelid tissue as well, or even to exenterate the whole orbit. A biopsy should be taken to confirm

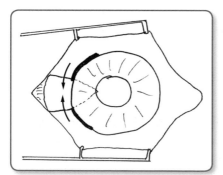

Figure 9.9 Advancing the adjoining conjunctiva to cover the bare area

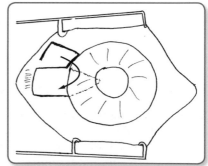

Figure 9.10 Rotating a flap of adjoining conjunctiva to cover the bare area

the diagnosis before planning any extensive surgery. Extensive surgery is not indicated if the tumour has spread to the regional lymph nodes or elsewhere.

Conjunctival reconstruction

The conjunctiva may be scarred or there may be adhesions between the eyelids and the eye (symblepharon) after severe conjunctival inflammation or burns. If possible an attempt should be made to reconstruct the conjunctiva using a flap graft of conjunctiva from the same eye.

It is possible to use a free conjunctival graft from the other eye, but the surgeon should be very hesitant about using tissue from the only good eye to repair the damaged one. A mucous membrane graft from the mouth can also be used to reconstruct the conjunctiva but it is not entirely satisfactory. The best place to remove the mucous membrane is from the bottom of the lower lip near the gum. For an eye which has been severely burnt with gross corneal scarring, a small graft of limbal tissue from the unaffected eye may greatly improve the scarring by bringing healthy limbal stem cells into the damaged eye. The technique is the same as described for a pterygium.

Removal of a sub-conjunctival loa-loa worm

This is an occasional problem in West and Central Africa. The worm moves actively under the conjunctiva and causes considerable irritation although there is no risk to sight. If it dies and disintegrates there will be a marked inflammatory reaction in the orbit and eyelids. Therefore the worm should be removed if possible.

Method
1. Anaesthetise the conjunctiva with several applications of topical local anaesthetic drops and apply a speculum.
2. Grasp the body of the worm through the conjunctiva with non-toothed forceps and do not let go.
3. Cut a small hole in the conjunctiva with scissors alongside the worm and continue the dissection until the edge of the worm is exposed. At this stage some local anaesthetic can be injected subconjunctivally if the patient is feeling pain or if the worm is very active.
4. Using either a probe, a muscle hook or forceps, lever the worm out through the hole in the conjunctiva. Then grasp it and let go with the forceps which were holding it through through the conjunctiva.
5. Carefully pull the entire worm out of the tissues.

Surgery for corneal scars

Corneal scarring is very common in hot countries for the reasons already given. Surgical treatment can benefit many patients with corneal scars, and there are four possible treatment options, corneal grafting, corneal rotation, optical iridectomy and superficial keratectomy. Before even thinking about operating, the surgeon must make a good clinical assessment of the case and the patient's background.

- Is the scar permanent and inactive or is there still some inflammation in the cornea? If the cornea is still inflamed, medical treatment especially with topical steroids may help to clear the cornea.
- Does the other eye have good vision? If the other eye is healthy there is little to be gained from surgery.
- At what age did the scar develop? If the patient was young, the eye is likely to be amblyopic especially if the other eye is normal. Poor fixation, nystagmus and a squint are all signs that the eye is amblyopic.
- Has a careful refraction been done? Many eyes with corneal scarring have bad astigmatism which can be helped with glasses.

Corneal grafting

A corneal graft operation removes the central part of the cornea which is diseased and scarred, and a healthy cornea is used to replace it (see **Figure 9.11**). Nearly always the donor cornea comes from a person who has died. The surgery is very delicate and fine, although not particularly difficult. However the body tends to reject tissue from another person, so the patient needs to be followed up very carefully for a long time postoperatively to prevent graft rejection. There are many visually handicapped people in the world whose sight could be restored with a corneal graft (probably several million). Unfortunately there are many reasons why corneal grafting is not in practice going to be of much help to them.

- The patients who have the most dense and opaque corneal scars are the same ones who are most likely to reject the graft. If the scar is very dense it is likely to be vascularised, and it is the blood vessels which provoke the rejection.
- Corneal graft donor material is very scarce, especially in those places where corneal scarring is common.
- Good reliable donor material is very expensive, and most patients with corneal scarring are poor. Trying to prevent corneal scarring is much more cost effective than trying to treat it.
- Lengthy follow up postoperatively is essential.
- The conjunctiva and eyelids must be healthy for a corneal graft to succeed.

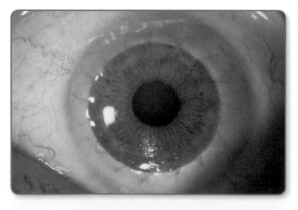

Figure 9.11 A successful corneal graft

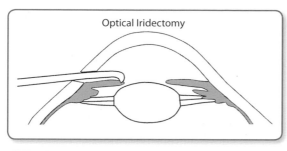

Optical Iridectomy

Figure 9.12 Optical iridectomy. The small hole in the iris enables the patient to see through the clear cornea and around the central corneal scar, which is opaque

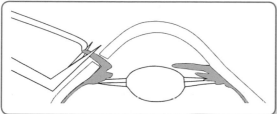

There are two types of corneal grafts; full thickness or penetrating grafts in which the full depth of the cornea is replaced, and lamellar grafts in which only the stroma and anterior part is replaced but the patient's own endothelium is preserved. Because of the complexity of corneal grafting it will not be described in any more detail.

Optical iridectomy

If there is a large central corneal scar, and a small piece of peripheral cornea is clear and transparent, it is possible by removing some of the iris to create an artificial pupil in line with the clear portion of the cornea (**Figure 9.12**). This is called an optical iridectomy. Ideally these patients should have a corneal graft operation but this is nearly always impossible. An optical iridectomy is a quicker and usually an easier operation. It requires very much less postoperative care, and the patients can be discharged after a few days. As described above there is little point in operating if the other eye is normal or if there is poor fixation.

The operative technique is basically the same as for a peripheral iridectomy (see page 205). However the hole in the iris is in a slightly different place. A peripheral iridectomy aims to place the hole in the periphery of the iris, but an optical iridectomy aims to make a much more central hole, and nearly always to divide the pupil margin. These eyes are often difficult to operate on because they have suffered a severe inflammatory disease. Besides the corneal scar, the iris is often adherent to the lens (posterior synechiae) and to the cornea (anterior synechiae). In severe cases the lens may also be damaged. So at every stage there may be difficulties:

- Place the incision to correspond with the clear gap in the cornea. Only a small iridectomy in the right place is necessary.
- It may be difficult to dissect a conjunctival flap because of scarring and adhesions between the conjunctiva and the sclera.

- The limbus may be very vascular because of previous inflammation in the eye.
- For an optical iridectomy the incision should enter the eye near the limbus but the aim is to grasp the iris with the iris forceps fairly near the pupil margin (**Figure 9. 13a**). The iris may not prolapse by itself from the eye because of adhesions to the cornea or the lens.
- Try to grasp the iris and pull it out through the wound, but great care must then be taken not to cause bleeding inside the eye. This usually comes from pulling too hard on the iris which is stuck down in the eye, and so detaching the base or root of the iris from the ciliary body and rupturing the main artery of the iris. Bleeding may come from adhesions between the iris and the lens or cornea.
- Take care not to damage the lens capsule which will cause a cataract to develop.
- Once the iris is out of the eye, use iris scissors to perform the iridectomy (**Figure 9.13b**).
- Plan to place the iridectomy hole in line with the clear cornea. Nearly always the sphincter of the pupil should be divided.
- In some cases it may be better to use intraocular scissors to cut a hole in the iris inside the eye, rather than try to prolapse a stuck down iris out of the eye. Again take great care not to damage the lens capsule.
- Having done the iridectomy, the surgeon may discover a cataract or a dense fibrous membrane which is the remains of a cataract behind the iris. It may be necessary to convert the operation to a cataract extraction, or to use intraocular scissors or a needling knife to make a hole in a dense fibrous membrane or thickened lens capsule lying behind the iris.
- If there has been intraocular bleeding, try to wait a few minutes for this to stop before closing the wound. It doesn't matter too much if a small blood clot is left in the eye, but it does matter if there is still active bleeding into the eye at the end of the operation.
- The wound may need one or two fine sutures for secure closure.

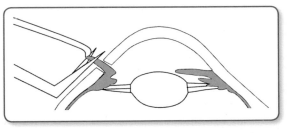

Figure 9.13a Grasping the iris near the pupil margin

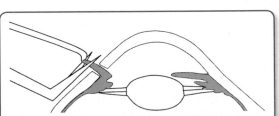

Figure 9.13b Excising the iris with De Wecker's scissors

Postoperative care

This is the same as for other intraocular surgery: topical antibiotics, steroids and mydriatics. A subconjunctival injection at the end of the operation may be helpful. The patients can be discharged after a few days.

Remember that all optical iridectomy patients need a careful refraction post-operatively. They often have severe astigmatism.

Corneal rotation

This is a possible alternative to an optical iridectomy. An optical iridectomy creates an artificial pupil to be in line with the clear cornea. A corneal rotation moves the cornea round so that the clear part comes into the centre to be in line with the normal pupil (**Figure 9.14**). This is a type of corneal graft, but it does not require a donor cornea because the patient's own cornea is being used, and there is no possibility of the cornea being rejected. It therefore avoids the two most important problems of corneal grafting. *However the operation should only be attempted by someone who has some experience of corneal grafting.* The steps of the operation are in outline as follows:

1. The anterior chamber is filled with visco-elastic fluid or air to protect the iris or lens, and a trephine of 8 or 8.5 mm is cut eccentrically to include the clear cornea and the scar at the centre. A sharp knife or scissors may be needed to complete the trephine.
2. If there is also a cataract, it may be removed at this stage and an intraocular lens inserted.
3. The cornea is then replaced with the clear cornea in the centre of the eye, and carefully sutured with interrupted monofilament 10-0 sutures with the knots buried.

Postoperatively topical steroids and antibiotics should be given for a few weeks and mydriatics for a few days. By carefully removing one or two of the sutures after about 8 weeks, post operative astigmatism which is very common can be much reduced.

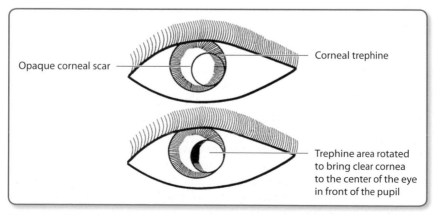

Opaque corneal scar

Corneal trephine

Trephine area rotated to bring clear cornea to the center of the eye in front of the pupil

Figure 9.14 Corneal rotation. The cornea is trephined eccentrically and then rotated so that the clear cornea comes to the centre of the eye and the scarred cornea goes to the periphery. If needed, a cataract extraction and intraocular lens implant can be performed at the same time.

For an experienced surgeon this is a slightly better operation than an optical iridectomy, because the post operative astigmatism can be better controlled. It also enables a cataract extraction and IOL implant to be done as well which is not possible with an optical iridectomy. However it is a more difficult operation than an iridectomy, and there are more risks of surgical mistakes occurring.

Superficial keratectomy

Sometimes the corneal opacity is located only in the very superficial layers of the cornea and merely by shaving off the anterior layers of the cornea the vision will improve. There are two distinct conditions in which this may happen.

Solar keratopathy affects people who are exposed to very high levels of sunlight such as desert dwellers, and fishermen who receive direct sunlight and also reflected sunlight from the sea surface. They develop degenerative changes in the anterior layers of the exposed central and lower parts of the cornea. As well as the opacity, the surface of the cornea becomes very irregular. After applying topical anaesthetic drops a sharp knife blade is used to excise the opaque and irregular surface layers of the cornea. The corneal epithelium regenerates very quickly in a day or two and there may be significant improvement in the vision.

Sub-epithelial band calcification of the cornea may occur but the cause is uncertain. A thin layer of opaque calcium salts is deposited just under the corneal epithelium and will affect the vision. The treatment is to apply topical anaesthetic drops, to scrape away the corneal epithelium, and then try to scrape off the calcified layer using the flat side of a scalpel. Irrigation of the cornea with a chelating agent which dissolves calcium helps this deposit to dissolve much more quickly and easily. Sodium versenate or EDTA is the usual agent. The epithelium grows again very quickly.

Tissue glues to seal perforated corneal ulcers

As an alternative to a conjunctival flap operation, it is possible to use tissue glue and a soft bandage contact lens to seal perforated corneal ulcers. This treatment is only recommended if the ulcer is not heavily infected with bacteria, and if bandage contact lenses are available.

The glue used is cyanoacrylic "superglue" which hardens instantly on contact with tissues or fluid. After applying local anaesthetic drops, the perforation and the area around it must be thoroughly and firmly scraped and dried to remove debris, mucus and fluid, so that the glue can stick to the tissues. A scalpel blade and a small dry swab are used for this. A very tiny amount of glue is then applied on to the ulcer, and immediately a soft bandage contact lens placed over the entire cornea.

Routine topical and systemic treatment for the ulcer should then be given, and the eye left without a pad if possible. After about 10 days the contact lens can be removed. The plug of glue will usually come off as well and the perforation should have healed.

Objectives
- Probing of the nasolacrimal duct
- Dacrocystectomy
- Dacrocystorhinostomy
- Obstruction of the common canaliculus
- Lacrimal punctal occlusion

The lacrimal drainage system drains the tears from the conjunctival sac into the nose. Obstruction in the lacrimal passages may occur at various sites (**Figure 10.1**). In all cases there will be watering of the eye called epiphora.

1. *The nasolacrimal duct.* This is the most common site for obstruction. As a consequence the lacrimal sac often enlarges (a mucocoele) and becomes infected (dacryocystitis). This causes chronic conjunctivitis and a muco-purulent discharge from the eye. Dacryocystitis is found particularly in communities where chronic eye and nose infections such as trachoma are common. It appears to be more prevalent amongst Caucasians and people from the Indian sub-continent, probably because of the shape of their nasal bones and their narrower nasal bridge.
2. The *punctum and* 3. *The common canaliculus.* Obstruction at either the punctum or the common canaliculus will result in epiphora but there will be no enlargement or infection of the lacrimal sac. Therefore the eye waters but is free from infection.'

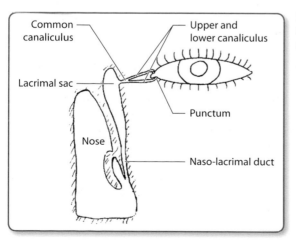

Figure 10.1 To show the anatomy of the lacrimal drainage system

Probing of the nasolacrimal duct

Indications

The main indication is for congenital obstruction of the duct in young children. This is usually caused by a thin membrane which obstructs the lower end of the duct. This membrane often ruptures spontaneously as the baby grows. If the symptoms of epiphora and discharge have not improved spontaneously by the age of 18 months to 2 years, then probing of the duct should be carried out under general anaesthetic. The success rate is about 80%.

Probing can also be done in adults under local anaesthetic, but in adults it has a much lower success rate.

Method

1. Dilate the punctum with a punctum dilator. Then pass a fine probe along the canaliculus to enter the upper part of the lacrimal sac. This can be done through either the upper or the lower punctum. It is better to use the upper punctum but it is easier to use the lower punctum.
2. Make sure that the tip of the probe is definitely in the lacrimal sac. The tip should rest against the lateral side of the nasal bone and the hard bone can be felt against the tip of the probe (a "hard stop") (**Figure 10.2**). If the tip is not resting against something hard and bony then it has not reached the lacrimal sac (a "soft stop") (**Figure 10.3**). In this case it is harmful to proceed further as it will only create a false passage through the tissues. This is a very serious complication and can cause permanent damage to the common canaliculus which is the narrowest part of the lacrimal passages. Therefore the child may have a watering eye for the rest of its life. If you do not feel a "hard stop" with the probe you should not proceed any further.
3. Keep the tip of the probe resting against the bone and rotate the probe to point down and very slightly out (laterally) and back (posteriorly)

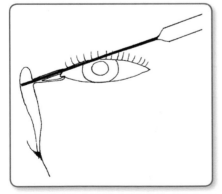

Figure 10.2 Probing through the upper punctum. The tip of the probe has entered the lacrimal sac and rests against the hard nasal bone

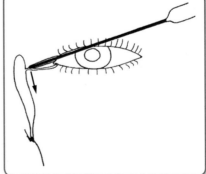

Figure 10.3 Probing through the upper punctum. The tip of the probe has not reached the lacrimal sac. Any attempt to proceed with probing will cause a false passage through the tissues as shown by the arrow

(**Figure 10.4**). In this direction it can be advanced from the lacrimal sac down into the nasolacrimal duct. There will usually be some resistance at the lower end of the nasolacrimal duct from the congenital membranous obstruction. Then the probe tip will enter the nose and hit the hard bone of the palate (**Figure 10.5**).

4. Some people like to confirm the success of the probing by then syringing the nasolacrimal passages, but be careful that the fluid does not go into the lungs of an anaesthetised baby.

Dacryocystectomy

The infected lacrimal sac is excised. This removes the source of infection and therefore cures the secondary conjunctivitis, relieving most of the symptoms. However the lacrimal passages are destroyed by the operation, so the eye continues to water.

Indications

Dacryocystitis in adults where surgical facilities are not good. It is a fairly simple and easy operation, although there may be quite brisk bleeding from the superficial facial veins under the skin. Dacryocystectomy is particularly suitable for elderly patients who do not produce so many tears.

Method

1. Inject around the lacrimal sac with local anaesthetic and adrenaline. It is helpful to block the infratrochlear and infraorbital nerves as well (**Figure 10.6**). The infra trochlear nerve carries the sensory nerve fibres from most of the lacrimal sac area. It can be blocked by injecting either through the skin in the upper and inner corner of the orbit, or through the conjunctiva just above the caruncle. Advance the needle about

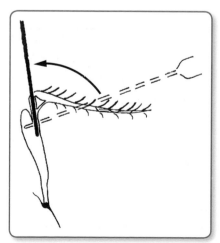

Figure 10.4 The probe is rotated across the forehead to point downwards and very slightly outwards and backwards

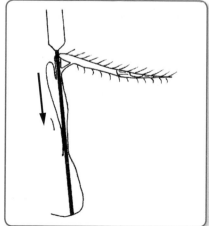

Figure 10.5 The probe is advanced down the naso-lacrimal duct, through the obstruction at its lower end till it hits the hard palate at the floor of the nose

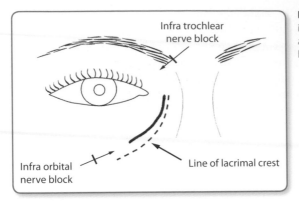

Figure 10.6 To show the incision for dacryocystectomy and the site of the nerve blocks

2 cm keeping close to the medial wall of the orbit and inject about 2 ml of local anaesthetic with adrenaline. The infra orbital nerve can be blocked where it emerges just below the infraorbital ridge.

2. An incision is made directly over the lacrimal sac, in the line of the skin crease (**Figure 10.6**). This incision should be just lateral to the lacrimal crest. This is the bony ridge which can be felt with the fingertip between the bridge of the nose and the orbit. The incision starts at the level of the medial canthus and passes downwards and outwards for about 2 to 3 cm. The skin on the two sides of the incision is held open either with sutures, a small self-retaining retractor, or by an assistant using two small retractors. The incision is deepened using blunt dissection through the Orbicularis Oculi muscle. There is often considerable bleeding from the angular vein and its branches. The bleeding points should be identified and secured in the usual way with ligature or diathermy.

3. Identify the lacrimal sac. This is usually enlarged and easy to find. If there is difficulty in finding it, then identify the bony lacrimal crest, and the lacrimal sac will be just lateral to the crest and a little deeper under a layer of fascia (**Figure 10.7**). Grasp the lacrimal sac with artery forceps. Then by gently pulling and twisting on the artery forceps while dissecting carefully around the sac, remove the entire mucous wall of the sac and as much of the nasolacrimal duct as is easily accessible. The lacrimal sac may rupture or leak mucopurulent

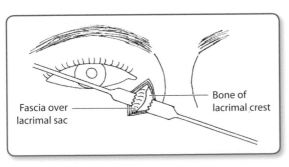

Figure 10.7 The skin and orbicularis muscle have been retracted to show the bony lacrimal crest and the fascia lying over the lacrimal sac

material and it may be necessary to remove the mucous wall of the sac in several pieces rather than in one piece. If there is doubt about whether some pieces of the lacrimal sac mucosa are still present, these can be destroyed with chemical cautery. A swab stick moistened in phenol can be applied to the tissues, and after a short pause the phenol residue is then irrigated away.

4. Close the skin incision with one or two interrupted sutures.
5. Use a canaliculus rasp if it is available to scrape the mucous membrane from the canaliculi. This is an optional extra and not essential (**Figure 10.8**).
6. Although the lacrimal passages are destroyed the operation will greatly reduce the symptoms by removing the source of infection from the conjunctiva and lacrimal sac.

Dacryocystorhinostomy

This is an operation in which the lacrimal sac is anastomosed to the nasal mucous membrane. It is a better operation for dacryocystitis than a dacryocystectomy because the patient is not left with a watering eye. The success rate should be about 90% and it successfully cures all the symptoms. However the operation is much more difficult and takes much longer than a dacryocystectomy. Special instruments are required (**Figure 10.9a–c**) and there is often considerable bleeding.

A dacryocystorhinostomy (DCR) can be done under local anaesthetic if the patient is cooperative, but a general anaesthetic is more acceptable.

The aim of the operation is to excise the bone between the lacrimal sac and the middle meatus of the nose, and then suture the lacrimal sac mucosa to the nasal mucosa of the middle meatus. **Figures 10.10** and **10.11** show in outline what the operation is trying to achieve.

Principle

The aim of the operation is to remove part of the lacrimal crest and all the thin bone separating the lacrimal sac from the middle nasal meatus (**Figure 10.12**). The mucosa of the lacrimal sac is then joined to the nasal mucosa so it forms part of the lateral wall of the nose (**Figures 10.10** and **10.11**).

Method

First check that the patient is not hypertensive because of the risk of excessive bleeding.

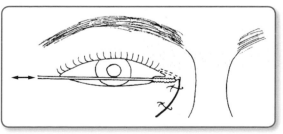

Figure 10.8 Using the canaliculus rasp

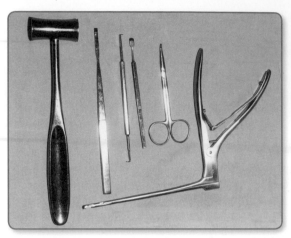

Figure 10.9a The instruments required for a dacryocystorhinostomy. A hammer, a chisel, Traquair's periosteal elevator, a straight periosteal elevator, right angled scissors and a bone punch

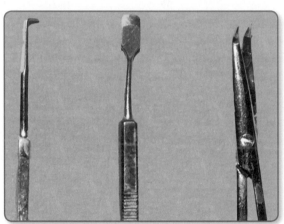

Figure 10.9b A picture to show the tips of the lacrimal bone trephines

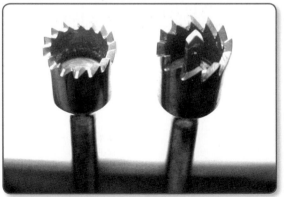

Figure 10.9c A small suture (arrowed) to bring down the conjunctiva incision

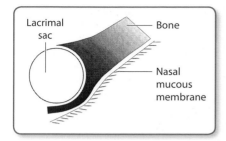

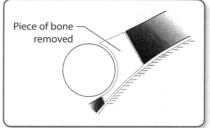

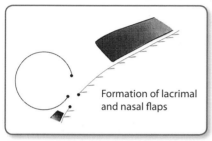

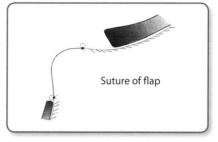

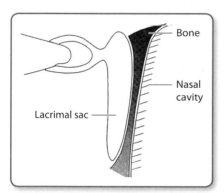

Figure 10.10 A diagram in cross section to show how to perform a dacryocyststorhinostomy

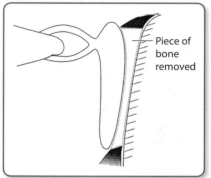

Figure 10.11 A diagram in vertical section to show how to perform a dacryocyststorhinostomy

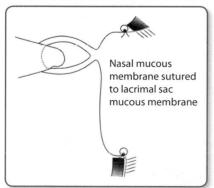

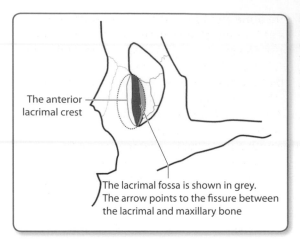

The anterior lacrimal crest

The lacrimal fossa is shown in grey. The arrow points to the fissure between the lacrimal and maxillary bone

Figure 10.12 The dotted line shows the bone removed for a dacryocystorhinostomy. This is the floor of the lacrimal fossa and the anterior lacrimal crest, and some bone in front of it

1. *Anaesthetic.* If the operation is under local anaesthetic the nose should be packed with ribbon gauze soaked in a mixture of 2 to 4 % lignocaine with adrenaline. This helps to vasoconstrict the very vascular nasal mucous membrane. (If available, cocaine 4% is both a local anaesthetic and a vasoconstrictor). The pack in the nose must be inserted above the inferior turbinate bone and into the middle meatus of the nose. To do this the pack should be pushed upwards in the nostril. It is an easy mistake to push the pack backwards below the inferior turbinate bone into the inferior meatus, so it does not reach the correct area in the middle meatus of the nose, which is above the inferior turbinate bone.

2. Local anaesthetic with adrenaline should be injected over the lacrimal crest and both the infratrochlear and infraorbital nerves blocked (see **Figure 10.6**).

    If the operation is under general anaesthetic the nose should still be packed with adrenaline because this lessens bleeding during the operation. Placing the patient with head slightly elevated on the operating table also helps to lessen the bleeding.

3. *Skin incision* (see **Figure 10.6**). This should be medial to the bony ridge of the lacrimal crest. (The incision for dacryocystectomy in **Figure 10.6** is just lateral to the lacrimal crest.) It should start at the level of the medial canthus and pass downwards and slightly laterally for 2 to 3 cm. The incision should not be over the lacrimal sac itself as this might damage it.

4. The incision is deepened down to the periosteum of the bone over the lacrimal crest and any bleeding from the angular facial vein is stopped with ligature or diathermy. This can bleed quite heavily. The skin flaps can be retracted by "cat's paw" retractors held by an assistant. Alternatively a self retaining retractor can be used or sutures can be placed in the wound edges and traction placed on the sutures with artery forceps secured to the drapes.

    The periosteum, which is a thin fibrous sheet over the surface of the bone, is then divided and the rest of the dissection carried out on the surface of the bare bone and underneath the periosteum (**Figure 10.13**). This is a safe tissue plane where no damage can be done to the lacrimal sac or to any blood vessels or nerves. At the top of the incision the medial canthal tendon can be seen as shining white fibres and it is separated from its insertion into the medial wall of the orbit. The periosteum is incised with a knife starting at the insertion of the medial canthal tendon and passing downwards, staying just medial to the anterior lacrimal crest. Dissect the periosteum off the bone with a periosteal elevator, moving towards the sharp lacrimal crest and then down into the lacrimal fossa, still separating the periosteum from the bone. Take great care to keep the periosteal elevator always just under the periosteum and right on the surface of the bone. The lacrimal crest can have quite a sharp angle and the dissection continues backwards to the floor of the lacrimal fossa.

5. The next stage is to remove the bone of the anterior lacrimal crest and the bone at the floor of the lacrimal fossa which separates the lacrimal sac from the nasal mucous membrane (see **Figures 10.10–10.12**). There are various ways of doing this:

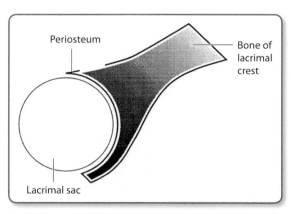

Periosteum

Bone of lacrimal crest

Lacrimal sac

Figure 10.13 To show how the periosteum is elevated and stripped off the bone of the lacrimal crest and the lacrimal fossa

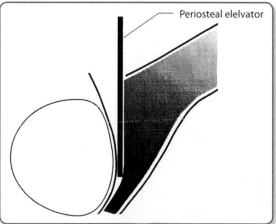

Periosteal elelvator

Method A

In the floor of the lacrimal fossa there is a thin vertical bony fissure, where the maxillary bone joins the lacrimal bone (**Figure 10.12**). Force a bent Traquair periosteal elevator into this suture line and enlarge the opening enough to allow the jaws of a bone punch through the hole. Use the Traquair's elevator to separate the nasal mucous membrane from the inside of the bone and to push it away from the bone. Then use a small bone punch to remove all the bone of the lacrimal fossa and the anterior lacrimal crest. Take great care to preserve intact the nasal mucous membrane which may easily get caught in the tip of the punch (**Figure 10.14**). To avoid catching the nasal mucous membrane in the punch, first take the local anaesthetic pack from the nose so that nasal mucous membrane is not being pushed outwards. Also advance the punch very carefully so it just catches the bone and does not catch the nasal mucous membrane. Also use the Traquair's elevator as described. Bone removal should continue until an area the size of a finger-tip has been removed. This should be about 1.5 cm in diameter and should include all the bone of the lacrimal fossa and the anterior lacrimal crest.

Method B

If the fissure between the maxillary bone and the lacrimal bone cannot be found or if there is not a good sharp bone punch available, a small chisel or osteotome or a circular bone drill should be used to remove the bone. It is best to remove a small piece of bone to include the lacrimal crest at first and then enlarge the hole in all directions. By holding the chisel tightly and by making gentle taps with the hammer it is possible to ensure that the chisel cuts through the bone without going

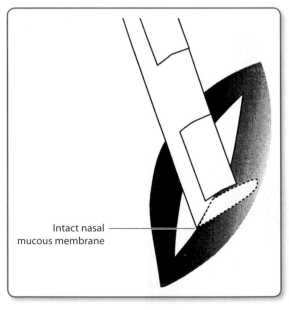

Figure 10.14 The use of the bone punch to remove the bone

Intact nasal mucous membrane

on to cut into the nasal mucous membrane underneath the bone. Some surgeons prefer to use a small round drill to make the first opening in the bone These usually come in pairs, one has a central spike and the other does not (see **Figure 10.9c**, page 294). First use the one with the central spike to mark a round groove on the bone, and then the other one to penetrate through the bone. As soon as one feels the pressure of the bone beginning to become less, then stop drilling to avoid damaging the nasal mucous membrane.

6. The flaps of the lacrimal and nasal mucosa are now prepared. These should now be lying next to each other because all the bone separating them has been removed. First the naso-lacrimal duct is cut through at the lower end of the lacrimal sac using the small right angled scissors (**Figure 10.15**). Then by inserting one blade of the scissors into the sac and the other blade outside the sac, the medial wall of the sac is opened up from the bottom to the top forming an anterior and a posterior flap. Confirm that the lacrimal sac has been properly opened by passing a lacrimal probe down from the punctum along the canaliculus (**Figure 10.16**). The tip of the probe will appear in the opened up lacrimal sac. If right angled scissors are not available then a scalpel blade and straight scissors can be used, but scissors with a small right angled bend make this delicate part of the dissection easier.

The nasal mucous membrane must now be opened. Hopefully it is still intact but sometimes the process of bone removal may have made a small hole in it. Cutting the nasal mucous membrane is easier if it is put under slight tension by placing a curved artery forceps or the tip of the sucker up the nostril so it presses the mucous membrane outwards into the space from where the bone has been removed. The nasal mucous

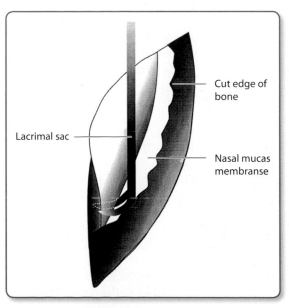

Figure 10.15 Use of right angled scissors to divide the naso-lacrimal duct

Cut edge of bone

Lacrimal sac

Nasal mucas membranse

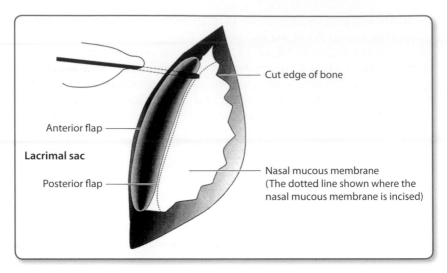

Figure 10.16 The lacrimal sac has been opened up and a probe inserted into the sac

membrane should be incised to make a large anterior flap but only a small posterior flap (see the dotted line in **Figure 10.16**). The reason for this is the anatomical relationship between the lacrimal sac and the nasal mucous membrane. **Figure 10.10** shows how the posterior part of the lacrimal sac is very close to the nasal cavity but the anterior part is separated by quite a large width of bone. Therefore the anterior nasal mucous membrane flap must be large to bridge this gap.

7. The lacrimal sac and nasal mucous membrane flaps are now sutured to each other. The posterior flaps should be lying very close to each other and there is usually little or no need to suture them. They are right down at the bottom of the incision and access is in any case difficult. It is important to suture the anterior flaps with at least two sutures. Absorbable material is best but if this is not available fine non-absorbable sutures can be used. A very curved needle makes the access and suturing of the flaps much easier. Try to keep the anterior and posterior flaps well apart so that the lacrimal sac drains well into the nose. This may be helped by tying the sutures of the anterior flap to the orbicularis oculi muscle so as to pull the anterior flap forwards.

8. Wound closure. The subcutaneous layers should be sutured if possible with interrupted absorbable sutures, and the skin closed. Post-operatively some people advise packing in the nose but providing it is not bleeding excessively it is best not to pack the nose for several reasons:
   • it is uncomfortable.
   • it may cause the very delicate mucosal anastomosis to break down.
   • when the pack is removed after 24 hours it may then provoke bleeding.

9. Postoperatively the skin sutures should be removed after 5-7 days. Antiobiotic drops or ointment should be applied to the conjunctiva,

and if the lacrimal sac is particularly infected a short course of systemic antibiotics is probably advisable.

The biggest problem during dacryocystorhinostomy is bleeding. This is often worse under general anaesthetic than local anaesthetic. In order to minimise bleeding during surgery it is essential to pack the nose well and pack it correctly so that the middle meatus above the inferior turbinate bone is vasoconstricted. It is also essential to stop all bleeding from the angular vein and its branches before proceeding with the rest of the operation. Slightly raising the head of the operating table will also diminish bleeding both under local anaesthetic and general anaesthetic. A good sucker is essential for a dacryocystorhinostomy.

In recent years there has been considerable interest in alternative methods of relieving dacryocystitis without open surgery. A dacryocystorhinostomy operation can be performed endoscopically through the nose without making any skin incision. Alternatively it is a possible to have a balloon dilatation of the obstructed nasolacrimal duct by passing a very fine catheter down the duct and then using high pressure to rupture the obstruction. However, both these operations require expensive equipment, and the results even in the best of hands are still no better than a dacryocystorhinostomy operation through the skin.

There is an alternative and simpler method of dacrocystorhinostomy. It is worth considering if the facilities are not available for a standard dacrocystorhinostomy, and the surgeon is unwilling to destroy the lacrimal drainage passages by a dacrocystectomy. The aim of the operation is to insert a short flanged plastic tube from the lacrimal sac into the nose to by-pass the obstructed naso-lacrimal duct.

The long term success rate is only about 50%.

Method

1. The anaesthetic blocks are the same as for dacrocystorhinostomy.
2. The lacrimal sac is exposed as for dacrocystectomy and then cut open from it its front surface.
3. A trocar is used to make a hole through the floor of the lacrimal sac and the thin lacrimal bone into the middle meatus of the nose (**Figure 10.17**).
4. A short flanged plastic tube is then forced tightly and securely into this hole (**Figure 10.18**). This tube can be made from firm plastic tube which is heated and pressed against a flat surface to create a flange.
5. The anterior wall of the lacrimal sac is closed with one or two catgut sutures and the skin sutured.

Obstruction of the common canaliculus

An obstruction here can only be relieved by a standard dacryocystorhinostomy operation and passing a soft silicone tube down the lacrimal canaliculi into the nose. The silicone tube has a short silverprobe at each end. These are passed down each canaliculus and into the opened up lacrimal sac after stage 6 of the dacryocystorhinostomy. They are then passed down into the nose and the two ends of the tube tied to each other, and the ends cut short.

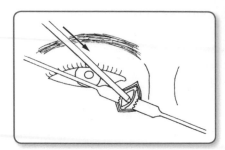

Figure 10.17 Pushing a trocar through the floor of the lacrimal sac and bone into the nasal cavity

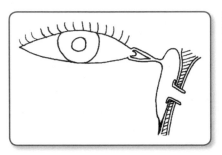

Figure 10.18 To show the position of the flanged tube

Lacrimal punctoplasty

Obstruction or stenosis of the lower lacrimal punctum is easy to cure with a punctoplasty procedure. Punctal stenosis should be suspected if the patient complains of epiphora, but after dilating the punctum and syringing the nasolacrimal passages there is a free flow of fluid down to the nose. (Sometimes the punctum does not rest against the eye due to ectropion. In such a case an operation to correct the ectropion is necessary).

The aim of the operation is to open up the punctum by excising a triangle on its posterior surface facing the globe of the eye.

Indications

Stenosis or occlusion of the punctum. The rest of the lacrimal passages must be patent for the operation to succeed.

Method

1. Inject local anaesthetic with adrenaline around the lower punctum.
2. Dilate the punctum with a punctum dilator.
3. Insert one blade of very fine scissors into the punctum with the other blade in the conjunctival sac. Make a vertical cut about 2 mm long (**Figure 10.19b**).
4. Again insert one blade of fine scissors into the canaliculus and cut medially (**Figure 10.19c**).
5. Make a third cut so as to excise a triangle of conjunctiva opening out the punctum on to the posterior surface of the lid (**Figure 10.19d**).

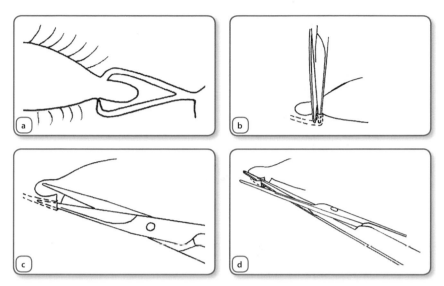

Figure 10.19 The lower eyelid is seen from its conjunctival (posterior) surface and a small triangle of conjunctiva excised to open up the punctum

Occlusion of the lacrimal punctum for dry eye patients

There are some patients who do not have enough tears, particularly patients with chronic rheumatoid arthritis. Their symptoms are often considerably helped by blocking off their lacrimal passages to preserve the small amount of tears that they have. This can very easily be done by using a cautery to seal off the lacrimal punctum. First inject local anaesthetic near the lacrimal punctum. Then dilate the punctum and pass a small cautery deep down into the punctum and turn the cautery on. This will burn the mucosa inside the punctum and seal it off permanently. Both the lower and the upper punctum should be sealed off in this way.

Evisceration, enucleation and exenteration

Objectives
- Indications for evisceration and enucleation
- Evisceration
- Enucleation
- Cosmetic implants
- Exenteration

This chapter describes three operations that either remove the contents of the eye (evisceration), the eye itself (enucleation) or the whole orbital contents (exenteration). Each operation has specific indications which are important to understand. In many cultures the removal of an eye, even if blind, is resisted. If an eye is very painful or grossly disfigured an operation will be accepted more readily. However, if the eye looks normal the patient or their family may be very reluctant to accept its removal. Therefore tact, compassion and patience are needed when recommending these operations.

Enucleation and evisceration

There are several reasons why either of these destructive operations may be necessary:

1. **Malignant tumours in the eye**. In the case of a malignant tumour or suspected malignant tumour the eye should be removed by enucleation and not evisceration. There are two important intraocular tumours, retinoblastoma and melanoma and for both of them the basic treatment is enucleation.

   Retinoblastoma is a relatively common tumour in early childhood. At first the growth is confined to the eye. Enucleation must be carried out at this stage and will probably save the child's life. It is vital not to delay or postpone surgery. If a child under 6 has a blind eye and the possibility of a tumour cannot be ruled out, it is best to remove the eye. Always examine the other eye very carefully under anaesthetic as well. It may contain an early retinoblastoma which could be treatable and still save the eye.

   Retinoblastoma spreads along the optic nerve to the brain. It also spreads by metastasis to other parts of the body and will break through the sclera into the orbit. Once proptosis has occurred the disease is almost always fatal within a short time unless the patient has access to advanced radiotherapy and chemotherapy treatment.

Most people consider there is no point in heroic or mutilating surgery for a child who will shortly die.

Melanoma of the choroid is the most common primary intraocular tumour in adults. It is however rare in Afro-Carribeams. As well as enlarging within the eye, the tumour will sometimes metastasize through the blood stream to the liver.

Rarely it may pass directly through the eye into the orbit. Removing an eye with melanoma may not prevent distant metastases from occurring. If a suspected melanoma is found in an eye which still has sight, it is better not to remove the eye but refer the patient to an expert. However most people would advise enucleation for an eye which is blind and may contain an intraocular tumour.

Secondary tumours of the choroid may occur as metastases from a primary elsewhere. These are often multiple, the primary site is usually the breast, the prostate or the lung, and surgery does not have any part to play in their management and treatment.

In centres where advanced methods of treatment are available it is possible to save an eye with early retinoblastoma or melanoma which still has vision. The tumour can be treated with chemotherapy, local irradiation or possibly photocoagulation or cryotherapy. A small melanoma can be excised and the eye preserved.

2. **Blind, painful eyes**. The patient may request the removal of the eye for relief of pain. If possible try to identify the cause as this may affect the management. For instance, if the cause is a possible intraocular tumour, enucleation and not evisceration should be performed. If the patient is very anxious for the eye not to be removed it may be possible to relieve the pain with a retrobulbar injection of phenol or alcohol. These selectively destroy the fine nerve fibres which carry pain sensation.

   Technique of retrobulbar injection

   Retrobulbar phenol. A local anaesthetic is not required, because the phenol itself acts a local anaesthetic Give a slow retrobulbar injection of 2 ml. of 5% phenol. The injection may be repeated after a few days. Retrobulbar alcohol is often used rather than phenol. However the injection can be very painful and so a local anaesthetic retrobulbar nerve block must be given first. Give a 1 ml. retrobulbar injection of local anaesthetic, and then 1-2ml.of 50% alcohol through the same needle. Therefore phenol is preferable to alcohol. Retrobulbar Chlorpromazine is a safe and effective alternative for the management of pain in blind eyes. The eye is sterilised and 1 to 2 ml retrobulbar injection of Lignocaine 2% is given; using the same needle, the syringe is switched to inject 1 to 2 ml of Chlorpromazine (dose 25 mg per ml).

3. **Very unsightly eyes such as staphyloma.** The patient may request removal for cosmetic reasons with the insertion of an artificial eye.

4. **A severe intraocular infection (endophthalmitis).** Removal of an eye for infection should only be carried out if the infection has failed to respond to a full course of antibiotic treatment and there is no doubt at all that the eye is totally blind.

5. **Following a penetrating injury** (see page 318).

Evisceration or enucleation?

Enucleation must be performed for a suspected intraocular tumour and also when removing a traumatised eye to prevent sympathetic ophthalmitis. Evisceration and not enucleation is generally recommended for endophthalmitis. The reason is that enucleation may risk spreading the infection along the ophthalmic veins into the cavernous sinus or along the cerebrospinal fluid into the meninges. For all other cases the eye may either be enucleated or eviscerated. The advantage of enucleation is that the socket heals much quicker and without pain. Following evisceration there is more post-operative pain and swelling of the conjunctiva. The sclera contracts to a fibrous mass in the floor of the socket with the extraocular muscles attached to it. Therefore the socket is not so empty and the floor of the socket moves better. An artificial eye therefore looks more natural after evisceration.

Evisceration

Principle

The removal of the contents of the eye leaving only the scleral shell.

Method

1. The operation can be performed under local anaesthetic using a retrobulbar block. If the tissues are inflamed more anaesthetic than usual will be required. It is advisable to give some additional systemic analgesia and sedation as well e.g. Pethidine 100 mg i.m. If facilities for general anaesthesia are available a general anaesthetic is probably better in cases of endophthalmitis.
2. A speculum is inserted to part the lids.
3. Using a scalpel a stab incision is made through the limbus (**Figure 11.1**). The cornea is then removed with scissors (**Figure 11.2**).
4. The contents of the eye are removed with a sharp curette or spoon (**Figure 11.3**). A fair amount of bleeding is common. It is extremely important to make sure that all the black choroid is removed leaving

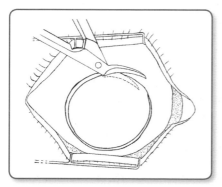

Figure 11.2 Evisceration. Excising the cornea with scissors

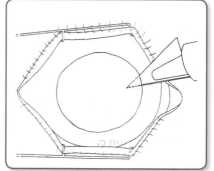

Figure 11.1 Evisceration. A stab incision with a scapel at the limbus

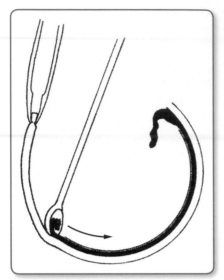

Figure 11.3 Evisceration. Using a curette to remove all the ocular contents. Try to separate the choroid gently from the sclera

bare white sclera. If any choroidal tissue is left there is a risk of sympathetic ophthalmitis occurring later. Cleaning the scleral cavity with a swab soaked in 5% phenol helps to lessen post-operative pain.

5. The sclera can be left open to drain. This is advisable in endophthalmitis, but otherwise the sclera can be closed with catgut, and the conjunctiva closed over it as another layer.
6. Antibiotic ointment is applied under a double pad and a firm bandage.

Post-operative care

-   The socket is usually left for 2 days before inspection. There is often considerable swelling of the conjunctiva which may protrude between the eyelids. This will settle after some days.
-   Antibiotic ointment is applied regularly and the patient can be discharged if feeling well.
-   Once the swelling and inflammation has settled an artificial eye can be inserted.

Enucleation

Principle

The removal of the whole intact eye by cutting the six extraocular muscles and transecting the optic nerve.

Method

1. The operation can usually be performed fairly easily under local anaesthetic with a retrobulbar block. For children general anaesthetic is obviously necessary.
2. A speculum is inserted.

3. Using forceps and scissors an incision in the conjunctiva is made right round the limbus to separate the conjunctiva from the cornea.
4. Using scissors the conjunctiva is separated from the globe in the four quadrants between the insertions of the extraocular muscles (**Figure 11.4**). This is an easy dissection but must be carried out back to the equator of the eye.
5. Use a muscle hook (strabismus hook) to catch each of the four rectus muscles in turn. Pass the hook back under the conjunctiva between the rectus muscles and then twist it so that the tip passes under the muscle and catches it (**Figure 11.5**). Each muscle should be divided about 1–2 mm from the globe. It may be helpful to use an artery forceps or a strong stitch to grasp the attachment of each muscle to the eye.
6. Heavy scissors are now passed round the eye either nasally or temporally until the optic nerve is felt as a tight cord against the scissors (**Figure 11.6**). The blades are opened and the nerve is cut. When the

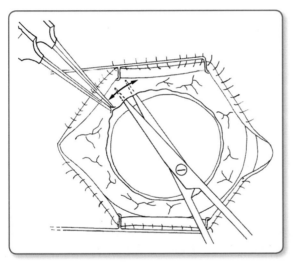

Figure 11.4 Enucleation. Separating the conjunctiva from the globe back to the equator of the eye using scissors

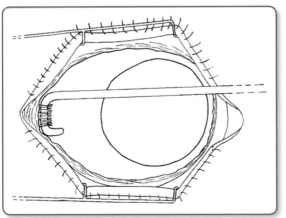

Figure 11.5 Enucleation. Catching the rectus muscle with a strabismus hook

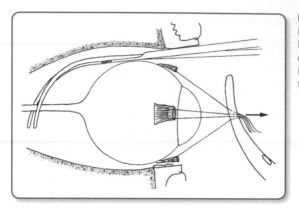

Figure 11.6 Enucleation. Dividing the optic nerve with heavy curved scissors. Traction on the rectus muscles makes it easier to cut the nerve near the apex of the orbit

operation is being performed because of a suspected retinoblastoma, it is very important to cut the optic nerve as far back in the orbit as possible. This is done by strong traction on the insertions of the four extra-ocular muscles with artery forceps or sutures so as to pull the eye forwards and stretch the optic nerve. There is usually profuse bleeding at this stage.

7. The eye can now be prolapsed forwards from the orbit and the remaining oblique muscles and attachments divided. The socket is packed with gauze swabs and pressure applied for 5 minutes. On removing the swabs the bleeding should have almost stopped.

8. Ideally the wound should be closed in 2 layers, first the Tenon's capsule and then the conjunctiva, using continuous or interrupted absorbable sutures. Antibiotic ointment and a firm pad and bandage are applied.

Post-operative care

- The socket should be examined on the second post-operative day.
- If well the patient can then be discharged with instructions to apply antibiotic ointment.
- An artificial eye can usually be inserted fairly soon as the socket heals quickly.

Cosmetic implants

If a plastic implant is left in the orbit after evisceration or enucleation, the final cosmetic result is much better. The artificial eye will be thinner and smaller, it will fit much better, it will not sag in the socket, and it will move much better when the other eye moves. After evisceration a small plastic ball can be placed in the scleral cavity, and then the sclera and the conjunctiva carefully closed in 2 layers. After enucleation a similar plastic ball can be placed in the orbit, and the ends of the four rectus muscles sewn to each other in front of the implant. (There are more sophisticated implants to which the extraocular muscles can actually be attached.) The Tenon's capsule and conjunctiva is then carefully closed in two layers.

Implants are not advised if the eye has been removed for a suspected tumour or for severe endophthalmitis.

Exenteration

Principle

The entire orbital contents down to the bone are removed. This is often covered with a skin graft. Exenteration is a mutilating operation and the only indication is in the treatment of some malignant tumours in the orbit.

A brief description of how to manage orbital disease will help to explain the indications for exenteration. Orbital diseases are nearly always difficult to manage.

- The diagnosis is usually difficult. There are many different types of tumour, benign or malignant as well as inflammatory masses and cysts which can occur in the orbit.
- Deciding the correct type of treatment is usually difficult.
- Operations on the orbit are usually difficult to carry out.

Symptoms	Cause	Treatment
Gradual proptosis or a slowly growing orbital mass	Benign tumour or cyst	Either leave untreated or excise completely. This is usually done through a lateral orbitotomy removing the bone of the lateral orbital wall
Fairly rapid proptosis often with some pain or inflammation	Chronic inflammation Pseudo tumour or malignant tumour	Biopsy Systemic steriods for pseudotumour Exenteration, chemotherapy or radiotherapy for malignant tumour
Very rapid proptosis with fever and malaise	Acutue orbital cellulitis	Systematic antibiotics

The following is a very simplified outline of the management of orbital lesions.

Remember thyroid eye disease is also a common cause of proptosis. An orbital biopsy may be performed through the eyelid or the conjunctiva. Inflammatory lesions are usually treated with steroids. Malignant tumours may be exenterated or treated with chemotherapy.

Many malignant tumours of the orbit spread quite early to other parts of the body. If metastatic spread has occurred exenteration will not save the patient's life. However exenteration may completely cure some tumours like a conjunctival carcinoma or an advanced basal cell carcinoma of the skin. Also the patient may have a hideous fungating smelly mass in the orbit and to remove it may make the last few months of the patient's life very much more pleasant.

Before performing a mutilating operation like an exenteration the surgeon should be as certain as possible of the diagnosis, and the patient should be adequately counselled. It is important not to confuse the marked proptosis that may occur with some cases of endophthalmitis or pseudotumour (an inflammatory condition of the orbit) with proptosis from a tumour.

Method

1. The operation must be performed under some sort of general anaesthesia, preferably with endotracheal intubation.

2. A firm incision is made right down to the bone along the line of the orbital rim (**Figure 11.7**). There will be considerable bleeding and this may be lessened by injecting very dilute adrenaline into the tissues just before operation. Firm pressure on the wound edge also controls this bleeding. The bleeding points are secured with artery forceps and then either ligated or diathermied.

3. The periostium is incised right round the orbital rim so that the dissection is now on bare bone. The periosteum is then stripped and separated from the bone passing back towards the orbital apex (**Figure 11.8**). The periosteum is very closely attached to the bone at the rim of the orbit, and it is hard to separate it from the bone, but further back in the orbit it is quite easy to separate the periosteum from the bone right back to the apex of the orbit. Particular care is needed over the medial orbital wall which is thin. The dissection is completed as far back as possible to the apex of the orbit. The tissues at the orbital apex are then divided using heavy curved scissors or a scalpel blade. There will be very profuse bleeding at this stage and it is best to control this with firm pressure for 5 minutes or more. If bleeding still persists pressure with a hot pack may control it. If possible hot packs should be avoided as they

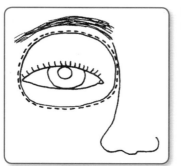

Figure 11.7 Exenteration. The skin incision is at the edge of the bony orbital rim

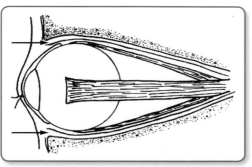

Figure 11.8 Exenteration. To show the plane of the dissection between the orbital bone and the periosteum

cause thrombosis of the small vessels within the bone and will delay healing.

4. The orbit may be left packed and a delayed skin graft performed, or it may be left to granulate and skin will gradually cover it from the edge. If the haemostasis is very good a split skin graft can be applied at the time of surgery. It is better to use a mesh graft with holes in it or a few small patches of skin as this allows drainage and is more likely to "take". The graft is applied over a damp pack which is pushed into the orbit. Vaseline gauze is best avoided as it prevents serous exudate draining into the pack. The edges of the graft may be stitched to the skin at the orbital rim. The graft will usually take even though it is applied directly to bone and if areas do fail they will re-epithelialise quite quickly.

5. *Modified exenteration*. In some cases it may be possible to preserve one or both of the eyelids. Alternatively some of the eyelid skin may be preserved and turned inwards to help cover the bare bone of the orbit.

Post-operative care

- Analgesia and a course of systemic antibiotics are required.
- The orbit is usually left for about 10 days until the pack is removed. This must be done with great care so as not to pull off any skin graft which is present and not to provoke bleeding from granulation tissue. If possible it is best to leave the donor site covered up for 10 days as well.
- Secondary skin grafting may be applied if necessary.
- The patient should be provided with a patch and taught how to remove keratin which will accumulate in the socket.

Objectives
- General management of eye trauma
- Penetrating eye injuries
- Blunt ocular trauma
- Minor superficial eye injuries
- Eyelid injuries
- Burns
- Orbital fractures

Every trauma patient is a special challenge to the surgeon because each case is different. The patient usually arrives as an emergency and may have other injuries as well. The medical staff may neither be fully prepared nor equipped to treat eye injuries. This chapter will describe the general management of any patient with ocular trauma. Then details of the treatment of the more common and important injuries will be given.

General management of eye trauma

The injuries must first be assessed in just the same way as for any other patient.

History taking

An accurate and detailed history must be taken. Two questions in particular are important: how long ago did the injury occur and what was it that injured the eye? Unfortunately there may be a long delay between the injury and treatment. The patient may already have received some treatment either from a doctor, a nurse, or a traditional healer.

Examination

A systematic detailed eye examination is absolutely vital. This may be not be easy if the eyelids are very swollen or bruised. It may be necessary to part the swollen eyelids with a lid retractor after applying local anaesthetic drops to the eye. If this fails an examination under anaesthetic is necessary especially in children.

The examination of the eye should follow an organised routine. Particular attention should be paid to the following:
1. Measure the visual acuity carefully and in each eye.
2. Examine the eyelids looking particularly for lacerations.
3. Palpate the orbital rim for any notches, tenderness or abnormal mobility, that would suggest a fracture of the orbit.

4. Examine the ocular movement to check for diplopia. Also check for proptosis if the eye is pushed forwards, or enophthalmos if it is displaced backwards.

5. Examine the cornea and conjunctiva. A laceration of the conjunctiva may indicate a deeper laceration in the underlying sclera, and lacerations to the cornea may be full thickness into the anterior chamber. If available, instill sterile fluorescein drops or use a filter paper impregnated with fluorescein to help to identify corneal abrasions and wounds. If there is a small corneal wound leaking aqueous, this will become very obvious when the eye is examined with fluorescein especially in a blue light (Seidel's test see plate 3 and 4).

6. Examine the anterior chamber to check whether or not any blood is present (hyphaema). Occasionally the whole anterior chamber is full of dark clotted blood which can easily be missed in a patient with a dark iris (see plate 8). Look also for inflammatory cells in the anterior chamber (hypopyon) which is evidence of infection in the eye (see plate 9).

7. Examine the pupil, its size, shape and reaction, and whether any iris, ciliary body, or choroid has prolapsed out of the eye through the wound.

8 Check the intraocular pressure. This is often forgotten and should always be done unless there is damage to the cornea or an obvious penetrating injury.

9. If indicated, dilate the pupil to examine the lens, vitreous, retina and optic nerve head.

Special tests

Following the eye examination, skull X-rays may be indicated if any orbital fractures are suspected. A soft tissue orbital X-ray may identify a suspected foreign body in the eye or orbit.

Treatment

There are three possible types of treatment:

1. First-aid treatment only

Penetrating eye injuries are difficult to repair well, and referral elsewhere may be the best choice. There are many factors to consider: the experience of the surgeon and the equipment available, the distance, time and money involved in referral, and the patient's circumstances. Sometimes the patient has other more serious injuries such as a head injury or serious body injuries which take precedence over the eye injury. First-aid treatment usually means applying antibiotic ointment and a sterile pad to the eye.

2. Medical treatment

Antibiotics –The first priority is to prevent bacterial infection with antibiotics.The eyelids are very vascular, so eyelid injuries may not require antibiotics. However all penetrating injuries to the eye must receive antibiotics.

Anti-fungal agents – These are indicated for injuries to the cornea with vegetable matter in hot and humid climates, as these favour the growth of fungi.

Anti-tetanus treatment – This is necessary, especially if there is a risk of contamination to the wound by soil or faecal matter. The importance of anti-tetanus treatment is often forgotten.

Other medical treatment – For injuries to the eye itself mydriatics are used to treat iritis. Steroids are used both to prevent and treat iritis and inflammation in the cornea.

3. Surgical treatment

The basic aim of trauma surgery is to try to perform a primary repair of the damaged tissues as an emergency operation. This gives the best chance of restoring the function of the damaged tissues. Lacerations should be resutured so that they can heal with minimal scar formation. It may be necessary to excise dead or infected tissues and to remove foreign bodies. Sometimes primary repair may not be possible. A conjunctival flap to cover the eye may be advisable, or even enucleation of a severely damaged eye may be indicated. Delayed or secondary surgery when the wound has healed may be beneficial in some cases.

Summary of general management of eye injuries

1. History taking, when and how the injury occurred
2. Assessment
   Careful routine examination:
   - especially visual acuity
   - fluorescein dye
   - intraocular pressure
3. Treatment/first-aid
   Medical:
   - antibiotics
   - antifungal agents
   - anti-tetanus
   - steroids
   - mydriatics
   Surgical:
   - primary wound repair
   - debridement and excision of damaged tissue
   - foreign body removal
   - conjunctival flap
   - removal of the eye
   - secondary (delayed) surgery

Types of eye injury

There are a great variety of possible eye injuries but they tend to fit into the following basic types.

   Penetrating eye injuries
   Non-penetrating eye injuries
   Minor superficial eye injuries:
   - corneal abrasions
   - corneal and conjunctival foreign bodies
   - conjunctival lacerations
   Eyelid injuries

Orbital injuries and fractures
Cranial nerve injuries affecting the eye
Burns to cornea, conjunctiva and eyelid

Naturally it is possible to have more than one of these injuries at the same time.

Penetrating eye injuries

These are the most serious eye injuries with a great risk of total or partial sight loss. They are also common injuries. It is often difficult to decide how to treat them, and carrying out any surgical operation may also be difficult. Therefore most of this chapter concerns penetrating eye injuries. There are basically two different types of penetrating eye injury:

1. *Full thickness lacerations or rupture of the cornea or sclera.* With these injuries the corneal or scleral wounds need to be repaired. Treatment is also necessary for any damage to the eye contents.
2. *Puncture wounds.* With these injuries the wound itself is small and seals off spontaneously. However treatment is still necessary to prevent damage inside the eye.

Full thickness corneal or scleral lacerations

An accurate history must be obtained and examination performed as already described.These injuries are usually easy to diagnose but in certain circumstances can be missed.

- A severe blunt injury to the eye may cause a posterior scleral rupture, which is not obvious from external eye examination. Suspicion should be aroused if the eye is soft and confirmed by examination of the fundus. A vitreous or choroidal haemorrhage will be seen.
- A conjunctival laceration may go deeper and also involve the sclera. Lacerations to the conjunctiva can easily be sutured, but the eye and wound must be examined carefully to exclude a scleral rupture.
- If the eyelids are swollen it may be difficult to examine the eye properly.

When the injury has been fully assessed a decision must be made about the basic management. There are 5 possibilities.

1. First-aid treatment and referral elsewhere.
2. Surgical repair of the wound and replacement or excision of extruded intraocular contents.
3. A conjunctival flap procedure.
4. Medical treatment only.
5. Immediate evisceration or enucleation.

Surgical repair of the wound and excision or replacement of the intraocular contents

This is the best choice of treatment and will give the best results. The corneal wound edges should be brought together and held in place by fine, non-irritant sutures. In this way the cornea will heal well, scarring will be minimized, and the regular curvature of the cornea which focuses light on the retina will be preserved. Scleral wounds should also be repaired with direct sutures. However the sclera is opaque, does not transmit light into the eye and is covered by the conjunctiva. Suturing of the sclera need not be so accurate, nor are such fine sutures required. However the exposure of a scleral laceration may be difficult, especially if it extends backwards behind the equator of the eye. Any uveal tissue (the iris, ciliary body and choroid) which has prolapsed through the wound should be excised or replaced, and damaged lens or vitreous may also need surgical treatment.

There are problems in carrying out a primary surgical repair if the patient's arrival at hospital after the injury is delayed. With the passage of time various changes occur in a wound which is left untreated. An inflammatory reaction develops in the injured tissues so that the cornea swells and becomes softer and less easy to suture. The uveal tract (the iris, ciliary body and choroid) is very vascular. These blood vessels will dilate and new vessels grow from the uvea into the wound. The wound will be sealed off with fibrin at first, and later fibroblasts and fibrous tissue as well as blood vessels will grow into the wound to form an opaque fibrous scar. This whole process of healing is often complicated by infection. Penetrating eye wounds often become infected, and the bacteria secrete toxins which cause further inflammation both in the wound and inside the eye.

Once a wound is several days old, any attempt to carry out a primary repair will cause various problems. The iris will not separate from the wound edges and attempts to separate it will only cause bleeding. The tissues become soft, difficult to suture and bleed easily. Any manipulation is likely to spread infection in the eye. Injuries seen within the first 2 days should normally be treated by direct suture. If there is no obvious infection, direct suture can sometimes be carried out up to 4 or 5 days after an injury. After this period, direct suture becomes increasingly difficult and less effective.

Conjunctival flap procedure

Covering a corneal wound with a flap of conjunctiva is often a better choice for infected wounds or injuries over 4 days old. The wound itself and the tissues are not disturbed by the surgery. The conjunctiva covers the bare iris and provides epithelial cover which acts as a barrier against infection and prevents leakage of aqueous. The blood vessels of the conjunctiva bring in antibodies and white cells to fight against infection, and fibroblasts to help form a scar. The technique of a conjunctival flap procedure is described on pages 274–77. Conjunctival flaps are suitable for all penetrating corneal wounds, but especially for wounds in the peripheral cornea.

Medical treatment only

For very old wounds, which are more than two weeks old, even a conjunctival flap may not be of much benefit. Once the wound has become epithelialised (this is shown by a failure to stain with fluorescein dye) there is little to be gained by any form of emergency surgery. It is best to give medical treatment only and consider secondary surgery later.

Enucleation or evisceration

Some years ago this was recommended as primary treatment for many injured eyes, because of the risk of a disease called *sympathetic ophthalmitis*.

This causes iritis in the other eye some weeks or months after a penetrating injury in the first eye. Nowadays the use of local steroids and better surgery has made sympathetic ophthalmitis extremely rare. However enucleation should be carried out if there is *definitely* no perception of light in the eye, and it has been very severely damaged with no hope of a good cosmetic repair. Once this decision has been made the enucleation should be carried out as an emergency.

Primary evisceration should only be carried out if there is *definitely* no perception of light in the eye and it is grossly infected.

Another advantage of enucleation or evisceration is that the wound heals up quickly, and so it avoids lengthy hospital treatment which is not going to restore any sight to the eye.

Surgical repair of penetrating wounds

There are two aspects to the surgical repair of a penetrating eye wound. Firstly, how to manage the intraocular contents and secondly, how to close the wound.

The intraocular contents

It is likely that the uveal tract will prolapse through the wound. The iris prolapses through corneal wounds, and the ciliary body and choroid through scleral wounds. The prolapsed uveal tissue can either be excised or replaced. Replacement gives a better chance of restoring the function of he eye but risks introducing infection in the eye. Excision has less risk of infection, but will cause bleeding from the cut edge of uvea. The following factors will influence the choice of either excision or replacement:

1. *How recent and how dirty was the injury?* It is usually safe to replace the uvea in a clean injury treated within 24 hours. With increasing delay or with a contaminated wound the risk of introducing infection increases. The uvea becomes so stuck to the wound edges that it is difficult to free and replace it.
2. *How much tissue destruction has occurred?* A small knuckle of uvea can be replaced and will function normally. Badly damaged tissue will be difficult to replace and will not function normally in any case.
3. *Which part of the uvea has prolapsed – the iris, ciliary body or choroid?* An iris prolapse is likely to get infected quickly, and the iris can be excised without excessive bleeding. Therefore an iris prolapse should be excised if there is any doubt. Prolapsed ciliary body or choroid is usually covered by the conjunctiva and so is less likely to be infected. The choroid and ciliary body will bleed excessively if excised, and excision may also damage the retina, vitreous or suspensory ligament of the lens.Therefore the choroid and ciliary body should be replaced in the eye unless it is essential to excise it.

Technique for excising uveal tissue (usually the iris)

Lift the uvea gently with fine forceps. If possible try to free it carefully from the edges of the wound with an iris repositor, then cut it flush with the surface of the wound using de Wecker's scissors (**Figure 12.1**). If the uvea is firmly adherent to the wound edges and cannot easily be freed, it is better to

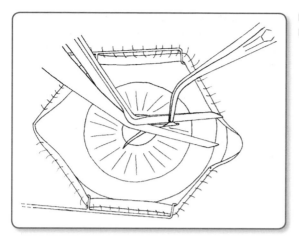

Figure 12.1 Excising an iris prolapse

leave it sticking to the cornea or sclera rather than provoke bleeding and risk spreading infection by trying to separate it. However, there must be no uveal tissue prolapsing when the corneal or scleral wound is finally sewn together.

Technique for replacing uveal tissue in the eye

First try to separate any adhesions between the uvea and the wound edge with an iris repositor or similar blunt instrument. Use the side of an iris repositor or blunt irrigation cannula to slide the uveal tissue back into the eye rather than poking it back. The assistant may need to press very gently on the uvea with an iris repositor to hold it back while the cornea or sclera is being sutured. The iris repositor should only rest between the lips of the wound and not enter the eye. The iris is a very delicate tissue and the choroid even more delicate. The choroid will bleed profusely if damaged in any way during the surgery.

If the iris is adherent to the back of the corneal wound but is not present in the lips of the wound, it is best just to suture the wound and not make any attempt to free the iris from the back surface of the cornea. The iris is often firmly adherent to the cornea and the manipulation will do more harm than good.

Penetrating injuries may also involve the lens, the vitreous and the retina. As a general rule there is little to be gained by any other manipulation inside the eye. It is likely to spread infection, provoke haemorrhage and cause further damage especially to the lens. It is a good principle simply to excise or replace the prolapsed uvea, and close the corneal or scleral wound. Other secondary procedures can be carried out once the eye has healed.

Blood clot in the anterior chamber is best left alone. Trying to remove it by grasping it or irrigating it from the eye is likely to cause damage and may provoke fresh bleeding.

There are two occasions when further intraocular surgery is indicated at the time of the emergency wound repair:

- *Vitreous prolapse*, especially through a corneal wound, should be treated like vitreous loss at cataract surgery (see page 129). Every attempt should be made to clear the vitreous from the anterior chamber and prevent adhesions of vitreous to the cornea.

- *Damage to the lens*. If there is extensive damage to the lens especially in a young person, the lens protein will break up and cause severe uveitis. Extensive damage to the lens is best treated by immediate extracapsular cataract extraction. The lens matter should be irrigated out of the eye with a two-way cannula hopefully preserving the posterior capsule. If the lens is only punctured, it should be left for cataract extraction later.

In countries where penetrating wounds are seen early and advanced instrumentation is available, severe penetrating wounds are often treated more aggressively. A vitrectomy and extensive intraocular surgery may well be done at the time of the emergency wound repair. In developing countries where injuries are often seen late, and less sophisticated equipment is available, it is better to adopt a more conservative approach; to do as little as possible as long as the wound is closed carefully either by direct suture or a conjunctival flap. Providing that the wound is properly closed and the eye does not become infected, there is a possibility of further surgical treatment later.

Corneal wound closure

The aim in repairing corneal wounds is to bring the 2 edges of the wound as close together as possible, so as to minimise any distortion of the cornea and prevent the formation of an opaque scar. Because the suture material is a foreign body, it will itself cause some scarring and irritation. Therefore sutures should be as fine and as non-irritant as possible. Usually the wound is closed with interrupted sutures.

The best suture material is 10-0 or 11-0 monofilament nylon, mersilene or polypropylene. These are so fine that an operating microscope is almost essential, but it is just possible to use them with operating glasses. Ideally this suture should be placed up to three-quarters of the depth of the cornea. It is a common mistake not to put the stitches deep enough. The stitches should be carefully aligned and the same depth on both sides of the wound (**Figure 12.2**). The needle should pass from the centre of the cornea outwards

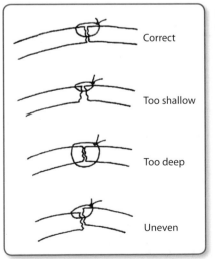

Correct

Too shallow

Too deep

Uneven

Figure 12.2 Correct and incorrect sutures for a corneal wound

to the periphery. The technique of tying the knot is described on pages 47–8. It is best to bury the knot, or the suture ends on the surface of the cornea will irritate the eye. Burying the knot is done by rotating the stitch with suture tying forceps after tying the knot and cutting the ends. The knot should be buried so that it passes into the periphery of the cornea. Alternatively the knot can be buried by starting and finishing the suturing with the needle in the wound.

If 10-0 or 11-0 suture material or good magnification is not available, 9-0 nylon is the best alternative and failing that virgin silk. However the knot will be too bulky to bury by rotating the stitch, and if it is buried it will be difficult to remove the knot from the cornea when removing the stitch. Therefore leave the knot on the surface, but place it at the peripheral side of the wound and cut the stitch ends very short. If neither 9-0 nor virgin silk sutures are available then use the finest sutures that are available.

In ideal circumstances the sutured corneal wound should be "water-tight". The anterior chamber may reform spontaneously during the operation. Alternatively it should be reformed when balanced salt solution is irrigated into the anterior chamber through a fine cannula placed in the wound between 2 sutures (**Figure 12.3**). Sometimes it is impossible to get a "water-tight" wound in which case an "air-tight" wound is satisfactory. A small bubble of air is injected into the anterior chamber through the fine cannula. It is best not to completely fill the anterior chamber with air as this may occasionally obstruct the circulation of aqueous in the eye and cause glaucoma. Enough sutures should be placed to ensure that the wound is at least air-tight.

Removal of corneal sutures

The removal of corneal sutures is quite important, and unlike the removal of other sutures it is a task that cannot be delegated. Corneal wounds, especially in the centre of the cornea, take a long time to heal because the cornea has no blood vessels. If mono-filament sutures with buried knots have been used these will not cause any irritation, and they can be left in place for up to six months. However, if the knots are on the surface or the sutures come loose, they will act as a foreign body and cause inflammation to the cornea

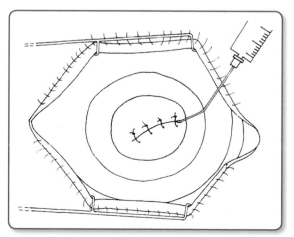

Figure 12.3 Reforming the anterior chamber

and provoke vascularisation and scarring. Thicker corneal sutures or those which do not have buried knots are usually removed about 4-6 weeks post-operatively because they irritate the eye. To remove corneal sutures:

- First apply local anaesthetic drops and reassure the patient that this is a painless procedure. The patient's cooperation is necessary to keep the head still and their eyes open.
- If available use a slit lamp, but if not lie the patient down and use magnifying glasses.
- Cut the suture with a scalpel blade and then pull on the cut end nearest the margin of the cornea with suture tying forceps (**Figure 12.4**).
- Apply topical antibiotic drops immediately before and for 2-3 days after removing corneal sutures to prevent any infection of the suture track.

Scleral wound closure

Scleral wounds are more difficult to expose and identify than corneal wounds. It may be necessary to incise and retract the conjunctiva to expose the scleral wound. For very posterior scleral wounds a muscle hook placed around a rectus muscle insertion may help exposure. However scleral wounds are easier to suture than corneal wounds, because very fine sutures are not required. Nor is it necessary to bring the two surfaces perfectly together as the sclera is vascular and heals much better than the cornea. 5-0 or 6-0 suture material, either absorbable or non-absorbable, can be used as the knots will in any case be buried under the conjunctiva. If a scleral wound extends backwards and is hard to expose, a useful hint to help exposure is to put an interrupted suture in the anterior end of the laceration. Leave the suture end long and the assistant can retract on the stitch. This will rotate the eye so that the next suture can be placed further back and so on.

After the sclera has been repaired, the conjunctiva should be sutured as a separate layer.

Puncture wounds of the eye

Puncture wounds the are usually small and seal off spontaneously, but extensive damage may be caused inside the eye. Puncture wounds are usually caused by thorns, splinters of wood or glass, or by tiny high velocity fragments of stone or metal which may be retained inside the eye. Careful history taking and examination are very important. The patient may not realise they have sustained a puncture wound, and often the doctor does not detect

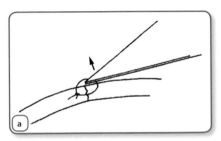
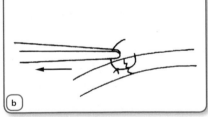

Figure 12.4 Removing the corneal sutures

it unless a very careful examination is made. Soft tissue X-rays may be helpful to confirm the presence of a foreign body inside the eye and to locate its
position. Puncture wounds do not usually require suturing. Wounds in the
periphery of the cornea will often become plugged with iris, but this does not
require treatment as long as the iris does not prolapse through the wound.
Wounds, especially in the central cornea, may leak aqueous. If the anterior
chamber is formed they do not need repairing. Even if the anterior chamber
is not formed it may be better to apply a firm pad and bandage to a puncture
wound than to attempt to suture it. As the tissues swell with oedema and the
epithelium heals, the wound will often seal itself. If available, a sterile bandage soft contact lens will help a corneal puncture wound to seal off. Scleral
puncture wounds do not usually require surgical treatment, but if there is
any doubt about a scleral wound the conjunctiva should be incised and the
wound examined to make sure it does not extend.

If a thorn or similar fragment is still embedded in the cornea it should be
removed. If there is a possibility that the thorn has gone right through the cornea into the aqueous, apply pilocarpine drops to constrict the pupil before
attempting removal. There may be a gush of aqueous humour with collapse of
the anterior chamber, and constricting the pupil prevents the lens becoming
damaged by the foreign body.

If a tiny fragment remains inside the eye, removal is difficult. These tiny fragments may be difficult to locate and even harder to remove. Usually it is best
to leave them, but magnetic foreign bodies must be removed as they will rust
and become toxic to the eye. Fortunately they can usually be extracted with a
powerful magnet. This is specialised surgery which can wait for a few days, so
referral is best. The post operative care and complications of penetrating injuries are basically the same whether they are lacerations or puncture wounds.

Post operative care of penetrating injuries

It is usual to keep the eye padded for 3 or 4 days to help the epithelium to
heal, but it should be examined every day.

Antibiotics

All penetrating wounds should be given antibiotics whether they appear infected or not. The choice of antibiotic depends upon availability and any information that may be available about the organism from culture or gram stain. A
sub conjunctival antibiotic injection is routinely given at the end of any surgical
repair and after puncture wounds (see page 176 for method and details of doses). A course of systemic antibiotics should be given as well. The first dose may
be given by injection but oral antibiotics are perfectly satisfactory. It is usual to
apply topical antibiotic drops and ointment until the wound is healed.

Mydriatics

These are given routinely to prevent post operative iritis. Atropine 1% daily is
usually recommended for at least a week.

Steroids

There are several reasons for using steroids after penetrating injuries:
- Steroids will reduce scarring and vascularisation of the cornea.

- Steroids will treat the uveitis which always occurs to some extent after penetrating injuries.
- Steroids will lessen the very slight risk of sympathetic ophthalmitis developing.

The usual recommendation is that steroids should be started about 3-4 days after any surgical treatment, so allowing the antibiotics and the body's defences against infection to work. Some surgeons like to start topical steroid treatment immediately to try to prevent inflammation in the eye from the beginning, as the antibiotics should be effective against the risk of infection. Steroid drops or ointment are usually prescribed every 2-4 hours for about two to three weeks.

Complications of penetrating injuries

There are many complications and only brief guide-lines about their management will be given here.

Infection

If the infection does not seem to be responding to treatment after a few days, the antibiotics should be changed. If there was loss of vitreous or the lens at the time of injury, an intra-vitreal injection of antibiotic may be indicated (see page 178). If there is no perception of light and the eye is still infected, evisceration is probably the best course.

Iritis

There is always some degree of iritis especially in severe injuries. Fortunately sympathetic ophthalmitis (see page 319) is very rare as long as penetrating injuries are treated promptly with topical steroids and effective surgery.

Hyphaema and vitreous haemorrhage

These may occur and should be left to absorb, unless the hyphaema is total.

Cataract

Cataract is very common after penetrating injuries and always occurs if the lens capsule has been damaged. Cataract may appear very rapidly after the injury or there may be a delay of some months or even years. There may be swelling of the lens causing angle closure glaucoma, or lens matter may leak into the anterior chamber causing secondary iritis and glaucoma. Therefore if a cataract develops after a penetrating injury, cataract extraction should be carried out without delay. If fragments of lens are seen in the anterior chamber immediately after a penetrating injury, the eye should be treated with intensive topical steroids because these lens fragments can cause severe uveitis. It may be best to wash out the lens matter with a two-way cannula.

Traumatic cataract is quite common in young children and these are good cases for an IOL implant. However the operation is often difficult because the lens may be degenerate and the eye damaged in other ways.

Corneal scarring and astigmatism: After corneal injury the patient may have quite marked astigmatism which can sometimes be corrected with spectacles. Where available, contact lenses may help.

Glaucoma and retinal detachments: These are also complications of penetrating eye injuries. Indeed every patient after an eye injury should be seen and thoroughly examined 2 to 3 months after the injury to check for these complications.

Sometimes after a primary repair of an eye injury it becomes obvious that the eye has no hope of vision. If it is also very inflamed an early decision to enucleate the eye is best. Delay means lengthy treatment for an eye which will never see, and also risks the possibility of sympathetic ophthalmitis. However if the eye is neither painful nor inflamed there is no point in removing it except for cosmetic reasons.

Blunt injuries to the eyeball

Blunt injuries occur when the eye is struck and deformed but the cornea and sclera remained intact. These injuries may severely damage the eye by disrupting the delicate intraocular structures, (see **Figure 12.5**) but for most of this damage emergency surgical treatment is not required.

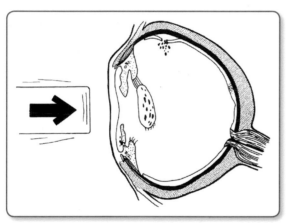

Figure 12.5a How an eye can be damaaged from a blunt injury

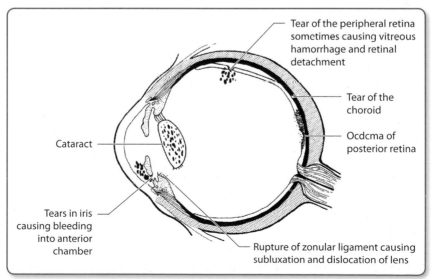

Tear of the peripheral retina sometimes causing vitreous hamorrhage and retinal detachment

Tear of the choroid

Ocdcma of posterior retina

Cataract

Tears in iris causing bleeding into anterior chamber

Rupture of zonular ligament causing subluxation and dislocation of lens

Figure 12.5b Results of a blunt injury

The only common indication for emergency surgery is to treat severe bleeding in the anterior chamber (hyphaema). This occurs from tears in the iris particularly the root of the iris, where the main iris blood vessels are found. Under normal circumstances fluid blood or blood clot will absorb from the anterior chamber without complications. The treatment is simply to rest the patient because sudden eye movements may provoke further haemorrhage. Blood should be evacuated from the anterior chamber only if there is a very severe hyphaema with raised intraocular pressure. There must be a total and complete hyphaema, so that the whole anterior chamber is full of thick dark blood obscuring any view of the iris. This is sometimes called a "black ball" hyphaema. If the intraocular pressure is raised, degenerate blood cells permanently stain the cornea and also block up the drainage angle, therefore this type of hyphaema should be evacuated.

Evacuation of a hyphaema

Method

1. Make an incision about 4 mm long in the peripheral cornea (**Figure 12.6**). Then slowly deepen the incision using a scalpel or a razor blade fragment and go right through the cornea into the anterior chamber. Try to decompress the eye slowly.
2. The important step is to allow thick treacle-like fluid blood to be washed out of the anterior chamber. Formed blood clot is likely to be stuck to the iris and trying to remove it may well provoke further bleeding. Gently irrigate the anterior chamber with Ringer's solution or similar irrigating fluid, attempting to remove as much as possible of the thick treacle-like blood and any blood clot which comes easily out of the eye. Close the wound with one corneo-scleral suture and reform the anterior chamber with Ringer's solution or saline.
3. Treat the patient post operatively with mydriatics and topical steroids. Check the intraocular pressure. The patient should be rested until the remaining blood clot and hyphaema have absorbed.

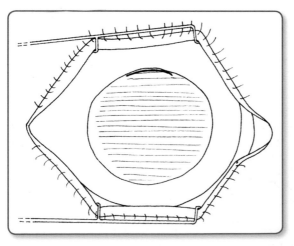

Figure 12.6 The incision to evacuate a hyphaema

An emergency trabeculectomy operation (see page 208) is an alternative way of treating a hyphaema with raised intraocular pressure. This is recommended if the hyphaema is not total and complete but the intraocular pressure is raised. The operation will drain the blood out of the anterior chamber and control the pressure for the next few weeks. Nearly always the drainage bleb will then become fibrosed and cease to function, but hopefully by that time the pressure will have returned to normal.

Complications of blunt injuries

These are numerous and may occur soon after the injury or even years later. The most common are:

- Mydriasis from damage to the iris muscle
- Glaucoma from damage to the anterior chamber angle
- Cataract
- Dislocated lens
- Vitreous haemorrhage
- Choroidal and retinal tears and haemorrhages
- Retinal detachment
- Optic atrophy

Minor superficial eye injuries

These are very common. Various types of injury may occur.

Foreign bodies

These are often blown into the eye and may lodge on the cornea or become trapped inside the eyelids particularly in the groove near the eyelid margin. Always evert the upper eyelid when examining a patient who may have a foreign body in the eye. Most superficial foreign bodies are very easy to remove.

A conjunctival foreign body can usually be wiped off with a sterile swab or cotton bud, after applying local anaesthetic drops.

A corneal foreign body can usually be lifted off with the edge of a small hypodermic needle. Occasionally a high velocity foreign body may become deeply impacted in the cornea. It may then be necessary to use the tip of a hypodermic needle to pick the foreign body out of the corneal stroma. Sometimes the entry point may have to be enlarged with a blade to aid the removal of a foreign body deeply embedded in the cornea. After removal of a foreign body, topical antibiotic drops or ointment should be given to prevent corneal infection. If the patient has come for treatment very late, and there is evidence of established infection in the cornea around the foreign body, then a sub conjunctival injection of antibiotic should also be given. If the foreign body was vegetable matter and injury occurred in a hot and humid climate, an antifungal preparation is also advisable. Natamycin (Pimaricin) has been widely used as an antifungal drop or ointment. If there is superficial damage to the cornea, mydriatics should also be used for 2-3 days, and the eye should be padded until the corneal epithelium has healed.

Corneal abrasions

These are caused by sharp objects striking or scratching the cornea and breaking the epithelium. The eye is very painful, but the abrasion is hard to recognise until fluorescein is applied, and the damaged cornea will be then outlined with fluorescein stain. Always make sure that there is no foreign body still in the cornea or lodged under the eyelid. The treatment is the same as for a corneal foreign body: topical antibiotics, possibly topical antifungal agents, mydriatics and an eye pad until the corneal epithelium has healed.

Conjunctival lacerations

These should be explored to make sure that the sclera is intact. Conjunctival lacerations usually heal very quickly. If the wound is gaping the edges of the conjunctiva should be brought together with one or two interrupted fine sutures. If the conjunctiva is not sutured, Tenon's capsule may prolapse through the conjunctival wound and delay healing.

Sub-conjunctival haemorrhages

These are common particularly after blunt injuries. The blood will absorb without complications and no treatment is necessary. However a sub conjunctival haemorrhage may be a sign of an underlying scleral rupture so a full eye examination is necessary. It may be a sign of a fracture of the anterior cranial fossa of the skull, if there is no posterior limit to the haemorrhage, but it spreads right back into the orbit.

Eyelid injuries

The eyelids are commonly injured because of their exposed position. Eyelid skin easily lacerates because it is so thin. Haematomas occur frequently because the eyelids are so vascular. The eyelids easily swell with oedema or blood because the connective tissue is so lax and secondary infection in the wound will cause further swelling. In spite of eyelid swelling, an attempt must be made to examine the eye itself for damage. The surgical management of eyelid lacerations is essentially the same as any other wound:
- Cleaning and debridement
- Primary repair
- Post-operative management
- Secondary reconstruction

Most eyelid repairs can be carried out under local anaesthetic infiltration with added adrenaline.

Cleaning and debridement

Cleaning the wound from dirt, debris or foreign bodies is most important. A good scrub with a fine brush may be helpful although this may provoke some bleeding. Make a very thorough search right to the depths of the wound for dirt or foreign bodies before starting the repair. The eyelid blood supply is so good that debridement of eyelid tissue is not usually necessary. If it is decided to excise severely damaged tissue, only the barest minimum should be removed.

Primary repair

Primary repair of eyelid lacerations should be carried out within 48 hours. The eyelids usually heal very well because of their good blood supply. Closure should be in 2 layers to prevent tethering of the skin.

The tarsal plate and the conjunctiva form the deep layer, and this should be closed with absorbable 5-0 or 6-0 sutures. Make sure that the knot is buried in the tissues and does not rest on the surface of the conjunctiva where it will irritate the cornea. If the laceration involves the eyelid margin take particular care with the suture at the lid margin, so that the two edges come together without a notch or an overlap. If the orbital fat has prolapsed through the orbital septum it can be replaced or carefully excised. The orbital septum joins the tarsal plate to the bony margin of the orbit.

The skin and orbicularis muscle form the superficial layer. Small lacerations require only the skin to be closed using 5-0 or 6-0 non-absorbable sutures. In a large laceration with gaping of the wound and separation of the muscle fibres, one or two subcutaneous sutures using absorbable material will help bring muscle fibres together. Take particular care in closing the lower eyelid skin if the wound is irregular and ragged as it is very easy to end up with skin contracture and an ectropion. If there is any loss of lower lid skin the risk of ectropion is lessened by suturing these irregular wounds vertically rather than horizontally (see page 288–99).

Lacerations through the medial end of the lower lid involving the lacrimal canaliculus require special care. Often the canaliculus becomes scarred leaving a persistently watering eye. It is best not to attempt a major repair of the canaliculus, but if an operating microscope is available, try to suture these wounds so that the two cut edges of the canaliculus are correctly aligned.

Tissue loss Sometimes large amounts of the eyelid may have been avulsed. If the margins of the wound cannot be brought together without excess tension, then the wound must be left to granulate and eventually epithelialise. If necessary an eyelid reconstruction can be carried out later. What is at first a large defect often shrinks by means of the natural healing processes. If there is a major eyelid defect particularly in the upper lid, the cornea must be very carefully observed to make sure an exposure ulcer does not develop. Plenty of lubricant drops and antibiotic ointment should be applied. A transparent plastic shield taped to the rim of the orbit may help to preserve the cornea whilst waiting for eyelid reconstruction.

Post-operative management

Eye pads are not usually necessary unless there are exceptional circumstances. Eyelid wounds very rarely become infected because of the good blood supply. However if the wound is badly contaminated, or has penetrated into the orbit, or the patient comes to hospital very late, then systemic antibiotics are a good precaution.

Skin sutures can usually be removed early (within 7 days) because the skin will heal rapidly.

Secondary reconstruction

This may be necessary after some eye lid injuries, but should be delayed if possible until the scar is inactive. This may take at least 3 months. The most common reasons for secondary reconstruction are notches of the lid margin, ectropion or tethering of the lower lid. These complications can usually be avoided by a careful primary suture with attention to basic principles.

Burns

Burns usually occur in small children at home or in adults from accidents at work. They may have various causes. The most common are:

- Direct heat from a fire.
- A scald from hot fluids.
- Acid burns, the most common is the acid in car batteries.
- Alkali burns, the most common cause is lime or cement used in building. There are of course many other chemicals or hot objects which may cause a burn.

There are 3 different tissues which may be burnt: the eyelids, conjunctiva and cornea. Burns from a fire usually involve the eyelids. The protective blink reflex occurs so rapidly that the conjunctiva and cornea are often partly or completely preserved.

Acid and alkali burns and indeed any chemical burn is much more likely to involve the conjunctiva and cornea because the fluid enters the eye before the blink reflex can occur. Alkali burns can be particularly severe. Alkalis are not so irritant to the skin, but spread deeply into the cornea causing severe inflammation.

First aid treatment of burns

A chemical burn of any sort should be treated with immediate and prolonged irrigation of the eye. Even if the patient comes for treatment some hours after the injury, it is still worth irrigating the conjunctival sac with saline or water. Topical anaesthetic drops will help by relieving the pain and blepharospasm. Prolonged irrigation (15 to 30 minutes) is especially important in the treatment of alkali burns. Obviously with increasing delay irrigation becomes less beneficial but it is never harmful. Other first-aid measures are to apply topical antibiotics and a sterile or clean pad and to give the patient analgesics. Solid particles may be embedded in the conjunctiva or cornea and will need removing.

Definitive treatment

This has 3 aims:

1. *Prevention of infection.* All burns destroy the epithelial cells which form a barrier against the infection, and so all burns have some secondary infection.
2. *Preservation and protection of the cornea.* The eyelids and the conjunctiva protect the cornea. If these are damaged the cornea is at risk of becoming ulcerated and scarred.

3. *Prevention of scarring, particularly in the cornea.* If the cornea becomes scarred the sight will be affected.

Eyelid burns

These are usually treated by exposure so that a firm scab develops and the eye itself can be examined. If the eyelids are padded the eye cannot be examined and the dressings may become very sticky and messy from exudate. Topical antibiotics should be applied to the burnt area and severe cases may require systemic antibiotics. In partial thickness burns when the scab finally separates, the underlying eyelid will be reasonably normal. In full thickness burns eyelid contractures will develop. If the eyelid contracture is causing exposure of the cornea, then the scab (burn eschar) must be excised and a skin graft applied. In severe burns repeated skin grafts may be required. As long as the cornea and conjunctiva remain healthy, skin grafting can be postponed until most of the inflammation in the burnt tissues has settled.

Conjunctival and corneal burns

Assessment

Once first-aid and emergency treatment has been given, try to get as good an assessment of the injury as possible by careful clinical examination.

- Instill sterile fluorescein drops to see how much of the corneal and conjunctival epithelium has been destroyed.
- Examine the corneal stroma to see if it is transparent or hazy. A hazy corneal stroma means that the deep tissues of the cornea have been damaged, and the cornea is likely to become opaque.
- Examine the limbal blood vessels at the margin of the cornea. If there are areas where the limbal blood vessels appear whitened and constricted rather than red and dilated, the prognosis is poor. The absence of blood vessels indicates necrosis or destruction of the limbal tissues and the limbal stem cells. In these cases severe corneal scarring is likely to develop later.

Treatment

The immediate treatment of conjunctival and corneal burns is medical.

- *Antibiotics.* Topical antibiotic drops or ointment should be used frequently until the epithelium has healed. Healing may be delayed especially with alkali burns, but until the epithelium has healed there is a risk of secondary infection.
- *Padding.* Padding protects the eye and helps the epithelium to heal quicker, but unfortunately it may encourage the growth of micro-organisms. It is safe to leave the eye without a pad as long as the patient can be carefully observed in clean surroundings.
- *Mydriatics.* These help to prevent iritis whilst the eye is inflamed.
- *Steroids.* There is controversy about the use of steroids. They suppress inflammation and fibrosis and this helps to limit the scarring of the cornea. However they encourage the growth of micro-organisms, and there is also some evidence that they promote the release of enzymes from damaged cornea which cause further corneal destruction. The

generally accepted principle is that topical steroids should be given at least 4 times daily for the first week, but not for the second or third weeks when there is danger of enzyme release, and then again after 3 weeks.

- *Ascorbate.* Freshly prepared 10% potassium ascorbate drops given 2 hourly are thought to limit the tissue destruction from alkali burns to the cornea but they sting. Oral ascorbic acid (vitamin C) is also helpful.

Delayed treatment

Surgery may be helpful for the delayed complications of burns to the conjunctiva and cornea. Symblepharon (adhesions between the eye and the eyelid) and cicatricial entropion can be treated with a conjunctivoplasty or a conjunctival graft from the other eye. Corneal scars can be treated with limbal grafts from the other eye (see page 283) and corneal grafts from a donor. However the patient's only good eye must not be put at risk in an attempt to preserve a badly damaged one.

Orbital fractures and injuries

Fractures of the orbital margin most commonly involve the zygoma which lies in the lower and outer quadrant of the orbital rim. If there is significant displacement of the fracture, the bone should be replaced within 10 days of the injury. It may be necessary to hold it in place with retaining wires. After 2 weeks it is very difficult to replace the fractured displaced bone.

Fractures of the thin walls of the orbit usually occur from blunt pressure on the orbit such as a punch, and the thin orbital wall gives way. This results in a so-called "blow out" fracture (**Figure 12.7**) and nearly always it is the floor of the orbit forming the roof of the maxillary sinus which gives way. The following signs indicate a "blow out" fracture:

- Anaesthesia of the cheek occurs because the infraorbital nerve, which runs along the floor of the orbit, is damaged. Limitation of eye movement and double vision particularly on looking up. This occurs because the orbital fat and the inferior rectus muscle become trapped in the fracture site.

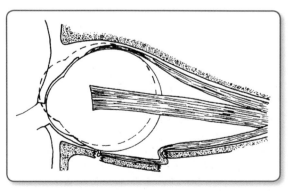

Figure 12.7 A "blow-out" fracture

- Enophthalmos occurs because some of the orbital contents prolapse into the sinus.
- The fracture itself is often not obvious on X-ray because the bone is very thin, but the maxillary sinus is often opaque containing either blood or some orbital contents.

These injuries frequently improve without surgical treatment, but if there is no sign of improvement after 10 days the damaged orbital floor should be explored surgically. The prolapsed orbital tissue must be freed from the fracture and the defect in the orbital floor repaired, usually with a silicone sheet implant.

Orbital haematomas are quite common. There is rarely any indication or need for surgically draining the haematoma.

Cranial nerve injuries

Head injuries can affect the cranial nerves which supply the eye. Paralysis of the 4th nerve (trochlear) and 6th nerve (abducent) are most common. These are thin nerves with a long intra cranial course inside the brain. The 3rd nerve (oculomotor) and 2nd nerve (optic) are less frequently damaged. A 3rd nerve palsy in an unconscious patient causing a dilated pupil is often a sign of raised intracranial pressure and urgent neurosurgery is required.

Cranial nerve palsies especially to the 3rd, 4th and 6th nerves often recover with time, but if there is no recovery after 6 months then surgery to the extraocular muscles may improve or cure the double vision.

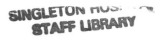

> **Objectives**
> - Cataracts in children
> - Glaucoma
> - Retinoblastoma
> - Trauma
> - Anaesthesia

This chapter provides an introduction to eye surgery in children. Certain conditions are much more common in children, such as retinoblastoma; and surgery for other common conditions such as cataract and glaucoma need special mention because the techniques and approach are very different to those used in adults. In some countries, a sub-specialist paediatric ophthalmologist may be available for referral of difficult cases and this may be ideal, but not always possible. We will also briefly discuss anaesthesia in children.

You may not come across as many children with potentially blinding conditions, as you do adult patients, in your clinic. But preventable or treatable childhood blindness is a priority for us all, as a person is saved from a lifetime of blindness. It is because of this that childhood blindness is a priority for Vision 2020: The Right to Sight.[1]

Cataracts in children

Cataracts in children are a special problem. Deciding the correct time to intervene is difficult and the technique varies from our adult surgical technique. If the operation has complications, the vision of the patient may be affected for their entire life. ***It is best for children with cataracts to be treated by experienced surgeons with special training in paediatric eye surgery.*** However, this may not always be possible. This section provides guidance for those who did not have a special paediatric training.

Even amongst experts there is some disagreement about aspects of paediatric cataract treatment. The following rules are generally accepted by all paediatric cataract surgeons:

1. Dense or mature bilateral congenital cataracts should be operated on as soon as possible, preferably within the first three months of life for proper visual development to occur. The definition of a dense or mature cataract is when the cataract is completely white obscuring the red reflex. If surgery is delayed, sensory deprivation amblyopia will develop; often the eyes will develop nystagmus. This means that the child will never see well in spite of successful surgery later. Rubella infection in

pregnancy is a common cause of bilateral congenital cataract. These children sometimes have retinal damage or microphthalmos as well as cataracts, and even with a successful operation may have poor vision. They may also suffer from deafness and congenital heart defects. Bilateral congenital cataracts may also be associated with other medical conditions such as diabetes, or genetic syndromes such as Down's.

2. Partial or immature cataracts often can have surgical treatment postponed until the child is older, depending on the size of the cataract. A partial or immature cataract is one in which some red reflex can still be seen when the pupil is fully dilated. These are usually lamellar cataracts when just one layer of the lens is affected with the central part of the lens and the peripheral part of the lens being fairly normal. Alternatively the cataract may affect just the very centre of the lens or the anterior or posterior pole of the lens just under the capsule, and there are other patterns of partial congenital cataract.

3. Uniocular congenital cataract with the other eye normal should not normally be treated. These eyes are nearly always very amblyopic. Trying to treat the amblyopia by putting an occlusive patch over the good eye is very disturbing for the child and the family and the benefit is uncertain. More paediatric experts do now treat uniocular cataracts and claim success.[1]

4. The post-operative aphakia must be corrected without delay either with spectacles or intra-ocular lenses (IOLs). Contact lenses in children are not usually possible unless there are expert contact lens fitting services available. The use of IOLs in children used to be controversial. Until a few decades ago IOLs were only inserted in adults. However in the last few years they have been inserted in children as well with encouraging results. Also there is the problem in less developed countries of getting small children to keep and wear aphakic spectacles. For these reasons IOLs are now recommended for young children as well. There remain however several problems with the use of IOLs in children:

    •   The posterior capsule will always become thickened and therefore requires a posterior capsulotomy and anterior vitrectomy, which may need to be repeated, and therefore requires vigilant observation and follow-up over time

    •   The age at which IOLs can be implanted is constantly being reduced. Nowadays most experts would recommend that IOLs should not be inserted in children under 6 months, although this is being done in some specialist centres. The eye is not fully grown until after the age of 12, therefore aiming for emmetropia in a child often results in myopia, or even high myopia, in later life.

    •   IOLs are harder to insert in children than in adults, given the size of the eye.

    •   Damage to the eye from a poorly inserted IOL can affect the child for the rest of their life.

Foldable acrylic lenses are considered by many to be very suitable for children, because they can be inserted through a much smaller incision.

Anterior chamber lenses should not be inserted in children, unless there is a very good reason, for example subluxed/dislocated cataracts (as in Marfan's syndrome, or some traumatic cataracts).

Traumatic cataracts should if possible be given IOL implants. The other eye will be normal and the full vision from the injured eye will not be used without an implant. However, if the eye has inflammation or scarring from the injury it is better to be safe and not insert an implant.

Surgeons with special paediatric training are inserting IOLs regularly. If a surgeon without paediatric training has to operate on a child because there is no possibility of referral, the decision about IOLs is very difficult. A successful result is so much better for the child, but complications can leave the child blinded for life. For a non-expert, it is probably better to be *"safe than sorry" and a cataract extraction without an IOL is a much simpler and safer option. There is no reason why an IOL cannot be inserted later when the child is older or improved facilities or expert treatment are available.* However you do have to balance this against the need for immediate post-operative aphakic spectacles (or contact lenses) to allow for continued visual development to occur.

The surgical treatment of congenital and juvenile cataracts

Both the lens and the eye of a child differs in several ways from an adult.

1. *The eye is smaller, especially in children under two, and the anterior chamber is more shallow.* Because the orbital bones of a child are not fully grown, there is much less space in the orbit for the eye. Therefore as soon as the eye is incised, it is very difficult to maintain the anterior chamber depth. This makes surgery much harder and risks damaging the corneal endothelium. Therefore all surgery in children should be done through very small tight oblique incisions so that the instrument seals off the incision.

   One very helpful instrument for this is an anterior chamber maintainer (see **Figure 6.55**). This is inserted obliquely into the anterior chamber through a small bevelled incision at the lower limbus. It is anchored at the lower limbus and attached to a drip bottle. It gives constant irrigation into the anterior chamber and maintains it at full depth. It also keeps the posterior capsule and vitreous well back throughout the operation.

   It is particularly useful when operating on children with either congenital, developmental or traumatic cataracts. With an anterior chamber maintainer providing irrigation, the aspiration can be done through a single one way cannula rather than a two way Simcoe cannula. This is also inserted into the anterior chamber through a small oblique incision to maintain a full depth anterior chamber (see **Figure 6.55**).

2. *The anterior capsule is very elastic.* Once it has been punctured it tears very easily towards the equator of the lens. The ideal method of anterior capsulotomy in children is the continuous capsulorexis (see page 120 and **Figure 6.26**) This removes the central part of the capsule and leaves

intact the peripheral capsule attached to the suspensory ligament. Unfortunately capsulorexis is extremely difficult to perform in young children as the capsule usually tears outwards towards the equator once it has been incised. Another problem in performing the anterior capsulotomy is that with white opaque cataracts the tear in the capsule is very difficult to see. Therefore in practice the most appropriate type of capsulotomy is to try to do a small "*can opener*" *capsulotomy* which will make a small tear in the centre of the anterior capsule (see page 119). The only way to actually remove any of the capsule is with a vitrectomy machine which takes very small "bites" from the anterior capsule (this is also called a 'vitrectorrhexis').

3. A child's lens does not have a hard nucleus. Therefore irrigation/ aspiration alone is sufficient to perform extracapsular extraction in children.

4. Posterior capsular thickening and opacification occurs in almost all cases. Therefore making a hole in the posterior capsule at the time of operation (a primary posterior capsulotomy) is recommended providing that the circumstances for this are suitable. Unfortunately new lens fibres grow very vigorously in young children. Even after a primary posterior capsulotomy new lens fibres may often grow across the anterior face of the vitreous, thus forming a new opaque posterior capsule. It is therefore much better to remove part of the posterior capsule and the anterior vitreous at the same time as the cataract extraction.

5. Just as in adults, cataracts in children can become degenerate. The capsule may be calcified, and the lens may liquefy or absorb by itself.

For all these reasons cataract extraction in a child can be performed much better with a vitrectomy suction cutter if it is available. Obviously general anaesthetic is essential. If ketamine is used as an anaesthetic agent, a local anaesthetic block should also be given to control eye movements. A superior rectus stitch makes the exposure easier.

Method for congenital or juvenile cataract extraction using a vitrectomy suction cutter

The only reliable way of removing some of the anterior capsule, some of the posterior capsule and the anterior vitreous is with a vitrectomy cutter. It can also remove the opaque lens matter itself. The operation is sometimes called a *lensectomy*.

1. The anterior chamber maintainer is inserted.

2. The vitrectomy probe is inserted through a small tunnelled incision at the upper limbus. Both these incisions should be self-sealing and not leak excessively during the operation nor require sutures post-operatively. If they do leak they can be sutured. Some vitrectomy machines have a an irrigation sleeve if an anterior chamber maintainer is not available.

3. The vitrectomy cutter is used to "nibble" a hole in the centre of the anterior capsule, and through this hole the lens matter itself is then cut

and aspirated. Finally a small hole is made in the centre of the posterior capsule and the anterior part of the vitreous also removed with the vitrectomy probe.

4. Alternatively the vitrectomy cutter can be inserted into the lens from behind the iris, through the pars plicata. The incision should be only 2 mm from the limbus. (Babies do not have a pars plana of the retina and so the incision must be close to the limbus to avoid the retina.) In this case the lens cortex is removed first, then the posterior capsule and the anterior vitreous and finally the anterior capsule.

Method for congenital or juvenile cataract extraction using conventional instruments

1. Insert the anterior chamber maintainer if available.
2. Make another very small bevelled incision at the limbus and through this carry out a small can opener capsulotomy (see page 119), or continuous curvilinear capsulorrhexis (CCC).
3. Through this same incision, aspirate the lens cortex with a single port aspirating cannula (see **Figure 6.55**).
4. If an anterior chamber maintainer is not available, the irrigation and aspiration must be done with a two way Simcoe cannula. This should be inserted through a very small bevelled incision at the limbus just large enough to fit the cannula. It is easier for the surgeon and safer for the eye if the anterior chamber remains formed throughout the operation. An incision which makes a small tunnel will ensure this, and is also self-sealing, however should still be sutured in case the child rubs the eye. The external opening is just in the sclera, and the internal opening just in the cornea. After light cautery or diathermy to the superficial scleral vessels, a knife is used to start the incision in the sclera. A tunnelling knife or a small angled keratome is then used to make the tunnel which enters the anterior chamber about 2 mm inside the limbus. (See **Figure 6.53** for the profile of a tunnelled incision.) The incision need only be large enough for a two way cannula. Whether using a one way or a two way aspirating cannula try to keep the anterior chamber deep all the time, and try to remove as much cortical lens matter as possible. If there are some hard pieces that will not be aspirated the incision may have to be slightly enlarged to wash them out of the eye by forceful irrigation, or captured by the use of forceps.
5. *The posterior capsulotomy.* Because of the high risk of posterior capsular thickening, many surgeons would recommend making a small hole in the posterior capsule at the time of cataract extraction. The posterior capsulotomy can be done with the point of the cystitome, By making a small cut in the centre of the capsule. Unfortunately if the anterior vitreous is not removed, posterior capsular thickening may still occur even after a posterior capsulotomy, because the lens fibres of children can grow across the anterior vitreous face to form another opaque membrane.

If a primary posterior capsulotomy is done the vitreous must not come forward into the anterior chamber. Therefore the incision must be watertight and the anterior chamber must be maintained at full depth all the time. The use of visco-elastic fluids or an anterior chamber maintainer may be very helpful for this. If the vitreous does come forward into the anterior chamber, the eye may develop pupil block glaucoma (see page 151). This may occur immediately after the operation or a long time later.

Sutures are not usually needed after cataract surgery in children, because a small tunnelled incision should be self sealing. If there is any doubt that the wound is water-tight, one or more sutures should be used to secure the wound.

Intraocular lens implants in children

If it has been decided to implant an IOL, these should almost always be posterior chamber implants. The basic method is the same as for an adult. Because of the small eye and the difficulty in keeping the anterior chamber deep, various other steps may be helpful.

- Always use a tunnelled incision to insert the lens, and try to use an anterior chamber maintainer as well. These both help to keep the anterior chamber deep.
- Foldable acrylic lenses are recommended because they can be inserted through a smaller incision and are said to cause less postoperative capsular opacification, although PMMA IOLs are more readily available.
- It is often helpful to insert the lens dialler through a very small separate incision rather than the main incision. This helps to keep the anterior chamber deep.
- If a primary posterior capsulotomy and anterior vitrectomy has been performed, some people advise placing the lens optic behind both the anterior and posterior capsule. This is called "optic capture". The haptics of course should be in the ciliary sulcus or the capsular bag. This is said to further reduce the risk of posterior capsular thickening.
- An alternative way is to insert the IOL with the posterior capsule intact. The vitrector is then used to carry out an anterior vitrectomy and a posterior capsulotomy through a pars plicata incision.
- If different diopter powers of lenses are available, it is important to give a power of lens that takes into account the child's biometry readings and age. As children grow and develop, the eye grows and becomes more myopic. Therefore a slightly hyperopic, or "plus", initial post-operative target refractive outcome should be chosen.

Postoperative care

This is basically the same as for an adult, but special precautions must be taken and much longer and more intensive follow-up care given.

- Posterior capsular opacification. This is extremely common after an ordinary extra-capsular extraction and may occur even after a primary posterior capsulotomy. It is obviously very unlikely following a lensectomy. If the capsule is thickened a capsulotomy should be done.

- Pupil block glaucoma. This is a particular risk after a posterior capsulotomy. Mydriatic drops may lessen the risk, and if it occurs an iridectomy may be needed.
- Retinal detachment. There is a risk of this occurring at any time in the child's future.
- Refraction and vision testing. This should be done every year, or preferably every 3 months if possible if they are young or are patching to prevent amblyopia. If the child does not develop good vision, educational advice and low visual aids may both be very helpful.

Glaucoma in children

Primary congenital glaucoma (PCG) is the second most common glaucoma seen in children after aphakic glaucoma, and is thankfully quite rare. Surgery is the primary treatment for PCG. Different surgical techniques have been used for the treatment of PCG, and these including goniotomy, trabeculotomy, trabeculectomy, and drainage implant procedures.

Angle surgery

Angle surgery, a goniotomy or a trabeculotomy, can be considered the procedure of choice for PCG; as long as the cornea is relatively clear.

A - Goniotomy:

1. A small limbal incision is made in the eye
2. Fill the eye with viscoelastic
3. Place a large gonioscopy lens, with a wide angle of view, on the cornea.
4. Using a fine MVR blade (or a needle on a syringe), incise 90 to 120 degrees of the angle.
5. Take special care to ensure that all of the viscoelastic is washed out at the end of the procedure, otherwise there will be a high risk of a post-operative spike in IOP and hyphaema.

Trabeculectomy

If the cornea is very cloudy, you have no experience of goniotomy, a previous goniotomy procedure has failed, in cases of advanced PCG, or in most cases of secondary paediatric glaucoma, trabeculectomy is the surgical procedure of choice.

Trabeculectomy in children is essentially the same as for adults (described in chapter 6), except with a few very important considerations. The sclera is often very thin and soft in the buphthalmic eye, which increases the chances of complications during and after surgery. Children have a thicker Tenon's capsule, and show a more aggressive healing response after surgery which leads to a higher failure rate of trabeculectomy. The use of antimetablites such as MMC are controversial. Thin avascular cystic blebs are well known to be associated, and great care should be taken. Specifically, you should follow the following modifications to the adult technique:

1. Use a fornix-based flap (where the incision is made at the limbus). This is said to reduce the chance of posterior scarring which would restrict

aqueous diffusion. In children especially it is important to aim for a diffuse elevated drainage bleb without any restricting scar.

2. Create a large (wide) scleral flap with shorter side incisions. This encourages posterior flow of aqueous.

3. Use anti-metabolite on a sponge to treat a *large* area of sclera. The aim is to end up with a large area for aqueous diffusion resulting in a diffuse drainage bleb.

Retinoblastoma in children

This is a treatable childhood tumour, which sadly often presents late, and may be bilateral. In any situation where a child presents with a white pupil (leukocoria) it is essential to thoroughly examine **both** eyes and specifically both retinas for any signs of retinoblastoma. If you diagnose retinoblastoma, it is important to always examine the other eye thoroughly.

In many cases where chemotherapy is not available, and the tumour is confined to the eye, the only treatment to save the child's life is enucleation. When retinoblastoma is diagnosed, it is vital not to delay surgical treatment. If left untreated, retinoblastoma will spread along the optic nerve to the brain, and may also metastasise to other parts of the body. It will also spread through local tissues and break through the sclera and orbit. Once proptosis has occurred the disease is almost always fatal within a short time, unless the patient has access to advanced chemotherapy and radiotherapy treatment. Most people consider there is no point in heroic or mutilating surgery for a child who will shortly die.

Chapter 12 explains the details of an enuclation procedure.

Trauma

Detailed description of surgical management of eye and orbital trauma is given in Chapter 12. There are however a few important points to consider specifically for children and eye trauma.

An accurate and detailed history should be taken from the child and parent or guardian. This may be a challenge, but it is important to try to find out at least how long ago the injury happened, and what caused the injury.

A detailed and systematic examination is very important, but may be very difficult or impossible If the child is distressed or in pain. It is very important that you **do not put any pressure on the eye itself**.

If you suspect a penetrating eye injury, or that you will need to perform an examination under anaesthesia (EUA), then you must find out when the child last ate food and drank liquids. Tell the child and parents/guardian that he/she should not eat or drink anything at all before going to theatre. Communicate with the anaesthetist and theatre staff to coordinate a time to start the EUA/surgical repair.

Place a **shield** over the eye, after instilling antibiotic drops. You should consider starting oral antibiotics as well, and also consider giving a tetanus shot if needed and available.

Anaesthesia in children

General anaesthesia is required for most ophthalmic operations in children. Ketamine is a very popular drug for the induction and maintenance of general anaesthesia in children, especially for procedures of shorter duration.[2, 3] It can be administered intravenously or intramuscularly. In fact ketamine is the mainstay of anaesthesia delivery in many rural hospitals in developing countries.[4]

Monitoring equipment may include a stethoscope, and pulse-oximetry may be life-saving. In reality, very few rural anaesthetic providors have access to full electronic monitors.

The ketamine dosage is:

- 2mg/kg if given intravenously   *or*
- 10mg/kg if given intramuscularly

The child should not have eaten anything for at least 8 hours, and not have drunk anything for at least 4 hours before any general anaesthesia.

References

1. Lambert SR, Buckley EG, Drews-Botsch C et al. A randomized clinical trial comparing contact lens with intraocular lens correction of monocular aphakia during infancy: grating visual activity and adverse effects at age 1 year. Arch Ophthalmol. 2010; 128:810-818.
2. Gilbert C, Foster A. Childhood blindness in the context of VISION 2020--the right to sight. Bull World Health Organ 2001;79:227-32.
3. Lin C, Durieux ME. Ketamine and kids: an update. Paediatr Anaesth 2005;15:91-7.
4. Roelofse JA. The evolution of ketamine applications in children. Paediatr Anaesth 2010;20:240-5.
5. Hodges SC, Walker IA, Bosenberg AT. Paediatric anaesthesia in developing countries. Anaesthesia 2007;62 Suppl 1:26-31.

Appendix

Surgeons working in developing countries are often professionally isolated and may have difficulty in locating reliable suppliers of equipment. In addition, most equipment manufactured in the West is extremely expensive for anyone who does not have access to hard currency. The purpose of this section is to try to provide some details of useful addresses where equipment can be purchased or helpful information can be obtained. The list is unfortunately far from comprehensive or complete. The authors have no commercial or personal association with any of the companies mentioned.

Manufacturing companies and suppliers in the developed countries of the Western World produce reliable and sturdy equipment of excellent quality but at high prices. Most equipment can be bought alternatively from manufacturers in developing countries, in particular India and China. Their prices are very much less, sometimes only 25% of Western prices or even less. In most cases the quality is perfectly acceptable.

The IAPB (International Agency for the Prevention of Blindness) have produced a very comprehensive Standard List of medicines, equipment etc., which is updated regularly. It is available from the International Centre for Eye Health (see page 350) and also available on-line. All users can access the catalogue of recommended products. Verified IAPB member organisations and their partners are entitled to access the full catalogue, complete with specially negotiated prices:

> **Website: http://iapb.standardlist.org**

Suppliers of equipment

Surgical instruments

Appasamy Associates
20, SBI Offices's Colony
First Street, Arumbakkam
Chennai (Madras) - 600 106
INDIA
Tel: +91 44 32980153

Fax : +91 44 23631208
E mail : info@appasamy.com
Provides instruments as well as
other eye care products

Website: www.appasamy.com

Aurolab
No: 1 , Sivagangai Main Road
Veerapanjan,
Madurai - 625 020, Tamil Nadu
INDIA
Tel: + 91 452 3096100
Fax: + 91 452 2446200
info@aurolab.com

Integral part of Aravind Eye Care
System, the world's largest eye care
service provider. Non-profit provider
of IOLs, instruments, consumables
and pharmaceuticals

Website: www.aurolab.com

Indo-German Surgical Corporation

123 Kaliandas Udyog Bhuvan, Near Century Bazar, Prabhadevi, Mumbai – 400025,
INDIA
Tel: +91 22 2422 1809
Fax: +91 22 2430 5894
Email: sales@indogerman.com

Indian manufacturer of ophthalmic surgical instruments and appliances. Recommended by experienced ophthalmic consultants.

Website: www.indogerman.com

Suzhou Medical Instrument Co

34 Darū Lane
Suzhou
Jiangsu
People's Republic of China 215005
Fax: +86 512 5244789

A Chinese company manufacturing surgical instruments, operating microscopes etc.

Operating microscopes

These must have co-axial illumination and preferably a variable magnification. Microscopes from Western Europe, America or Japan are extremely expensive. Much cheaper microscopes can be obtained from India through the Indo-German Surgical Corporation or from China through Suzhou Medical Instrument Company.

Scan Optics

Scan Optics
32 Stirling Street
Thebarton SA 5031
Adelaide AUSTRALIA
Tel: +61 (8) 8234 9120
Fax: +61 (8) 8234 9417
sales@scanoptics.com.au
Scan Optics manufactures medical equipment to help prevent blindness throughout the world, and

manufacture a reasonably priced and reasonably compact portable table-mounted operating microscope especially designed for rural and outreach work. Scan Optics also make a floor standing microsope.

Website: www.scanoptics.com.au

Magnifying operating spectacles

These are made by various companies both in the Western and developing world. Reliable manufacturers from the Western World include:

Keeler

Clewer Hill Road
Windsor
SL4 4AA
UK
Tel: +44 1753 857177
Fax: +44 1753 827145
Email: info@keeler.co.uk

Heine

HEINE Optotechnik
Kientalstrasse 7
D-82211 Herrsching,
GERMANY
Tel: +49 8152 380
Fax: +49 8152 38202
Email: info@heine.com

They are also available through the Indo-German Surgical Corporation and the Suzhou Optical Company (addresses above).

Operating theatre lights

Daray Lighting Limited

7 Commerce Way
Stanbridge Road
Leighton Buzzard
Bedforshire LU7 8RW
UK
Tel: +44 1525 376 766
Fax: + 44 1525 851 626
Email: sales@daray.co.uk

Daray manufacture a portable and very robust operating light which will run off both a car battery or a mains electrical supply.

Website: www.daray.co.uk

Portable cryoprobes

Bright Instrument Company Limited

St. Margarets Way
Stukeley Meadows
Huntingdon
Cambridgeshire PE18 6ED
UK
Tel: + 44 1480 454 528
Fax: + 44 1480 456 031

Email: sales@BrightInstruments.com
This company manufactures small cylinders of a gas substitute which is ozone-friendly for use with hand held cryoprobes

Website: www.brightinstruments.com

Cheap pocket electrolysis equipment

Runs off torch batteries and is also available through various suppliers. One unit is known as the 'One Touch' Epilation Unit and is manufactured by:

Inverness Corporation
Fairlawn

N.J. 07410
U.S.A

Autoclaves

These are manufactured both in developed and developing countries.

L.T.E. Scientific Limited
Greenbridge Lane
Greenfield
Oldham OL3 7EN
UK

Tel: +44 1457 876221
Fax: +44 1457 870131
Email: info@lte-scientific.co.uk
This company manufactures a wide range of high quality surgical autoclaves
Website: www.lte-scientific.co.uk

Organisations offering help and information

1. **ICEH (International Centre for Eye Health)**
   London School of Hygiene and Tropical Medicine
   Keppel Street
   London WC1E 7HT
   UK
   Tel: +44 20 7958 8359
   E Mail: iceh@iceh.org.uk

This is a research, training and information centre concerned with all aspects of ophthalmology in developing countries. It also has a Resource Centre which provides help, information and teaching materials and produces the Journal of Community Eye Health.

Websites: www.iceh.org.uk   www.cehjournal.org

2. **CBM**
   Nibelungenstrasse 124
   D6140 Bensheim
   GERMANY
   Phone: +49 6251 131-131
   Fax: +49 6251 131-165
   Email: contact@cbm.org

This is an international Christian development organization, committed to improving the quality of life of persons with disabilities in the poorest communities of the world. Based on its Christian values and over 100 years of professional expertise, CBM addresses poverty as a cause and consequence of disability, and works in partnership to create a society for all.

Website: www.cbm.org

3. **Sightsavers** (Formerly the Royal Commonwealth Society for the Blind)
   2a Halifax Road
   Melksham
   SN12 6YY
   UK
   Tel: +44 1444 44 66 00
   Email: info@sightsavers.org

Sightsavers works with partners in more than 30 countries in Africa, Asia and the Caribbean to help restore sight, prevent blindness and promote equality for people who are irreversibly blind.

Website: www.sightsavers.org

4. **The Fred Hollows Foundation**
   Level 2, 61 Dunning Ave.   Level 6, 12 Morgan Street

Rosebery
NSW 2018
AUSTRALIA
Telephone: +61 2 8741 1900
Fax: +61 2 8741 1999
Email: fhf@hollows.org

Newmarket,
Auckland 1023
NEW ZEALAND
Tel: +64 9 304 0524
Fax: +64 9 379 7178
Email: info@hollows.org.nz

The Fred Hollows Foundation is dedicated to eradicating avoidable blindness, aiming in particular to eradicate cataract blindness, to train surgeons in developing countries in appropriate methods of cataract surgery and provide low cost equipment and intraocular lenses. Their mission is to work with local partners and communities to ensure all people in the areas they work have access to high quality, comprehensive eye care.

Websites: www.hollows.org.au   www.hollows.org.nz

5. **International Council of Ophthalmology**
   945 Green Street #10
   San Francisco,
   California 94133
   USA
   Fax: +1 415 409 8403
   Email: info@icoph.org

The ICO works with ophthalmological societies and others to enhance ophthalmic education and improve access to the highest quality eye care in order to preserve and restore vision for the people of the world

Website: www.icophth.org

Other non-government organisations involved in blindness treatment and prevention are:

Brien Holden Vision Institute
Level 4 North Wing
Rupert Myers Building
Gate 14 Barker Street
 University of New South Wales
Sydney NSW 2052
AUSTRALIA
Tel: +61 2 9385 7516
Website: www.brienholdenvision.org

Website: www.cartercenter.org
Helen Keller International
352 Park Avenue South, 12th Floor
New York, NY 10010
USA
Tel: +1 212 532 0544
Fax: +1 212 532 6014
E-mail: info@hki.org
Website: www.hki.org

The Carter Center
One Copenhill
453 Freedom Parkway
Atlanta, GA 30307
USA
Phone: +1 404 420 5100
E-mail: carterweb@emory.edu

HelpAge International
PO Box 70156
London WC1A 9GB
UK
Tel: +44 20 7278 7778
email: info@helpage.org
Website: www.helpage.org

International Eye Foundation
10801 Connecticut Avenue
Kensington, MD 20895
USA
Tel: +1 240 290 0263
Fax: +1 240 290 0269
E-mail: ief@iefusa.org
Website: www.iefusa.org

Light for the World
Niederhofstrasse 26
1120 Vienna
AUSTRIA
Tel: + 43 1 810 13 00
Email: info@licht-fuer-die-welt.at
Website: www.light-for-the-world.org

**Lions Clubs International
Foundation**
300 W. 22nd St.
Oak Brook, IL 60523-8842
USA
Tel: +1 630 468 6901
Fax: +1 630 571 5735
Email: lcif@lionsclubs.org
Website: www.lcif.org

NABP
Postboks 5900
Majorstuen 0308
Oslo
NORWAY
Tel: +47 23 21 50 00
Email: info@blindeforbundet.no
Website:
www.blindeforbundet.no/internett/
english-info

Nadi Al Bassar
9 Boulevard Bab Menara
Tunis 1008
TUNISIA

Tel: +216 1 560 333
Fax: +216 1 561 737
E-mail: nadi.albassar@planet.tn
Website: www.nadialbassar.planet.tn

**Organización Nacional de Ciegos
Españoles (ONCE)**
José Ortega y Gasset, 18
28006 Madrid
SPAIN
Tel: +91 436 53 00
Fax: +91 436 53 53
Email: once@once.es
Website: www.once.es

Operation Eyesight Universal
4 Parkdale Crescent
NW Calgary
Alberta
CANADA T2N 3T8
Tel: +1 403 283 6323
Fax: +1 403 270 1899
Email: info@operationeyesight.com
Website: www.operationeyesight.com

Orbis International
520 8th Avenue, 11th Floor
New York, NY 10018
USA
Tel: +1 800 ORBIS US
Fax: +1 646 674 5599
Email: info@orbis.org
Website: www.orbis.org

**OPC – Organisation pour la
Prévention de la Cécité**
17 Villa d'Alésia
75014 Paris
FRANCE
Tel: +33 1 44 12 41 92
Fax: +33 1 44 12 23 01
E-mail: assistante2@opc.asso.fr
Website: www.opc.asso.fr

Essential medications

This section is a list of essential medications required for successful surgery. It is a summary of the various drugs recommended throughout the book.
1. **Disinfectants for chemical sterilisation of instruments and skin preparation**
   Chlorhexidine and Cetrimide (marketed as concentrated solutions called

Hibitane and Savlon).
Povidone iodine can be used for both chemical sterilisation and for skin preparation. Chemical sterilisation is most effective with alcoholic solutions but skin preparation must be done with aqueous solutions.

2. **Solutions for irrigating inside the eye**
Hartmann's solution or Ringer's solution are best but isotonic normal saline is acceptable. All solutions for irrigation in the eye must be guaranteed sterile and free of any preservative or contaminant.

3. **Topical preparations**
Drops are preferable to ointments because of the relative ease with which they can be produced locally. However, ointments have a longer shelf life which may be an advantage.

Antibiotics
Chloramphenicol 0.5%
Gentamicin 0.3%

Mydriatics
Cyclopentolate 0.5-1%
Atropine 1%
Tropicamide 1%
Phenylephrine 2.5–10%

Steroids
Prednisolone 0.5% or Betamethasone 0.1% or Dexamethasone 0.1%. Other anti-inflammatory drops are Ketorolac (Acular) 0.5%

Topical anaesthetic drops
Tetracaine 0.5%–1% or Oxybuprocaine 0.4% or Lignocaine 4%

4. **Drugs to lower intraocular pressure**
   i. Miotics
       Pilocarpine 1% 4%

   ii. Topical betablockers
       Timolol, Levobunolol or Carteolol

   iii. Carbonic acid anhydrase inhibitors
        Acetozolamide 250mg tablets, or 500mg by intravenous injection; or Dorzolamide drops 2%
        Brinzolamide drops

   iv. Prostaglandin analogues
       Latanoprost 0.05% drops

5. **Local anaesthetic for nerve blocks**
   Lignocaine 1%–2% with hyaluronidase and adrenaline as additives to improve the quality of certain nerve blocks.

6. **Antibiotics and steroids for subconjunctival injection**
   See page 180.
   Cefuroxime, gentamicin, and dexamethasone or betamethasone or pred-nisolone or hydrocortisone.

7. **Antibiotic for intracameral use**
   Cefuroxime. A very strict protocol must be used for dilution.

8. **Antibiotics for intravitreal use**
   Vancomycin
   Ceftazidine
   Amikacin
   (Gentamicin if others not available)

9. **Other medications**
   i. Viscoelastic fluids for injection into the anterior chamber: HPMC (highly purified methyl cellulose) or sodium hyaluronate.
   ii. Adrenaline injection 1/1000 for adding to infusion bottles and local anaesthetic solutions.

Index

Note: Page numbers in italic refer to figures.